Atlas of Tumor Pathology

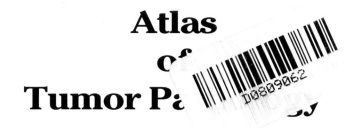

Tumors of the Gallbladder, Extrahepatic Bile Ducts, and Ampulla of Vater

by
Jorge Albores-Saavedra, M.D.
Donald Earl Henson, M.D.
and David S. Klimstra M.D.

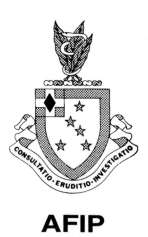

AFIP

ATLAS OF TUMOR PATHOLOGY

Third Series
Fascicle 27

TUMORS OF THE GALLBLADDER, EXTRAHEPATIC BILE DUCTS, AND AMPULLA OF VATER

by

JORGE ALBORES-SAAVEDRA, M.D.
Philip O'Bryan Montgomery Jr Professorship in Surgical Pathology and
Director, Division of Anatomic Pathology
Department of Pathology
University of Texas Southwestern Medical Center
Parkland Health and Hospital System
Zale Lipshy University Hospital
Dallas, Texas

DONALD EARL HENSON, M.D.
Early Detection Branch
Division of Cancer Prevention
National Cancer Institute
Bethesda, Maryland

DAVID S. KLIMSTRA, M.D.
Assistant Pathologist, Department of Pathology
Memorial Sloan-Kettering Cancer Center
New York, New York and
Assistant Professor of Pathology, Department of Pathology
Cornell University Medical College
New York, New York

Published by the
ARMED FORCES INSTITUTE OF PATHOLOGY
Washington, D.C.

Under the Auspices of
UNIVERSITIES ASSOCIATED FOR RESEARCH AND EDUCATION IN PATHOLOGY, INC.
Bethesda, Maryland
2000

Accepted for Publication
1998

Available from the American Registry of Pathology
Armed Forces Institute of Pathology
Washington, D.C. 20306-6000
www.afip.org
ISSN 0160-6344
ISBN 1-881041-58-1

ATLAS OF TUMOR PATHOLOGY

EDITOR
JUAN ROSAI, M.D.
Department of Pathology
Memorial Sloan-Kettering Cancer Center
New York, New York 10021-6007

ASSOCIATE EDITOR
LESLIE H. SOBIN, M.D.
Armed Forces Institute of Pathology
Washington, D.C. 20306-6000

EDITORIAL ADVISORY BOARD

EDITORS' NOTE

The Atlas of Tumor Pathology has a long and distinguished history. It was first conceived at a Cancer Research Meeting held in St. Louis in September 1947 as an attempt to standardize the nomenclature of neoplastic diseases. The first series was sponsored by the National Academy of Sciences-National Research Council. The organization of this Sisyphean effort was entrusted to the Subcommittee on Oncology of the Committee on Pathology, and Dr. Arthur Purdy Stout was the first editor-in-chief. Many of the illustrations were provided by the Medical Illustration Service of the Armed Forces Institute of Pathology, the type was set by the Government Printing Office, and the final printing was done at the Armed Forces Institute of Pathology (hence the colloquial appellation "AFIP Fascicles"). The American Registry of Pathology purchased the Fascicles from the Government Printing Office and sold them virtually at cost. Over a period of 20 years, approximately 15,000 copies each of nearly 40 Fascicles were produced. The worldwide impact that these publications have had over the years has largely surpassed the original goal. They quickly became among the most influential publications on tumor pathology ever written, primarily because of their overall high quality but also because their low cost made them easily accessible to pathologists and other students of oncology the world over.

Upon completion of the first series, the National Academy of Sciences-National Research Council handed further pursuit of the project over to the newly created Universities Associated for Research and Education in Pathology (UAREP). A second series was started, generously supported by grants from the AFIP, the National Cancer Institute, and the American Cancer Society. Dr. Harlan I. Firminger became the editor-in-chief and was succeeded by Dr. William H. Hartmann. The second series Fascicles were produced as bound volumes instead of loose leaflets. They featured a more comprehensive coverage of the subjects, to the extent that the Fascicles could no longer be regarded as "atlases" but rather as monographs describing and illustrating in detail the tumors and tumor-like conditions of the various organs and systems.

Once the second series was completed, with a success that matched that of the first, UAREP and AFIP decided to embark on a third series. A new editor-in-chief and an associate editor were selected, and a distinguished editorial board was appointed. The mandate for the third series remains the same as for the previous ones, i.e., to oversee the production of an eminently practical publication with surgical pathologists as its primary audience, but also aimed at other workers in oncology. The main purposes of this series are to promote a consistent, unified, and biologically sound nomenclature; to guide the surgical pathologist in the diagnosis of the various tumors and tumor-like lesions; and to provide relevant histogenetic, pathogenetic, and clinicopathologic information on these entities. Just as the second series included data obtained from ultrastructural (and, in the more recent Fascicles, immunohistochemical) examination, the third series will, in addition, incorporate pertinent information obtained with the newer molecular biology techniques. As in the past, a continuous attempt will be made to correlate, whenever possible, the nomenclature used in the Fascicles with that proposed by the World Health Organization's International Histological Classification of Tumors. The format of the third series has been changed in order to incorporate additional items and to ensure a consistency of style throughout. Close cooperation between the various authors and their respective liaisons from the editorial board will be emphasized to minimize unnecessary repetition and discrepancies in the text and illustrations.

To its everlasting credit, the participation and commitment of the AFIP to this venture is even more substantial and encompassing than in previous series. It now extends to virtually all scientific, technical, and financial aspects of the production.

The task confronting the organizations and individuals involved in the third series is even more daunting than in the preceding efforts because of the ever-increasing complexity of the matter at hand. It is hoped that this combined effort—of which, needless to say, that represented by the authors is first and foremost—will result in a series worthy of its two illustrious predecessors and will be a suitable introduction to the tumor pathology of the twenty-first century.

Juan Rosai, M.D.
Leslie H. Sobin, M.D.

PREFACE AND ACKNOWLEDGMENTS

Fourteen years have past since the publication of the second edition of the Fascicle, *Tumors of the Gallbladder and Extrahepatic Bile Ducts*. At that time, an effort was made to summarize the knowledge available about the pathologic and clinical features of these tumors. At the suggestion of the editor of the third edition of the Fascicles, Dr. Juan Rosai, we added tumors of the ampulla of Vater, a structure which is, partly, an extension of the terminal portion of the common bile duct. Since many of the tumors that arise in the terminal bile ducts, ampulla, and periampullary region share clinical and pathologic features, and are often diagnosed with the same tools, it seemed logical to discuss them together.

In this Fascicle we have tried to update the information regarding the clinical and pathologic characteristics as well as the biologic behavior of those tumors that arise in these three anatomic sites, emphasizing the useful diagnostic features revealed by light microscopy. However, results of electron microscopic, immunohistochemical, and molecular pathology studies are provided when considered appropriate.

We are indebted to the countless pathologists who during the last 14 years shared with us their material on tumors of the gallbladder, extrahepatic bile ducts, and ampulla of Vater, allowing us to broaden our knowledge about these neoplasms. Their contribution to this Fascicle is invaluable and cannot be overemphasized. Through the courtesy of Drs. Leslie Sobin and Linda Murakata we had access to interesting and rare tumors of these anatomic regions that were on file at the Armed Forces Institute of Pathology. We want to express our deep appreciation to both of them. We wish to thank Dr. Glenn Tillery, from Baylor University Medical Center, Dallas, Texas, for allowing Dr. Albores-Saavedra to review his rich material on these tumors. We would like to thank Drs. Oscar Larraza and Carlos Manivel for providing us with electron micrographs of adenocarcinomas and adenosquamous carcinomas of the gallbladder.

We acknowledge Mr. Ricardo Dreyfuss from the National Institutes of Health for his valuable assistance with the photomicrographs. The data included from the Survey, Epidemiology, and End Results Program of the National Cancer Institute were kindly provided by Lynn A. Ries. We also thank Mr. Jeffrey M. Aarons from the National Institutes of Health for the preparation of the drawings and diagrams. Finally, Dr. Albores-Saavedra would like to express his deep appreciation to his Administrative Assistant, Mrs. R. Nelly Murillo, for the typing and preparation of the text.

Jorge Albores-Saavedra, M.D.
Donald E. Henson, M.D.
David Klimstra, M.D.

Permission to use copyrighted illustrations has been granted by:

Academy of Sciences Hungary:
   Acta Morphol Acad Sci Hung 1979;27:107–14. For figure 1-11

American Roentgen Ray Society:
   Am J Roentgenol Rad Ther Nucl Med 1972;116:393–5. For figure 9-2.

College of American Pathologists:
   Arch Pathol Lab Med 1995;119:1173–6. For figures 10-18 and 10-19.

Georg Thieme Publishers:
   Efficiency and Limits of Radiologic Examination of the Pancreas. For figure 1-14.

John Wiley & Sons:
   Cancer 1976:37;2448–54. For figures 8-21 and 8-22.

Lippincott-Raven:
   Am J Surg Pathol 1995;19:91–9. For figures 13-25 and 13-26.
   Am J Surg Pathol 1985;9:31–41. For figure 21-24.
   Ann Surg 1925;82:584–97. For figure 1-13.

Springer-Verlag:
   TNM Atlas. For figure 20-54.

W.B. Saunders:
   Ann Diagn Pathol 1999;3:75–80. For Table 13-2.

Contents

❖❖❖

TUMORS OF THE GALLBLADDER, EXTRAHEPATIC BILE DUCTS, AND AMPULLA OF VATER

1
NORMAL ANATOMY

For reasons of anatomy alone, tumors arising in the extrahepatic biliary tree offer a challenge to the physician and heightened anxiety for the patient. The separation of benign from malignant conditions, the treatment of cancer, and even the histologic diversity of malignant tumors require an understanding of the anatomic relations and their frequent variations. In contrast to the liver and pancreas, which are also foregut derivatives, the extrahepatic tree is primarily a ductal system. Therefore, its anatomy and histology are described to underscore the effect of structure on pathology.

GALLBLADDER

A pear-shaped saccular organ, the gallbladder is normally found under the right lobe of the liver near the quadrate lobe. Traditionally, it has been divided into three parts: a fundus, a body, and a neck. The neck tapers into the cystic duct, which connects the gallbladder to the common hepatic duct. A small projection or diverticulum, Hartmann's pouch, named after the nineteenth century German anatomist, is often located at the junction of the neck and cystic duct. Originally considered a fourth part of the gallbladder, the pouch is now thought to be the result of chronic inflammation.

The superior surface of the gallbladder is firmly adherent to the liver, while the inferior surface is covered with peritoneum. Occasionally, the gallbladder is freely suspended from the liver by a mesentery or completely buried in its substance. Gallbladders attached by a mesentery, the so called floating gallbladders, are prone to torsion. Those buried in the liver, intrahepatic gallbladders, are predisposed to the formation of calculi. The inferior surface of the gallbladder lies near the pylorus, duodenum, and hepatic flexure of the colon.

Histology

Histologically, the wall of the gallbladder has four layers: 1) a mucosa composed of epithelium and underlying lamina propria; 2) a smooth muscle layer; 3) perimuscular connective tissue; and 4) serosa (fig. 1-1). The muscle layer, which is most prominent near the neck of the gallbladder, is embryologically equivalent to the muscularis mucosa of the small intestine. A muscularis propria is not present. As a consequence, the gallbladder does not have a submucosa. The perimuscular connective tissue contains nerves, blood vessels, lymphatic channels, and scattered paraganglia. These paraganglia are usually found adjacent to nerve fibers and ganglion cells (figs. 1-2, 1-3). Ganglion cells are occasionally found in the lamina propria, among the smooth muscle bundles, and in the perimuscular connective tissue; they are most numerous in the neck of the gallbladder (10). Along the hepatic surface, no serosa exists, and the perimuscular connective tissue is continuous with the interlobular connective tissue of the liver. This continuity facilitates extension of malignant tumors directly into the liver.

The mucosa forms multiple irregular folds that flatten as the gallbladder fills and its lumen expands. During contraction, these folds come together and increase in height (11). The epithelium consists of a single layer of tall, uniform, columnar cells aligned along a periodic acid–Schiff (PAS)-positive basement membrane. The cells have ovoid basal nuclei and a pale cytoplasm that may contain small vacuoles. Functionally, the cells secrete sulfoglycoproteins, some of which are related to the glycoproteins secreted by the intestine (25). Interspersed among the columnar cells are narrow, dark-staining cells that have been described as penciloid (fig. 1-4) (60). These cells are considered modified columnar cells, although

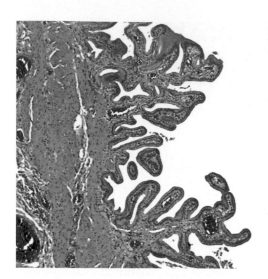
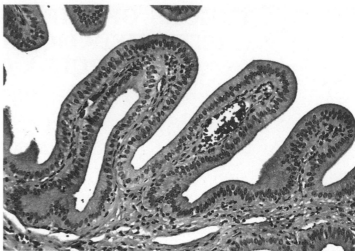

Figure 1-1
NORMAL GALLBLADDER

Left: The specimen was removed because of trauma to the liver. Except for congestion the gallbladder is normal. The mucosal folds are of different height and width. This section includes the lamina propria, muscle layer, and serosa.

Right: Higher magnification of normal columnar cells.

their nature and function are unknown. Because of their increased enzymatic activity, it is unlikely that these cells are effete or represent artifacts of fixation (63).

Basal cells, which are smaller than columnar cells, are located immediately above the basement membrane. They are usually round with elongated or ovoid nuclei whose long axis lies parallel with the basement membrane. These cells, which are not common, are usually scattered along the epithelium. Basal cells are always separated from the lumen by the taller columnar cells and should not be confused with the more common intraepithelial lymphocytes. As in the intestine, T lymphocytes are found among the columnar lining cells (fig. 1-5). A few intramucosal plasma cells are always seen in normal gallbladders.

Goblet cells have been described in the fetal human gallbladder, but are not found in the normal gallbladders of adults (33). Mucin-secreting glands, which differ morphologically and histochemically from pyloric type glands, are normally present only in the neck (34,35). In abnormal gallbladders showing intestinal metaplasia, argyrophil and argentaffin cells are found along the surface epithelium and in the metaplastic glands (1,36). These argyrophil and argentaffin cells are randomly distributed along the epithelium and within the glands (1).

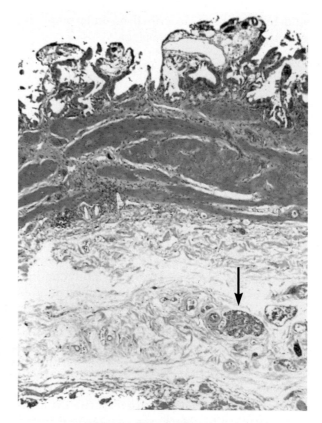

Figure 1-2
PARAGANGLION

Well-defined paraganglion located in the perimuscular connective tissue of the gallbladder.

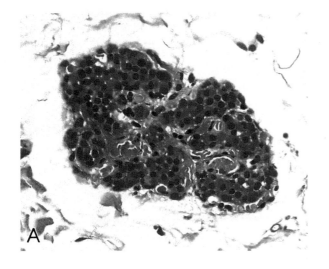

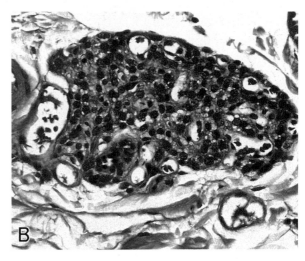

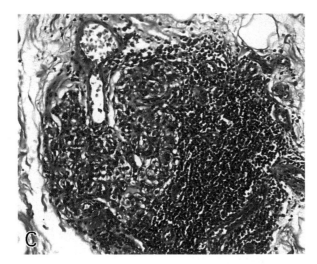

Figure 1-3
PARAGANGLIA
Under higher magnification, paraganglia are seen with a well-defined lobular pattern (A), with cells containing round hyperchromatic nuclei (B), and surrounded by lymphocytes (C).

Small aberrant bile ducts (Luschka's ducts), which are remnants of the embryonic primordium of the liver, are occasionally seen in the perimuscular connective tissue adjacent to the liver. Lined by a cuboidal type of biliary epithelium, they are found in 10 to 15 percent of gallbladders removed for cholelithiasis. The ducts are easy to recognize since they are usually surrounded by compressed fibrous connective tissue. Those located along the serosal surface may open into the peritoneal cavity. Leakage of bile through these ducts can lead to peritonitis.

Immunohistochemistry

The normal columnar cells of the gallbladder express low molecular weight cytokeratins (fig 1-6). In contrast, they are weakly positive for the high molecular weight cytokeratins. Although malignant epithelial cells are diffusely reactive for carcinoembryonic antigen (CEA), normal columnar cells are reactive only along the apical cytoplasmic border, especially with the polyclonal antibody (2). The reactivity in normal cells is now attributed to cross-reacting CEA-related antigens (38). Since the normal human gallbladder does not contain endocrine cells, immunostains for peptide hormones are uniformly negative. Immunohistochemistry has revealed that endothelin-1, a small peptide that causes contraction of smooth muscle cells, is produced by the gallbladder and bile duct epithelium (28). It is now thought that cholecystokinin causes contraction of the gallbladder by stimulating the release of endothelin from the lining epithelium.

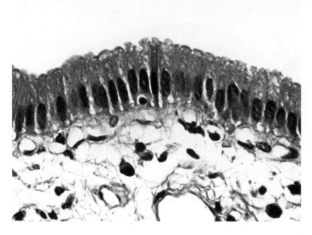 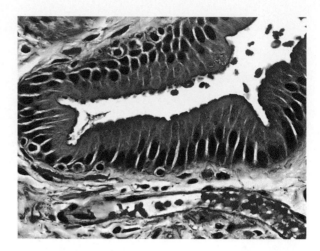

Figure 1-4
NORMAL EPITHELIUM

Left: The columnar cells rest on a basement membrane, and some contain small cytoplasmic vacuoles. A single penciloid cell, which is thinner and darker than surrounding columnar cells, is seen in the center of the field. A small intraepithelial lymphocyte is also present.

Right: Normal epithelium of the fundus of the gallbladder. The columnar cells contain round or ovoid, basally placed nuclei and rest on a basement membrane. Several small intraepithelial lymphocytes are visible.

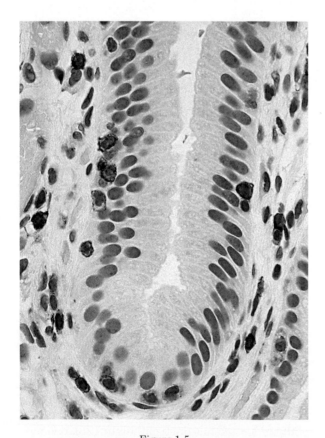 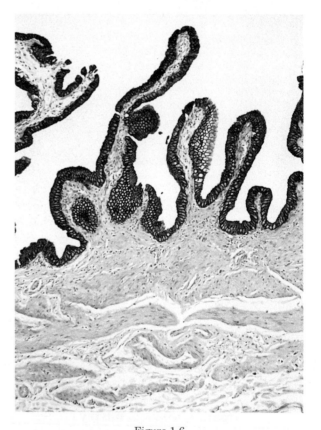

Figure 1-5
INTRAEPITHELIAL LYMPHOCYTES

The intraepithelial lymphocytes stain with the pan T-cell monoclonal antibody CD45RO. Adjacent cells are negative.

Figure 1-6
NORMAL EPITHELIUM

All columnar cells lining the mucosal folds show positive reactivity for low molecular weight cytokeratin.

Interstitial cells of Cajal, similar to those found in the gastrointestinal tract (28a,32a), occur in the muscle layer of the gallbladder and are immunoreactive with antibodies against Kit (CD117), a tyrosine kinase receptor (fig. 1-7) (Albores-Saavedra J. Unpublished observations, 1999). We assume that these cells, as their intestinal counterparts, function as pacemakers, are involved in muscle contraction, or act as mediators of neurotransmission (28a,32a).

The intraepithelial lymphocytes stain for leukocyte common antigen. They are also immunoreactive for the T-cell markers, such as the monoclonal antibodies CD45RO and CD3, in paraffin-embedded material. Intramucosal plasma cells usually contain IgA, while those found in the muscle layer contain IgM (24).

Ultrastructure

Three types of epithelial cells—ordinary light columnar cells, dark penciloid cells, and basal cells—are found in the normal gallbladder (17). The light columnar cells are the most common, comprising 98 percent of the epithelium. Both the columnar and penciloid cells are covered with microvilli and rest on a basal lamina similar to that found under all epithelia (figs. 1-8–1-10). The basal cells are confined to the region of the basal lamina and do not reach the lumen.

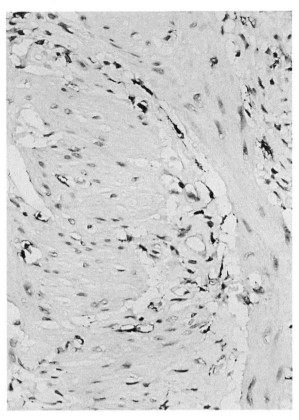

Figure 1-7
INTERSTITIAL CELLS OF CAJAL
Most CD117-positive dendritic cells are seen at the periphery of the muscle bundles.

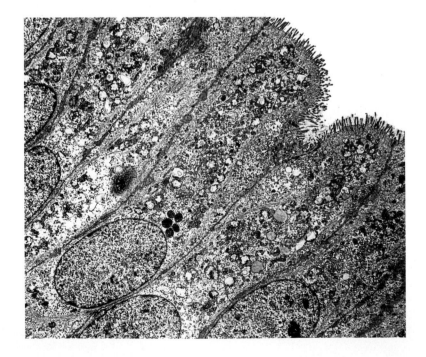

Figure 1-8
ULTRASTRUCTURE OF
NORMAL COLUMNAR CELLS
Several columnar cells are covered by microvilli and contain mucin droplets, mitochondria, and large electron dense bodies. Most cytoplasmic organelles are located above the nucleus.

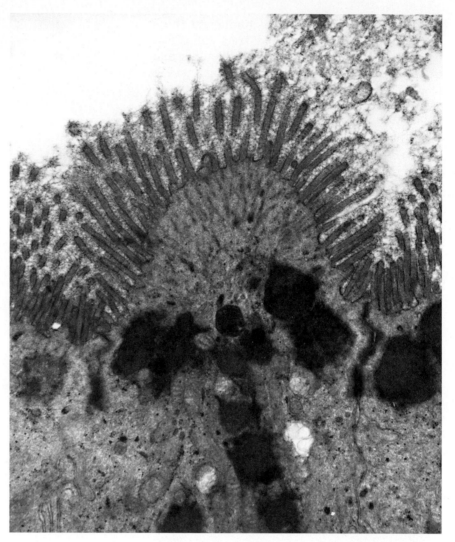

Figure 1-9
ULTRASTRUCTURE
OF NORMAL
COLUMNAR CELLS
Portions of three columnar cells showing microvilli with filamentous glycocalyx. The apical cytoplasm contains large electron dense granules which probably represent mucin. A junctional complex is also visible. (Fig. 4B from Fascicle 22, 2nd Series.)

Adjacent cells are connected by junctional complexes located at the apical ends of the lateral walls. These walls have complex membrane interdigitations and are separated by intercellular spaces. Fluid transport occurs through the junctional complexes and lateral spaces. These spaces enlarge according to the rate and direction of fluid transport (20,21).

Most cytoplasmic organelles are located in the supranuclear region and consist of mitochondria, rough endoplasmic reticulum, a prominent Golgi apparatus, lysosomes, and a variety of vesicles and granules. The vesicles and granules contain mucin or lipid material. Pinocytic vesicles that are found along the apical surface seem to provide morphologic evidence for another mechanism of

absorption. Mitochondria are most numerous in the supranuclear area and may be partially surrounded by rough endoplasmic reticulum. In the human, mucus production is not prominent, but becomes excessive in some pathologic conditions such as chronic cholecystitis (18), benign epithelial tumors, and adenocarcinomas. Mucous secretory granules are released by a process called reverse pinocytosis (33).

The penciloid cells are characterized by a narrow dark profile and a well-developed rough endoplasmic reticulum located above the nucleus. Comprising about 1 percent of all columnar cells, they can be recognized by light microscopy (26). These cells are dispersed along the epithelium, occurring singly, although often increasing in

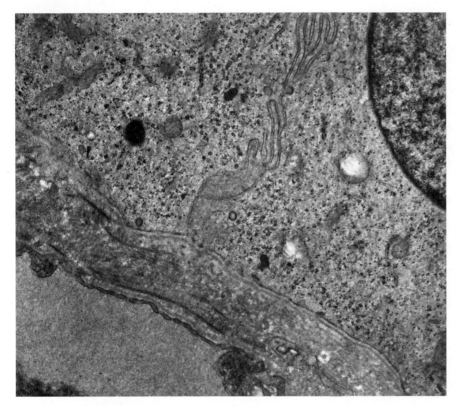

Figure 1-10
ULTRASTRUCTURE OF
NORMAL COLUMNAR CELLS
The basal cytoplasm of two cells rests on the basal lamina. Note the complex interdigitations of the lateral cell membranes. Many glycogen particles, some mitochondria, lysosomes, and some rough endoplasmic reticulum are also present. The lamina propria contains many collagen fibers and a capillary. (Fig. 5 from Fascicle 22, 2nd Series.)

chronic cholecystitis. Found in many species, these penciloid cells have also been described as peg or dark cells.

The basal cells are randomly distributed along the epithelium. They tend to be ovoid or elongated and have some mitochondria, which usually surround the nucleus, and little endoplasmic reticulum. The cytoplasm forms complex interdigitations with adjacent columnar cells. They are similar to the basal cells seen in other sites.

The intraepithelial lymphocytes contain the lobulated or cerebriform nuclei typical of T lymphocytes. They are located adjacent to the basal lamina and the basolateral aspect of the columnar cells.

Under the scanning electron microscope, the mucosal surface appears as rolling, branching folds lined with uniform epithelial cells (fig. 1-11) (34,52). The cells have regular, polygonal or hexagonal boundaries and a slightly convex surface covered with microvilli (fig. 1-12). This structural arrangement corresponds in many respects to the surface architecture of the stomach and small intestine. Mucosal changes, as seen by scanning electron microscopy, have been published for some pathologic conditions (43,52).

EXTRAHEPATIC BILE DUCTS

Of greater importance than the gallbladder are the extrahepatic bile ducts (fig. 1-13). Emerging from the liver, the left and right hepatic ducts join to form the common hepatic duct, which descends on the lateral aspect of the hepatoduodenal ligament. Connecting the gallbladder to the common hepatic duct is the cystic duct. Their union forms the common bile duct, which passes behind the first part of the duodenum and then traverses the head of the pancreas until it opens into the second part of the duodenum through the major papilla (papilla of Vater).

The common hepatic duct can vary from 0.8 to 5.2 cm in length, while the common duct, exclusive of the ampulla, varies from 1.5 to 9.0 cm. In general, the diameter of the common bile duct increases with age (39,59). The cystic duct varies from 0.4 to 6.5 cm in length (41). The structure of the proximal cystic duct is similar to that of the gallbladder (47), although prominent mucosal folds, the valves of Heister, give the duct a spiral appearance. These valves contain smooth muscle fibers that regulate the filling

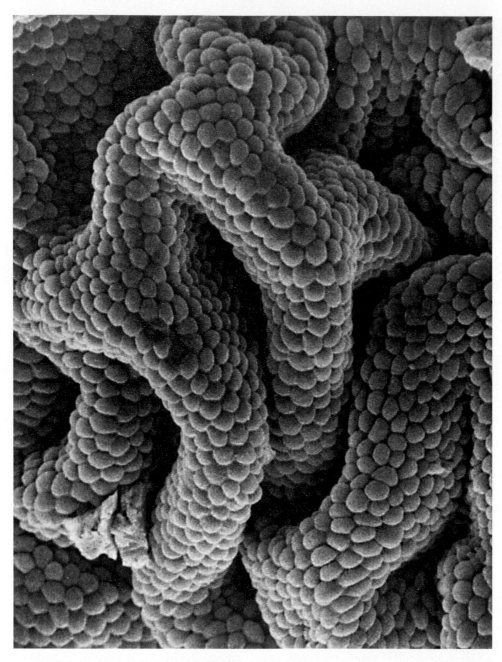

Figure 1-11
NORMAL MUCOSA
Scanning electron micrograph of gallbladder mucosa. The surface is composed of small, rolling folds covered by uniform epithelial cells (X1500). (Fig. 3 from Schaff Z, Lapis K, Csikos A. Scanning electron microscopic study of human gallbladder mucosa in cholelithiasis. Acta Morphol Acad Sci Hung 1979;27:107–14).

and emptying of the gallbladder according to the pressure in the biliary system. More than one left or right hepatic duct may be present.

The common bile duct is divided into four parts in relation to the duodenum and pancreas: supraduodenal, the longest part; retroduodenal; pancreatic; and intraduodenal. The supraduodenal segment is the most accessible portion of the common bile duct during laparotomy and the easiest to explore by the surgeon.

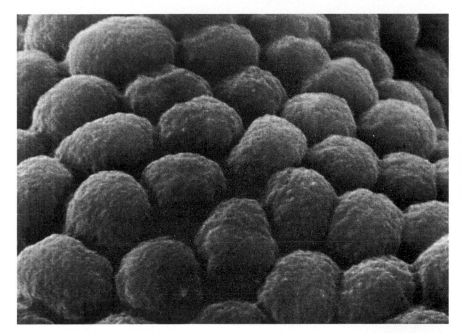

Figure 1-12
NORMAL MUCOSAL CELLS
Scanning electron micrograph shows normal epithelial cells. The cells, which are separated by deep intercellular clefts, have rounded tips and are nearly identical is size and shape. (Fig. 7 from Fascicle 22, 2nd Series.)

Histology

The hepatic, distal part of the cystic duct and the common bile duct are essentially identical in structure (9). Lined by a single layer of tall uniform columnar cells, the mucosa of the bile ducts usually forms irregular pleats or small folds that run longitudinally. An underlying subepithelial layer is composed of compact elastic and collagen fibers. Scattered small bundles of smooth muscle are found in the ductal wall. Usually aligned parallel with the lumen, they are generally absent or sparse in the upper portion of the bile ducts. The common duct often shows an interrupted or continuous muscle layer that is more prominent near the sphincter of Oddi (27a).

The periductal layer consists of loose areolar connective tissue. Small intramural mucous glands that increase in number toward the distal part open into the lumen in small pits, the sacculi of Beale. Developmentally, these glands reach their maximum number within the first year of life. Thereafter, the number remains relatively constant. In contrast, the lumen and wall of the common duct do not reach adult proportions until adult life (57). In small biopsy specimens, these mucous glands can be confused with carcinoma, especially in specimens distorted by inflammation.

Because the walls of the extrahepatic bile ducts are less than 1.5 mm in thickness, malignant

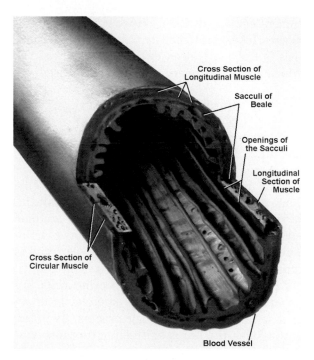

Figure 1-13
STRUCTURE OF THE NORMAL BILE DUCT
Diagrammatic representation of the common bile duct shows folds in the lining epithelium, the openings of the sacculi of Beale, and a cross section through the wall. Smooth muscle is most pronounced along the intrapancreatic segment of the common duct. It is usually sparse proximal to the intrapancreatic segment of the common duct. (Fig. 1 from Burden VG. Observation on the histology and pathologic anatomy of the hepatic cystic and common bile ducts. Ann Surg 1925;82:584–97.)

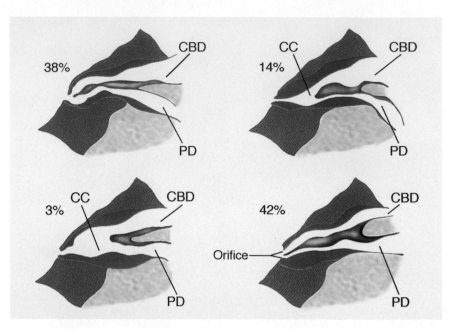

Figure 1-14
PAPILLA OF VATER
ANATOMIC VARIANTS
Anatomic variants of the papilla of Vater and the openings of the bile and pancreatic ducts. CBC = common bile duct; PD = pancreatic duct; CC = common channel. (Fig. 14 from Anacker H. Radiological anatomy of the pancreas. In: Anacker H, ed. Efficiency and limits of radiologic examination of the pancreas. 3rd ed. Stuttgart: Georg Thieme Pub., 1973.)

tumors can rapidly gain access to the periductal tissues. Invasion of small nerves and vascular channels is frequently seen in the periductal tissues, which are richly innervated and vascularized.

Immunohistochemistry

The columnar cells that line the extrahepatic bile ducts, the sacculi of Beale, and the intramural glands are immunoreactive for the low molecular weight cytokeratins. Endocrine cells, some containing immunoreactive somatostatin, have been observed in the surface and glandular epithelia of the ampulla and bile ducts (14,19). These endocrine cells may be widely scattered or may occur in clusters. However, it is often difficult to determine if such endocrine cells are normally present or develop secondarily in response to age or a pathologic process. As in the gallbladder, the lining epithelium contains lymphocytes, most of which are of the suppressor/cytotoxic T-cell phenotype (13).

VATERIAN SYSTEM

Located 7 to 10 cm from the pylorus, in the wall of the duodenum, the vaterian system is situated at the confluence of the common bile duct and the major pancreatic duct, the duct of Wirsung. In addition to the ducts, it includes the primary duodenal papilla, the ampulla of Vater (when present), the sphincter muscle (sphincter of Oddi) which controls the flow of bile, and fibrous coverings (16). The ducts usually open into the duodenum through the tip of the papilla.

Any consideration of the vaterian system is not complete without noting the variation in the connections between the pancreatic and common bile ducts (fig. 1-14). The ducts may open separately, form a common channel which is the most common arrangement (15), or have an intervening septum (fig. 1-15). The common channel, which varies from 1 to 12 mm in length, forms the ampulla of Vater. However, a true ampulla, defined as a dilated reservoir into which the ducts empty, is an infrequent finding (4). For this reason, it has been suggested that the term "ampulla" be abandoned and replaced by the more appropriate description "pancreaticobiliary duct" (16). Most often, the ducts join near the orifice in the tip of the papilla without forming a true ampulla. Located in the wall of duodenum, the sphincter muscle surrounds the ducts and the ampulla. Embryologically and functionally, the sphincter is not part of the muscle of the duodenum. Details regarding the complex anatomy of the sphincter muscle have been published (8). Because two major ducts come together, it is virtually impossible in this area to localize the precise origin of tumors after they have invaded adjacent tissue.

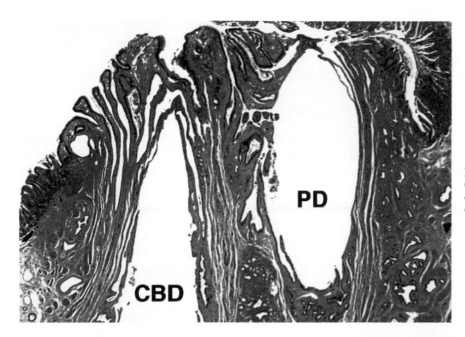

Figure 1-15
NORMAL AMPULLA
In this low-power view, the larger terminal common bile duct (CBD) and the smaller pancreatic duct (PD) drain separately into the duodenum.

Histology

As the pancreatic and common bile ducts approach the papilla, their lining epithelium becomes papillary, often with long, narrow fronds protruding toward the lumen. There is also transition from the ductal type epithelium of the distal ducts to the small intestinal type epithelium covering the papilla (fig. 1-16). Multiple mucin-secreting glands usually supported by a dense fibrovascular stroma empty into the terminal ducts or even into the ampulla. In addition, small accessory pancreatic ducts are often seen. Because of the normal papillary structure, tumors developing in this area often have a villous configuration

BLOOD SUPPLY

Following is a description of the normal vascular supply. Departures from normal, which occur frequently, are described in a later section, Anatomic Variations.

The gallbladder receives its main blood supply from the cystic artery, a branch of the right hepatic artery. In the neck of the gallbladder the cystic artery divides into two branches: a superficial and deep branch. The superficial branch supplies the serosal surface, while the deep branch supplies the gallbladder along the hepatic bed. As they

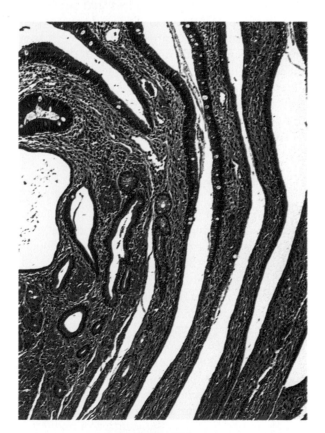

Figure 1-16
NORMAL AMPULLA
Transition from the normal biliary type epithelium to intestinal type epithelium is seen. This is the most common site for the development of malignant epithelial tumors of the ampulla.

course along the gallbladder toward the fundus, these branches give off, at right angles, four to eight pairs of smaller lateral branches that anastomose with the corresponding branches from the opposite side. This arterial pattern creates a bipinnate blood supply (23). Branches also arise that pass directly into the liver along the gallbladder fossa (46).

The common bile duct is supplied by the retroduodenal, gastroduodenal, cystic, and hepatic arteries. The supraduodenal segment is mainly supplied distally by the retroduodenal and proximally by the right hepatic arteries (45). The intraduodenal segment, however, is largely supplied by branches from the anterior and the posterior superior pancreaticoduodenal arteries.

From the gallbladder, venous blood drains through the cholecystic veins which arise from a network of small vessels located primarily in the perimuscular connective tissue. This network is continuous with a similar plexus that surrounds the extrahepatic bile ducts. The cholecystic veins usually pass directly into the liver, where they continually subdivide until they form the superficial and deep capillaries or, less frequently, empty directly into the portal system. This pattern of venous drainage allows for localized hematogenous tumor spread to the liver. Venous drainage from the common duct is usually through the portal system.

LYMPHATIC DRAINAGE

Important for the consideration of regional metastasis, the lymphatic drainage of the gallbladder is complex and follows three independent pathways (30): 1) the cholecystoretropancreatic, the main pathway, descends to the posterior surface of the head of the pancreas and enters the retroportal and retropancreatic lymph nodes; 2) the cholecystoceliac runs through the hepatoduodenal ligament to the celiac nodes; and 3) the cholecystomesenteric flows posterior to the pancreas to the origin of the superior mesenteric artery and connects with nodes at the superior mesentery root. Because of this complex drainage, the location of nodal metastases is often difficult to predict. There is also some variability in the distribution of specific lymph nodes (30). Located at the neck of the gallbladder in 74 percent of cases, the cystic node

primarily drains the anterior surface of the gallbladder. Lymph nodes most commonly involved with metastatic tumor include the cystic, pericholedochal, posterosuperior pancreatoduodenal, retroportal, right celiac, superior mesenteric, and interaortocaval (55).

Major lymph nodes that drain the extrahepatic bile ducts include those around the common hepatic artery, celiac trunk, hilus of spleen, splenic artery, and superior mesenteric artery, in the hepatoduodenal ligament, the posterior pancreaticoduodenal lymph node, along the middle colic artery, para-aortic nodes, anterior pancreaticoduodenal lymph node, and inferior body lymph nodes. The pericholedochal and posterior-superior pancreaticoduodenal nodes occupy important positions in the spread of carcinomas arising in the distal common duct (31).

EMBRYOLOGIC DEVELOPMENT

Embryologically, the derivatives of the foregut have a complex and interdependent development. The gallbladder originates in the fourth week of fetal life as a ventral-medial outgrowth that buds from the primitive endoderm, near the junction of the foregut and yolk sac, opposite the dorsal pancreatic bud. Pushing into the splanchnic mesenchyme, this outgrowth will eventually become the hepatic diverticulum. The cranial part differentiates into the liver and intrahepatic bile ducts, while the caudal part branches to form the gallbladder and cystic duct. A small bud, the ventral pancreas, which eventually becomes part of the head of the pancreas, arises from the hepatic diverticulum near its origin from the foregut. The original hepatic diverticulum then elongates to form the common bile duct. By the time the embryo reaches 5 mm, or 5 weeks, the gallbladder is a small tubular structure lined by epithelium and connected to the common duct by a short stem, the future cystic duct.

As the stomach rotates, causing torsion on the duodenum, the hepatic diverticulum comes to lie dorsal to the duodenum and the small ventral pancreas comes around to fuse with the larger dorsal pancreas, which is now ventral, to form the head and uncinate process. As a result of fusion, the ventral pancreatic duct becomes the proximal segment of the main pancreatic duct (duct of Wirsung) which, because of its origin from the hepatic diverticulum, usually opens into the duodenum through the terminal part of the common bile duct.

For the first 8 weeks, the choledochopancreatic junction is located outside the wall of the duodenum. But as a result of differential growth and migration the junction normally comes to lie within the wall of the duodenum. Failure to migrate may explain the development of an anomalous junction which allows bile and pancreatic juice to mix. This mix is considered important for the pathogenesis of choledochal cysts (62) and possibly acalculous gallbladder carcinoma.

By the eighth week of gestation, a lumen has been established throughout most of the biliary tract. The layers of the gallbladder are completely differentiated when the fetus reaches 15 to 18 weeks. Bile secretion by the fetal liver first takes place around the third month of gestation.

CONGENITAL ANOMALIES

Anomalies of the gallbladder, such as duplication, luminal septation, atresia, ectopia, and cysts, are rarely seen (40,58). Agenesis of the gallbladder occurs with a frequency less than 0.016 percent (5,40). Familial cases of agenesis have been documented. Many congenital anomalies are asymptomatic and incidentally found during radiologic procedures for other disorders (49).

Atresia, an anomalous choledochopancreatic junction, and cystic dilatation are among the most common anomalies of the extrahepatic bile ducts. Other anomalies include aberrant location and connection of the common hepatic duct to the gallbladder. Cases of agenesis have also been reported (54). Multiple anomalies of the foregut derivatives are occasionally observed (12,27,37). Anomalies of the biliary tract have been associated with congenital defects in other organs such as renal hypoplasia or agenesis, polycystic renal disease, and megaureter.

Of greater significance for the pathologist are those congenital anomalies associated with cancer. These include choledochal cysts and the premature union of the pancreatic and common bile ducts (3,32,42,44). An anomalous choledochopancreatic junction is found in more than 80 percent of patients with a choledochal cyst. Cystic dilatation of the extrahepatic bile ducts may be associated with dilatation of the intrahepatic ducts.

ANATOMIC VARIATIONS

Anatomic variations are more meaningful for the surgeon than for the pathologist. The important vascular and ductal variations encountered during surgery have been reviewed (6,16). Variations in the vascular supply are found in more than 50 percent of patients undergoing cholecystectomy. Variations of the ducts, on the other hand, are much less frequent, occurring in 14 percent of such patients. By combining these figures, it becomes obvious that a surgeon can expect some type of anatomic variation in every other operative case.

The most common vascular variations include an accessory cystic artery; anterior transposition of the cystic or right hepatic artery, or both; and a short cystic artery that arises from the right hepatic artery. The cystic artery may also arise from the superior mesenteric artery, hepatic trunk, left hepatic artery, or gastroduodenal artery. The cystic artery may also be doubled. Variations in the vascular supply to the bile ducts and their implications for postoperative strictures have also been described (45).

The two most common ductal variations include a long cystic duct fusing low with the common duct and high fusion of the cystic and hepatic ducts. Because anatomic variations are so common, some authors have questioned the meaning of the term normal as applied to the extrahepatic tree (16).

FUNCTION

The functions of the gallbladder are: 1) concentrating and storing bile (50) and 2) propelling the bile into the duodenum to facilitate digestion and absorption of fats (7,56).

By absorption of water against osmotic gradients, the gallbladder can concentrate bile to less than 20 percent of its original volume. Absorption is coupled to an electrically neutral sodium chloride influx process which is inhibited by agents that elevate intracellular levels of cyclic 3',5' adenosine monophosphate (20,21). The gallbladder epithelium has one of the highest rates of fluid absorption of all epithelia that have been studied (48). Physiologic studies indicate that the gallbladder mucosa, at least in normal animals, consists of a single functional cell type, capable of absorbing sodium chloride and water, but not sugars or amino acids.

Postprandial contraction of the gallbladder as well as relaxation of the sphincter of Oddi is largely mediated by cholecystokinin, a peptide hormone secreted by the duodenum and upper small intestine in response to a meal. In addition to stimulating the release of endothelin (28), cholecystokinin exerts its contractile effects in two other ways: binding to receptors on the smooth muscle cells of the gallbladder and interaction with cholinergic nerves (53,61). Relaxation of the gallbladder is caused by vasoactive intestinal peptide (51). Secretin, another peptide hormone secreted by the duodenum, inhibits the concentrating mechanism and stimulates secretion by the gallbladder epithelial cells (29). Somatostatin, a small peptide hormone secreted by D cells, inhibits gallbladder contraction and flow of bile. Excess production of somatostatin as found in D cell tumors (somatostatinomas) leads to bile stasis and stone formation. The actions of these peptide hormones are complex, since secretin and cholecystokinin also stimulate somatostatin release.

In addition to storage and contraction, the gallbladder is also a secretory organ. The epithelium secretes a colorless alkaline fluid that contains glycoproteins and electrolytes (22). Secretion tends to increase following a fatty meal or a lithogenic diet and decreases during fasting. Secretion is also increased after stimulation of the small cholinergic nerves that innervate the gallbladder. As a result of its secretory activity, the gallbladder epithelium also affects the composition of bile.

REFERENCES

1. Albores-Saavedra J, Nadji M, Henson DE, Ziegels-Wiessman J, Mones JM. Intestinal metaplasia of the gallbladder: a morphologic and immunocytochemical study. Hum Pathol 1986;17:614–20.
2. Albores-Saavedra J, Nadji M, Morales AR, Henson DE. Carcinoembryonic antigen in normal, preneoplastic and neoplastic gallbladder epithelium. Cancer 1983;52:1069–72.
3. Babbit DP. Congenital choledochal cysts: new etiological concept based on anomalous relationships of the common bile duct and pancreatic bulb. Ann Radiologie 1969;12:231–40.
4. Baggenstoss AH. Major duodenal papilla: variations of pathologic interest and lesions of the mucosa. Arch Pathol 1938;26:853–68.
5. Bennion RS, Thompson JE, Tompkins RK. Agenesis of the gallbladder without extrahepatic biliary atresia. Arch Surg 1988;123:1257–60.
6. Benson EA, Page RE. A practical reappraisal of the anatomy of the extrahepatic bile ducts and arteries. Br J Surg 1976;63:853–60.
7. Boyden EA. The effect of natural foods on the distention of the gallbladder, with a note on the change in pattern of the mucosa as it passes from distention to collapse. Anat Rec 1925;30:333–63.
8. Boyden EA. The anatomy of the choledochoduodenal junction in man. Surg Gynec Obstet 1957;104:641–52.
9. Burden VG. Observations on the histologic and pathologic anatomy of the hepatic, cystic, and common bile ducts. Ann Surg 1925;82:584–97.
10. Burnett W, Gairns FW, Bacsich BP. Some observations on the innervation of the extrahepatic biliary system in man. Ann Surg 1964;159:8–26.
11. Castelluci M, Caggiati A. Surface aspects of the rabbit gallbladder mucosa and their functional implications. J Submicros Cytol 1980;12:375–90.
12. Coughlin JP, Rector FE, Klein MD. Agenesis of the gallbladder in duodenal atresia: two case reports. J Pediatr Surg 1992;27:1304.
13. Dancygier H. Endoscopic transpapillary biopsy (ETPB) of human extrahepatic bile ducts—light and electron microscopic findings, clinical significance. Endoscopy 1989;21:312–20.
14. Dancygier H, Klein U, Leuschner U, Hubner K, Classen M. Somatostatin-containing cells in the extrahepatic biliary tract of humans. Gastroenterology 1984;86:892–6.
15. DiMagno EP, Shorter RG, Taylor WF, Go VL. Relationships between pancreaticobiliary ductal anatomy and pancreatic ductal and parenchymal histology. Cancer 1982;49:361–8.
16. Dowdy GS Jr, Waldron GW, Brown WG. Surgical anatomy of the pancreatobiliary ductal system. Arch Surg 1962;84:229–46.
17. Evett RD, Higgins JA, Brown AL Jr. The fine structure of normal mucosa in human gallbladder. Gastroenterology 1964;47:49–60.
18. Fox H. Ultrastructure of the human gallbladder epithelium in cholelithiasis and chronic cholecystitis. J Pathol 1972;108:157–64.

19. Frierson HF Jr. Gallbladder and extrahepatic biliary system. In: Sternberg SS, ed. Histology for pathologists. New York: Raven Press, 1992:639–55.

20. Frizzell RA, Dugas MC, Shultz SG. Sodium chloride transport by rabbit gallbladder. Direct evidence for a coupled NaCl influx. J Gen Physiol 1975;65:769–95.

21. Frizzell RA, Heintze K. Transport functions of the gallbladder, In: Javitt NB, ed. Liver and biliary tract physiology 1. International review of physiology, Vol 21. Baltimore: University Park Press, 1980:221–7.

22. Glickerman DJ, Kim MH, Malik R, Lee SP. The gallbladder also secretes. Digest Dis Sci 1997;42:489–91.

23. Gordon KC. A comparative anatomical study of the distribution of the cystic artery in man and other species. J Anat 1967;101:351–9.

24. Green FH, Fox H. An immunofluorescent study of the distribution of immunoglobin-containing cells in the normal and the inflamed human gallbladder. Gut 1972;13:379–84.

25. Hakkinen I, Laitio M. Epithelial glycoproteins of human gallbladder. Immunological characterization. Arch Pathol 1970;90:137–42.

26. Hayward AF. The structure of gallbladder epithelium. Int Rev Gen Exp Zool 1968;3:205–39.

27. Heij HA, Niessen GJ. Annular pancreas associated with congenital absence of the gallbladder. J Pediatr Surg 1987;22:1033.

27a. Hong SM, Kang GH, Lee HY, Ro JY. Smooth muscle distribution in the extrahepatic bile duct. Histologic and immunohistochemical studies of 122 cases. Am J Surg Pathol 2000;24:660-7.

28. Housset C, Carayon A, Housset B, Legendre C, Hannoun L, Poupon R. Endothelin-1 secretion by human gallbladder epithelial cells in primary culture. Lab Invest 1993;69:750–4.

28a. Huizinga JD. Pathophysiology of gastrointestinal motility related to interstitial cells of Cajal. Am J Physiol 1998;275:6381–6.

29. Igimi H, Yamamoto F, Lee SP. Gallbladder mucosal function: studies in absorption and secretion in humans and dog gallbladder epithelium. Am J Physiol 1992;263;G69–74.

30. Ito M, Mishima Y, Sato T. An anatomical study of the lymphatic drainage of the gallbladder. Surg Radiol Anat 1991;13:89–104.

31. Kayahara M, Nagakawa T, Ueno K, Ohta T, Takeda T, Miyazaki I. Lymphatic flow in carcinoma of the distal bile duct based on a clinicopathologic study. Cancer 1993;72:2112–7.

32. Kimura K, Ohto M, Saisho H, et al. Association of gallbladder carcinoma and anomalous pancreaticobiliary ductal union. Gastroenterology 1985;89:1258–65.

32a. Kindblom LG, Remoti HE, Aldenborg F, Meis-Kindblom JM. Gastrointestinal pacemaker cell tumor (GIPACT). Gastrointestinal stromal tumors show phenotypic characteristics of the interstitial cells of Cajal. Am J Pathol 1998;152:1259–69.

33. Koga A. Electron microscopic observations on the mucous secretory activity of the human gallbladder epithelium. Z Zellforsch Mikrosk Anat 1973;139:463–71.

34. Laitio M, Nevalainen T. Scanning and transmission electron microscope observations on human gallbladder epithelium. I. Adult structure. Z Anat Entwicklungsgesch 1972;136:319–25.

35. Laitio M, Nevalainen T. Gland ultrastructure in human gallbladder. J Anat 1975;120:105–12.

36. Laitio M, Nevalainen T. Ultrastructure of endocrine cells in metaplastic epithelium of human gallbladder. J Anat 1975;120:219–25.

37. Martinek V, Keller HW, Vossing R, Dolken W. Congenital duodenal stenosis in combination with ectopic gastric mucosa. Chirurg 1994;65:807–9.

38. Maxwell P, Davis RI, Sloan JM. Carcinoembryonic antigen (CEA) in benign and malignant epithelium of the gallbladder, extrahepatic bile ducts, and ampulla of Vater. J Pathol 1993;170:73–6.

39. Millbourn E. Calibre and appearance of the pancreatic ducts and relevant clinical problems. Acta Chir Scand 1960;118:286–303.

40. Monroe SE. Congenital absence of the gallbladder: a statistical study. J Int Coll Surg 1959;32:369–73.

41. Moosman DA, Coller FA. Prevention of traumatic injury to the bile ducts. A study of the structures of the cystohepatic angle encountered in cholecystectomy and supraduodenal choledochostomy. Am J Surg 1951;82:132–43.

42. Mori K, Nagakawa T, Ohta T, et al. Association between gallbladder cancer and anomalous union of the pancreaticobiliary ductal system. Hepatogastroenterology 1993;40:56–60.

43. Myllarniemi H, Nickels JI. Observations by scanning electron microscopy of normal and pathological human gallbladder epithelium. Acta Pathol Microbiol Scand [A] 1977;85:42–8.

44. Nagata E, Sakai K, Kinoshita H, Kobayashi Y. The relation between carcinoma of the gallbladder and an anomalous connection between the choledochus and the pancreatic duct. Ann Surg 1985;202:182–90.

45. Northover JM, Terblanche J. A new look at the arterial supply of the bile duct in man and its surgical implications. Br J Surg 1979;66:379–84.

46. Polyzonis MB, Tsikaras P, Hytiroglou P, Agios A. Further observations on the vascular system of the gallbladder in man. Bull Assoc Anat 1989;73:25–8.

47. Repassy G, Schaff Z, Lapis K, Marton T, Jakab F, Sugar I. Mucosa of the Heister valve in cholelithiasis. Transmission and scanning electron microscopic study. Arch Pathol Lab Med 1978;102:403–5.

48. Reuss L. Ion transport across gallbladder epithelium. Physiol Rev 1989;69:503–45.

49. Rizzo RJ, Szucs RA, Turner MA. Congenital abnormalities of the pancreas and biliary tree in adults. Radiographics 1995;15:49–68.

50. Rous P, McMaster PD. The concentrating activity of the gallbladder. J Exp Med 1921;34:47–73.

51. Said IS. Progress in gastroenterology V. Vasoactive intestinal polypeptide (VIP). Gastroenterology 1974;67:735–7.

52. Schaff Z, Lapis K, Csikos A. Scanning electron microscopic study of human gallbladder mucosa in cholelithiasis. Acta Morphol Acad Sci Hung 1979;27:107–14.

53. Schjoldager B, Molero X, Miller LJ. Functional and biochemical characterization of the human gallbladder muscularis cholecystokinin receptor. Gastroenterology 1989;96:1119–25.

54. Schwartz MZ, Hall RJ, Reubner B, Lilly JR, Brogen T, Toyama WM. Agenesis of the extrahepatic bile ducts: report of five cases. J Pediat Surg 1990;25:805–7.

56. Soloway RD, Balistreri WF, Trotman BW. The gallbladder and biliary tract. In: Recent advances in gastroenterology, No 4. New York: Churchill Livingstone, 1980.

57. Spitz L, Petropoulos A. The development of the glands of the common bile duct. J Pathol 1978;128:213–20.

58. Stolkind E. Congenital abnormalities of the gallbladder and extrahepatic ducts. Br J Child Dis 1939;36:115–31, 182–212, 295–307.

59. Takahashi Y, Takahashi T, Takahashi W, Sato T. Morphometrical evaluation of extrahepatic bile ducts in reference to their structural changes with aging. Tohoku J Exp Med 1985;147:301–9.

60. Togari C, Okada T. The minute structure of the epithelium of the human gallbladder. Okajimas Folia Anat Jpn 1953;25:1–12.

61. Tokunaga Y, Cox KL, Coleman BS, Conceptcion W, Nakazato P, Esquivel CO. Characterization of cholecystokinin receptors on the human gallbladder. Surgery 1993;113:155–62.

62. Wong KC, Lister J. Human fetal development of the hepato-pancreatic duct junction—a possible explanation of congenital dilatation of the biliary tract. J Pediatr Surg 1981;16:139–45.

63. Yamada K. Morphological and histochemical aspects of secretion in the gallbladder epithelium of the Guinea pig. Anat Rec 1962;144:117–23.

2
HISTOLOGIC CLASSIFICATION

The histologic classification of tumors of the gallbladder, extrahepatic bile ducts, and ampulla of Vater is shown below. Adopted by the World Health Organization (WHO) in 1991 (4), the classification is based on light microscopic features of hematoxylin and eosin–stained sections with recognition of the adjunctive value of immunohistochemistry and electron microscopy (3). This classification, which is the second WHO classification, includes lesions that were not listed in the first published in 1978 (7). The second classification is similar to the one recommended in the second edition of the Armed Forces Institute of Pathology (AFIP) Fascicle on this subject published in 1986 (1). Although based primarily on the histologic characteristics of the tumor, the classification also takes into account histomorphology and prognosis.

In the 1991 WHO classification, tubular adenomas are recognized as metaplastic tumors and subdivided into pyloric gland and intestinal types. Likewise, papillary adenomas are subdivided into intestinal and biliary types. Biliary cystadenomas are considered distinctive benign neoplasms which belong to a family of mucinous cystic tumors with a characteristic ovarian-like stroma. In addition to the biliary tract, they can also arise in the pancreas and in the retroperitoneum unattached to any organ. Although the term papillomatosis has been retained, it has recently been recognized that some cases metastasize and that both benign-appearing and obviously malignant cells are present in the metastatic deposits. It is possible, therefore, that papillomatosis may represent a low-grade, multifocal, intraductal papillary carcinoma similar to the intraductal papillary mucinous neoplasms occurring in the main pancreatic duct (2,10,11).

Pleomorphic giant cell adenocarcinomas and poorly differentiated carcinomas composed of small cells were considered separate entities in the AFIP Fascicle published in 1986 (1). These tumors are now included under the generic term "undifferentiated carcinoma." The term carcinosarcoma has been restricted to neoplasms with both carcinomatous and malignant mesenchymal components including heterologous elements such as cartilage, bone, and skeletal muscle. The mesenchymal components of carcinosarcomas lack immunoreactivity for epithelial markers.

The term small cell carcinoma is preferred over small cell undifferentiated carcinoma. Although some undifferentiated carcinomas are composed predominantly of small cells, these cells have vesicular nuclei, prominent nucleoli, and frequently, cytoplasmic mucin droplets. Moreover, small cell undifferentiated carcinomas do not show endocrine differentiation. The WHO does not recommend the use of the term "neuroendocrine carcinoma" for small cell carcinoma because of the confusion it has generated among oncologists and surgeons, which in turn may have therapeutic implications. Moreover, a variable proportion of small cell carcinomas lack evidence of endocrine differentiation by immunohistochemistry and electron microscopy.

At least one third of all adenocarcinomas of the gallbladder and extrahepatic bile ducts contain endocrine cells (5,12). Regardless of the number of endocrine cells, their presence does not justify the diagnosis of a carcinoid tumor, adenocarcinoid, or neuroendocrine carcinoma, an erroneous interpretation that may have prognostic implications. This endocrine cell population is present in both in situ and invasive carcinomas and is not unique to tumors of the gallbladder, extrahepatic bile ducts, or ampulla. Similar endocrine cells have been described in carcinomas arising in the colon, stomach, and pancreas (5,6,8,9).

We do not recommend the use of the term "cholangiocarcinoma" to designate the malignant epithelial tumors of the extrahepatic bile ducts. This term should be restricted to the malignant epithelial tumors of the intrahepatic bile ducts.

The widespread use of this classification, by pathologists and clinicians, will facilitate international comparative studies on the incidence, histologic distribution, and treatment of the tumors of the gallbladder, extrahepatic bile ducts, and ampulla.

HISTOLOGIC CLASSIFICATION OF TUMORS OF THE GALLBLADDER, EXTRAHEPATIC BILE DUCTS, AND AMPULLA OF VATER

Epithelial Tumors
  Benign
    Adenoma
      Tubular
      Papillary
      Tubulopapillary
    Cystadenoma
    Papillomatosis
  Premalignant Lesions
    Dysplasia
    Carcinoma in situ
  Malignant
    Adenocarcinoma
    Papillary adenocarcinoma
    Adenocarcinoma, intestinal type
    Adenocarcinoma, gastric foveolar type
    Clear cell adenocarcinoma
    Mucinous carcinoma
    Signet ring cell carcinoma
    Adenosquamous carcinoma
    Squamous cell carcinoma
    Small cell carcinoma (oat cell carcinoma)
    Large cell neuroendocrine carcinoma
    Undifferentiated carcinoma
      Spindle and giant cell type
      Small cell type
      With a nodular growth pattern
      With osteoclast-like giant cells
    Cystadenocarcinoma
    Other
Endocrine Tumors
  Carcinoid tumor
  Adenocarcinoid (goblet cell carcinoid)
  Tubular carcinoid
  Mixed carcinoid-adenocarcinoma
Tumors of Paraganglia
  Paraganglioma
  Gangliocytic paraganglioma

Nonepithelial Tumors
  Benign
    Leiomyoma
    Lipoma
    Hemangioma

    Lymphangioma
    Osteoma
    Granular cell tumor
  Neurogenic Tumors
    Neurofibroma
    Neurofibromatosis
    Ganglioneuromatosis
  Malignant Mesenchymal Tumors
    Rhabdomyosarcoma
    Malignant fibrous histiocytoma
    Angiosarcoma
    Leiomyosarcoma
    Kaposi's sarcoma
Miscellaneous Tumors
  Carcinosarcoma
  Malignant melanoma
  Malignant lymphoma
  Yolk sac tumor
Unclassified Tumors

Secondary Tumors

Tumor-Like Lesions
  Regenerative epithelial atypia
  Intestinal metaplasia
  Pyloric gland metaplasia
  Papillary hyperplasia
  Squamous metaplasia
  Rokitansky-Aschoff sinuses
  Adenomyomatous hyperplasia
  Luschka's ducts
  Mucocele
  Heterotopia
  Cholesterol polyp
  Inflammatory polyp
  Fibrous polyp
  Myofibroblastic proliferations
  Xanthogranulomatous cholecystitis
  Cholecystitis with lymphoid hyperplasia
  Malacoplakia
  Congenital cyst
  Amputation neuroma
  Primary sclerosing cholangitis
  Other

REFERENCES

1. Albores-Saavedra J, Henson DE. Tumors of the gall-bladder and extrahepatic bile ducts. Atlas of tumor pathology. 2nd series, Fascicle 22. Washington, DC: Armed Forces Institute of Pathology, 1986.
2. Albores-Saavedra J, Henson DE, Milchgrub S. Intraductal papillary carcinoma of the main pancreatic duct. Int J Pancreatol 1994;16:223–4.
3. Albores-Saavedra J, Henson DE, Sobin LH. The WHO histological classification of tumors of the gallbladder and extrahepatic bile ducts. A commentary on the second edition. Cancer 1992;70:410–4.
4. Albores-Saavedra J, Henson DE, Sobin LH. In: WHO histological typing of tumors of the gallbladder and extrahepatic bile ducts. Berlin: Springer-Verlag, 1991.
5. Albores-Saavedra J, Nadji M, Henson DE, Angeles-Angeles A. Enteroendocrine differentiation in carcinomas of the gallbladder and mucinous cystadenocarcinomas of the pancreas. Pathol Res Pract 1988;183:169–74.
6. Arends JW, Wiggers T, Verstijnen K, Bosman FT. The occurrence and clinicopathological significance of serotonin immunoreactive cells in large bowel carcinoma. J Pathol 1986;149:97–102.
7. Gibson JB. Histological typing of tumors of the liver, biliary tract and pancreas. Geneva: World Health Organization, 1978.
8. Mori M, Mimori K, Kamakura T, Adachi Y, Ikeda Y, Sugimachi K. Chromogranin positive cells in colorectal carcinoma and transitional mucosa. J Clin Pathol 1995;48:754–8.
9. Park JG, Choe GY, Helman LJ, et al. Chromogranin-A expression in gastric and colon cancer tissues. Int J Cancer 1992;69:2641–6.
10. Sessa F, Solcia E, Capella C, et al. Intraductal papillary-mucinous tumors represent a distinct group of pancreatic neoplasms: an investigation of tumour cell differentiation and K-ras, p53 and c-erβ-2 abnormalities in 26 patients. Virchows Arch 1994;425:357–67.
11. Solcia E, Capella C, Klöppel G. Tumors of the pancreas. Atlas of Tumor Pathology, 3rd Series, Fascicle 20. Washington, DC, Armed Forces Institute of Pathology, 1997.
12. Yamamoto M, Takahashi I, Iwamoto T, et al. Endocrine cells with extrahepatic bile duct carcinoma. J Cancer Res Clin Oncol 1984;108:331–5.

3

BENIGN EPITHELIAL TUMORS OF GALLBLADDER

ADENOMA

Definition and General Features. For many years adenomas of the gallbladder have caused diagnostic problems because of a lack of adequate histologic criteria and uniform nomenclature. Moreover, these tumors often coexist with hyperplastic and metaplastic lesions, contain a heterogenous cell population, and display a range of morphologic patterns, further complicating interpretation. In recent years, however, a better understanding of their microscopic features has resulted in a more accurate histologic classification.

Adenomas of the gallbladder are uncommon benign neoplasms of glandular epithelium which are typically polypoid and well demarcated. According to their pattern of growth, adenomas of the extrahepatic biliary tree are divided into three types: tubular, papillary, and tubulopapillary (1,2,23). Cytologically, they are classified as pyloric gland type, intestinal type, and biliary type. Adenomas are found in 0.3 to 0.5 percent of gallbladders removed for cholelithiasis or chronic cholecystitis (1). Some investigators have reported an incidence of 10 to 12 percent in cholecystectomy specimens, but they included a number of tumor-like lesions as adenomas. The malignant potential of these adenomas has been a source of controversy (6,7) and is discussed in the section, Adenoma-Carcinoma Sequence at the end of this chapter.

Clinical Features. Adenomas of the gallbladder are more common in women than men. In our series of 37 patients, 26 (70 percent) were females (3). The age of the patients ranged from 17 to 79 years, with a mean of 58 years. Rarely, gallbladder adenomas occur in children (12).

Adenomas are often small, asymptomatic, and usually discovered incidentally during cholecystectomy (3,4). However, when they arise in the neck, they may block the flow of bile, which leads to gallbladder distention. When larger than 2 cm, or when multiple and filling the gallbladder lumen they can produce symptoms similar to those of chronic cholecystitis. If pedunculated, they can undergo torsion, infarction, or self-am-putation and may be found free in the lumen of the gallbladder. If the stalk is long the polyp may act as a ball valve, leading to intermittent obstruction at the neck. The adenoma may become detached from the gallbladder wall, with subsequent lodgement of tumor fragments into the cystic and common bile ducts, resulting in obstruction (13). Clinical diagnosis often depends on imaging. Some are visualized as fixed radiolucent defects on cholecystograms; but the majority are now recognized by ultrasound or by computed tomography.

Occasionally, adenomas of the gallbladder occur in association with the Peutz-Jeghers (5, 18) or Gardner's syndrome (17,19). Some believe that both benign and malignant epithelial tumors of the biliary tree are in fact a rare component of Gardner's syndrome (19). Adenomas of the gallbladder have also been reported in patients with an anomalous union of the pancreatobiliary duct (11,21). Whether this association is coincidental or has a causal relationship is not yet known. The suggestion has been made that regurgitation of pancreatic juice leads to inflammation, metaplasia, and adenomatous growth. If this hypothesis is correct one would expect to find the adenomas in the extrahepatic bile ducts rather than in the gallbladder.

Gross Findings. Adenomas of the gallbladder are usually solitary, pedunculated or sessile, and generally measure less than 2 cm (14–16). They are most commonly located in the body, followed in frequency by the fundus and neck (figs. 3-1, 3-2). Approximately 10 percent are multiple (3,10). When multiple they may fill the gallbladder lumen (fig. 3-3). According to different series, 50 to 65 percent of adenomas are associated with cholelithiasis (3,4,20).

A tubular adenoma initially appears as a soft, nodular, pink elevation on the mucosa. As the lesion enlarges, it projects into the lumen. At this stage the adenoma resembles a lobulated, berry-like nodule similar to the tubular adenomas of the large intestine (fig. 3-2). Papillary adenomas exhibit the typical cauliflower-like appearance with a fine granular surface.

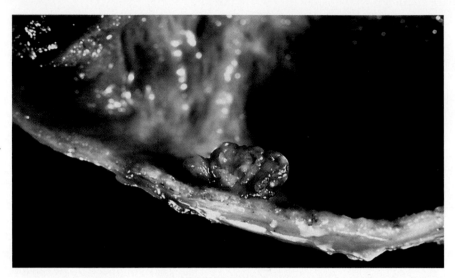

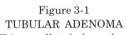

Figure 3-1
TUBULAR ADENOMA
This small tubular adenoma which has a fine nodular surface arose from the wall of the body of the gallbladder. Multiple stones had been previously removed from the gallbladder. The adenoma was an incidental finding.

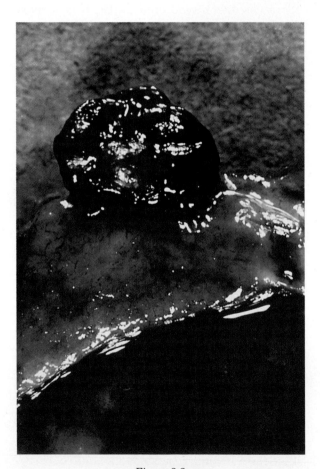

Figure 3-2
TUBULAR ADENOMA
A small sessile nodule is seen on the mucosal surface. The gallbladder has been everted to expose the nodule, which, histologically, was a tubular adenoma.

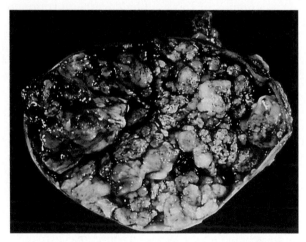

Figure 3-3
TUBULAR ADENOMAS
The gallbladder is filled and distended with innumerable tubular adenomas of different sizes.

Tubular Adenoma, Pyloric Gland Type

Definition. This is a benign tumor composed of closely packed, short tubular glands that are similar to pyloric glands and lined by mild to moderately dysplastic epithelium.

Pathologic Findings. In its early phase of development, pyloric gland type tubular adenomas appear as well-demarcated nodules embedded in the lamina propria and covered with normal biliary epithelium. They are composed of lobules that contain closely packed, pyloric type

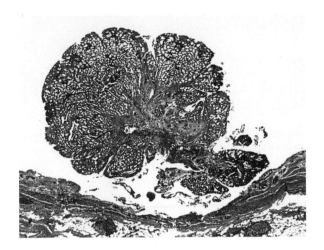

Figure 3-4
PYLORIC GLAND TYPE ADENOMA
Pedunculated pyloric gland type adenoma with well-defined lobular architecture.

glands, some of which may be cystically dilated (figs. 3-4, 3-5). The glands, which form lobules, are lined by columnar or cuboidal cells with vesicular or hyperchromatic nuclei and small nucleoli. A variable amount of cytoplasmic mucin is present (fig. 3-6). Nodular aggregates of cytologically bland spindle cells with an eosinophilic cytoplasm but without keratinization or intercellular bridges, known as squamoid morules (8,15), are present in about 10 percent of the cases, whereas frank squamous metaplasia is exceedingly rare (fig. 3-7). Approximately 20 percent of the tumors contain Paneth cells as well as endocrine cells (fig. 3-8).

By immunohistochemistry, serotonin and a variety of peptide hormones including somatostatin, pancreatic polypeptide, and gastrin, have

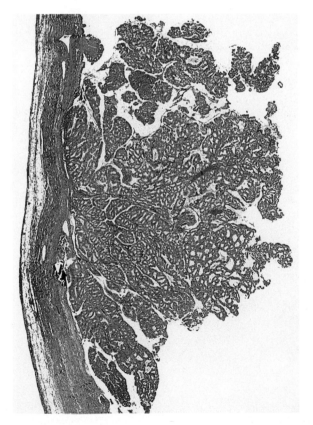
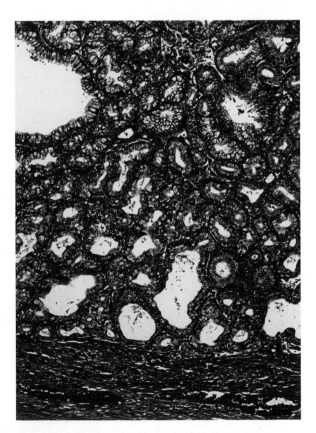

Figure 3-5
PYLORIC GLAND TYPE ADENOMA
Left: Low-power view of a sessile pyloric gland type adenoma containing some dilated glands.
Right: Sessile pyloric gland adenoma containing cystically dilated glands.

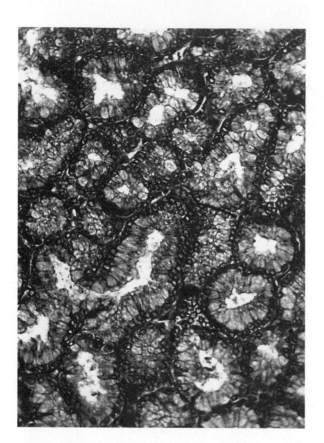 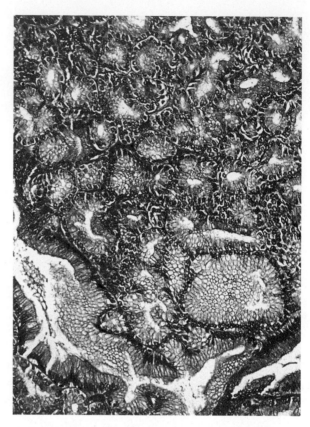

Figure 3-6
PYLORIC GLAND TYPE ADENOMA
Left: Higher magnification of pyloric type glands lined by cells with vesicular nuclei and mucin-containing cytoplasm.
Right: A lobule of closely packed tubular glands is lined by columnar cells with hyperchromatic nuclei. A dilated duct is seen in the center of the lobule.

Figure 3-7
SQUAMOID MORULE
IN A PYLORIC GLAND
TYPE ADENOMA

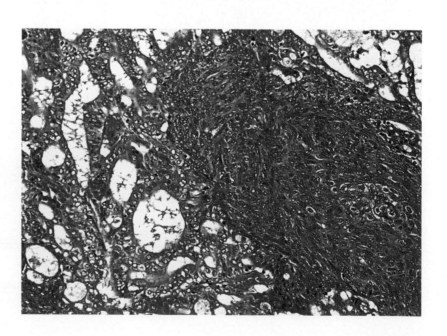

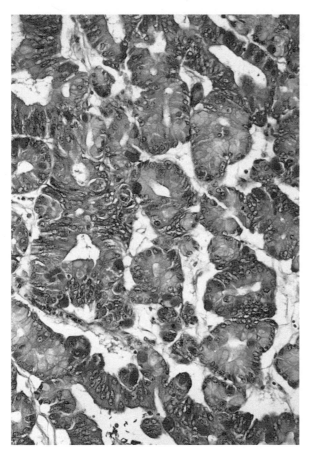

Figure 3-8
PYLORIC GLAND TYPE ADENOMA
Numerous Paneth cells are admixed with columnar cells in a pyloric gland type adenoma.

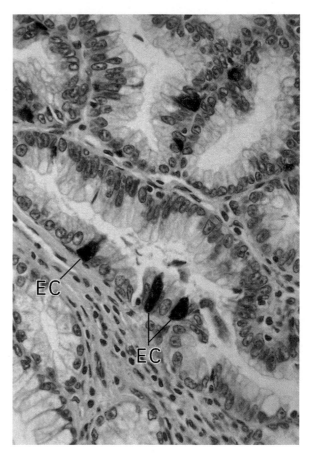

Figure 3-9
SEROTONIN-CONTAINING (EC) CELLS
IN A PYLORIC GLAND TYPE ADENOMA

been found in the cytoplasm of these cells (fig. 3-9). Dysplastic changes are more pronounced in larger adenomas. Foci of carcinoma in situ are seen in 7 percent of adenomas and invasive carcinoma in 7 percent (fig. 3-10). As they enlarge, most adenomas develop a pedicle and project into the lumen. Rarely, they extend into or arise from Rokitansky-Aschoff sinuses, a finding that should not be mistaken for carcinoma (fig. 3-11) (3,9). Adenomas that extend into or arise from these sinuses show the same morphologic features as mucosal adenomas, and do not infiltrate the muscle wall or serosa of the gallbladder. The sinuses containing the adenoma are markedly dilated and lined, at least in part, by histologically normal biliary epithelium. The stroma of pyloric gland type adenoma is usually minimal, but can become edematous or partially

hyalinized and may even contain lymphocytes. It is continuous with the connective tissue in the lamina propria. When the stroma is abundant and edematous and there are only scattered glands, the microscopic picture is reminiscent of a fibroadenoma of the breast.

Differential Diagnosis. Pyloric gland type adenomas often coexist with pyloric gland hyperplasia, suggesting that the latter is the precursor lesion. In contrast to the adenomas, however, pyloric gland hyperplasia is not well demarcated, often extending laterally to the lamina propria and vertically into the muscle layer. It usually lacks dysplastic changes. Pyloric gland type adenomas can also be confused with polypoid ectopic gastric mucosa which, in addition to pyloric glands, contains fundic mucosa with chief and parietal cells (22).

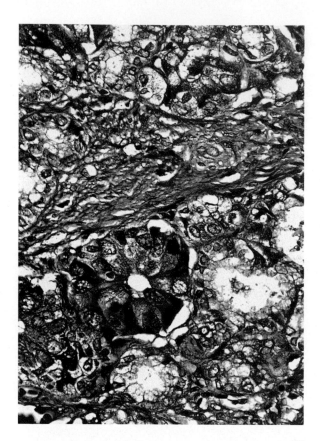
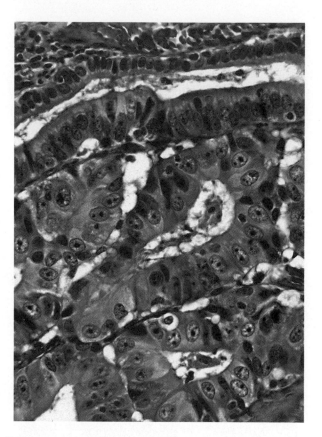

Figure 3-10
PYLORIC GLAND TYPE ADENOMA WITH CARCINOMA IN SITU
Left: Marked cellular atypia and large hyperchromatic nuclei are seen in one gland.
Right: The glands are lined by columnar cells with little or no mucin. Their nuclei are large, pseudostratified, and vesicular, and contain prominent nucleoli.

Figure 3-11
PYLORIC GLAND
TYPE ADENOMA
A pyloric gland type adenoma with tubular and papillary architecture extends into a Rokitansky-Aschoff sinus.

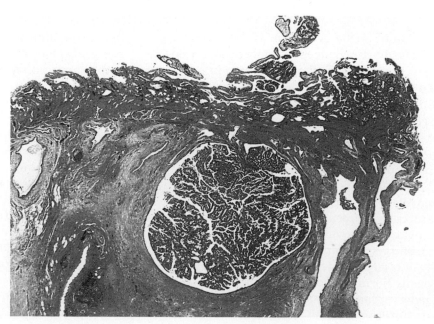

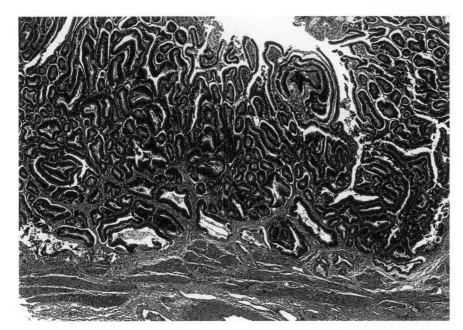

Figure 3-12
TUBULAR ADENOMA,
INTESTINAL TYPE
Low-power view showing glands of different sizes, some of which are cystically dilated.

Tubular Adenoma, Intestinal Type

This benign tumor is composed of tubular glands lined by cells with an intestinal phenotype. The lining cells characteristically show moderate to severe dysplastic changes (fig. 3-12). This type of adenoma closely resembles colonic adenoma. It consists of tubular glands lined by pseudostratified columnar cells with elongated hyperchromatic nuclei. The glands lack invasive properties and focally are arranged in well-defined lobules (fig. 3-13). The adenomatous epithelium may extend into the Rokitansky-Aschoff sinuses and should not be confused with stromal invasion. Clusters of goblet, Paneth, and endocrine cells are usually mixed with the columnar cells. Serotonin and, less frequently, peptide hormones have been identified in the endocrine cells by immunohistochemistry (fig. 3-14). Hyperplasia of metaplastic pyloric type glands is often seen at the base of the adenoma.

Papillary Adenoma, Intestinal Type

This benign tumor consists predominantly of papillary structures lined by dysplastic cells with an intestinal phenotype (fig. 3-15). The predominant cell is columnar, with elongated hyperchromatic nuclei and little or no cytoplasmic mucin. The cells are pseudostratified, mitotically active, and indistinguishable from those of papillary

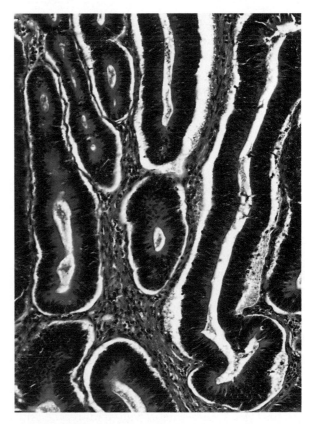

Figure 3-13
TUBULAR ADENOMA, INTESTINAL TYPE
Higher magnification of tumor shown in figure 3-12. The long tubular glands are lined by tall columnar cells similar to those of intestinal adenomas.

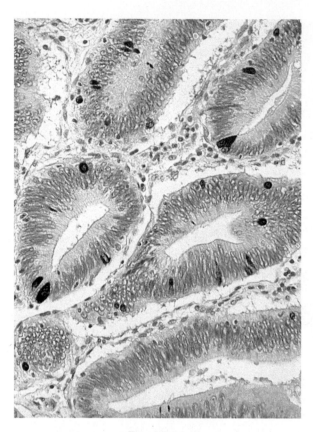

Figure 3-14
SEROTONIN-CONTAINING CELLS IN
A TUBULAR ADENOMA, INTESTINAL TYPE

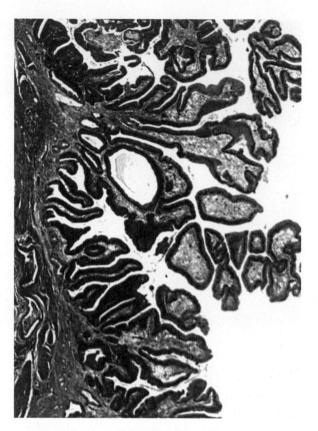

Figure 3-15
PAPILLARY ADENOMA, INTESTINAL TYPE
Low-power view.

adenomas arising in the large intestine (fig. 3-16). Tubular glands lined by the same type of epithelium but representing less than 20 percent of the tumor may also be found. Dysplastic changes are more extensive than in pyloric gland type adenomas. Also present are goblet, Paneth, and serotonin-containing cells (fig. 3-17). Some of the endocrine cells are immunoreactive for peptide hormones. These adenomas usually arise in a background of pyloric gland metaplasia. In our series, one of five papillary adenomas, intestinal type, progressed to invasive carcinoma (fig. 3-18).

Papillary Adenoma, Biliary Type

This type of adenoma is well demarcated and consists of papillary structures lined by tall columnar cells, which, except for the presence of more cytoplasmic mucin in the lining cells, show minimal variation from normal gallbladder epi-

thelium (fig. 3-19). In our experience, this is the rarest form of adenoma of the gallbladder; in fact, we have seen only one case. Endocrine or Paneth cells are not found in these adenomas. Only mild dysplastic changes are noted; in situ or invasive carcinoma has not been reported. Most papillary lesions composed of normal-appearing gallbladder epithelium are examples of hyperplasia secondary to chronic cholecystitis.

Tubulopapillary Adenoma

When tubular glands and papillary structures each comprise more than 20 percent of the tumor, the term tubulopapillary adenoma is applied. Two subtypes are recognized: one is composed of tubular glands and papillary structures similar to those of mixed intestinal adenomas; the other consists of tubular glands similar to pyloric glands and papillary structures often

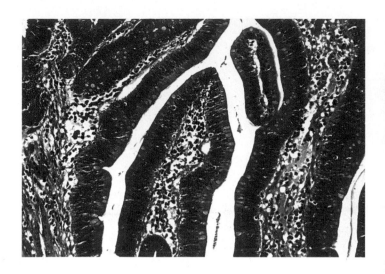

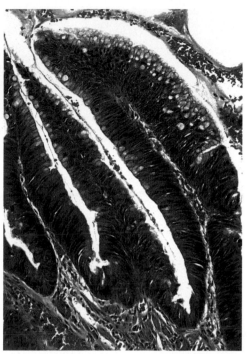

Figure 3-16
PAPILLARY ADENOMA, INTESTINAL TYPE
Above: Pseudostratified columnar dysplastic cells admixed with goblet cells line the papillary structures, which contain chronic inflammatory cells.
Right: The papillae are lined by tall columnar cells with elongated pseudostratified nuclei. Goblet cells are admixed with the columnar cells.

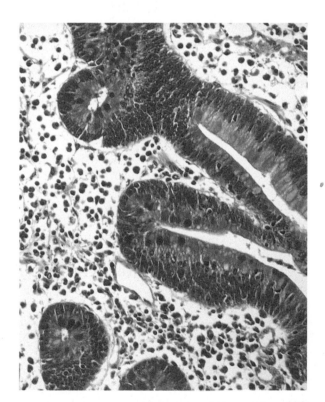

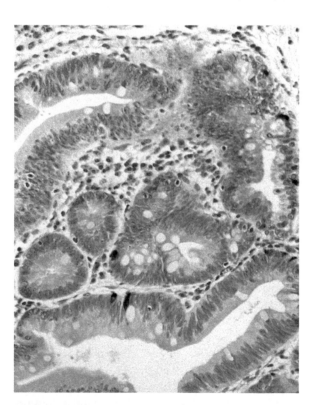

Figure 3-17
PAPILLARY ADENOMA, INTESTINAL TYPE
Left: Numerous Paneth cells in a papillary adenoma, intestinal type.
Right: A few serotonin-containing cells in a papillary adenoma, intestinal type.

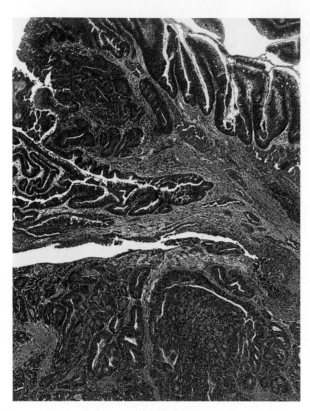

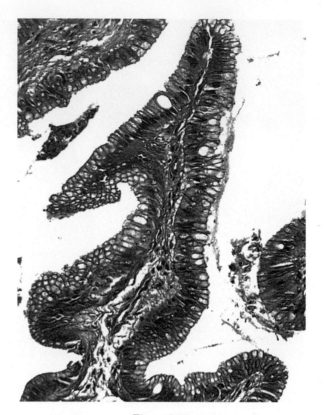

Figure 3-18
ADENOCARCINOMA ARISING AT THE BASE
OF A PAPILLARY ADENOMA, INTESTINAL TYPE

Figure 3-19
BILIARY TYPE PAPILLARY ADENOMA
A papillary adenoma is composed of fibrovascular stalks
that extend outward into the lumen of the gallbladder. They
are lined by tall, columnar, mucus-secreting cells.

lined by foveolar epithelium (figs. 3-20, 3-21). Paneth and endocrine cells are seen in some adenomas. Dysplastic changes are usually present. Rarely tubulopapillary adenomas arise from the epithelial invaginations of adenomyomatous hyperplasia (fig. 3-22).

Differential Diagnosis

The intestinal type of tubular adenoma should be separated from intestinal metaplasia and intestinal type adenocarcinoma. In contrast to tubular adenoma, intestinal metaplasia often preserves the gallbladder architecture and is poorly demarcated. In fact, this metaplastic lesion begins at the tip of the mucosal folds with replacement of the normal columnar epithelium by mature goblet cells that eventually extend down along the lateral surfaces. In more advanced cases, endocrine and Paneth cells make their appearance. Tubular glands eventually fill

and expand the lamina propria forming small, poorly defined nodules. Tubular adenomas are well demarcated and covered by normal biliary epithelium. The predominant columnar cell is dysplastic, having elongated, pseudostratified, hyperchromatic nuclei. Intestinal type adenocarcinomas show invasive properties and greater cytologic atypia than tubular adenomas.

The secondary type of papillary hyperplasia should be included in the differential diagnosis of the intestinal type of papillary adenoma since both lesions may contain goblet, Paneth, and endocrine cells. However, the former lesion is composed of tall mucosal folds lined by columnar cells which lack the elongated hyperchromatic nuclei characteristically seen in papillary adenomas with an intestinal phenotype. True papillary structures with fibrovascular stalks, as seen in adenomas, are not observed in secondary papillary hyperplasia.

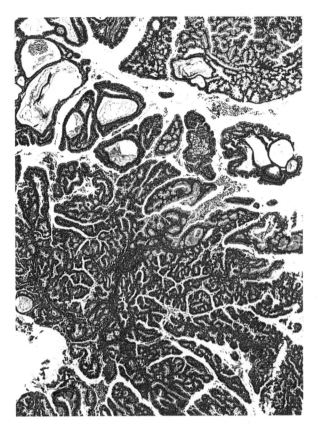

Figure 3-20
TUBULOPAPILLARY ADENOMA
Low-power view of papillary and tubular structures.

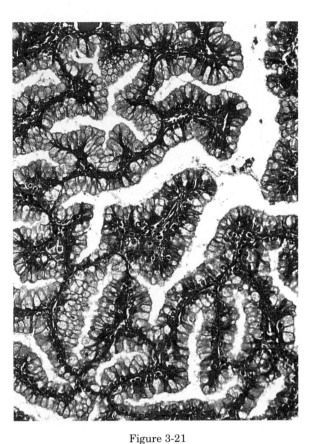

Figure 3-21
TUBULOPAPILLARY ADENOMA
Papillary structures are lined by foveolar type epithelium
in this higher magnification of tumor shown in figure 3-20.

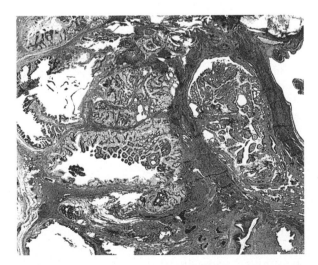

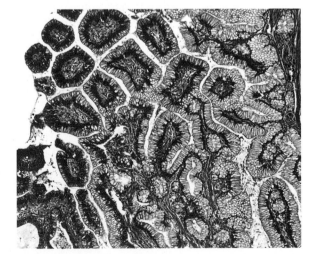

Figure 3-22
TUBULOPAPILLARY ADENOMA
Left: This tubulopapillary adenoma arose in a Rokitansky-Aschoff sinus of adenomyomatous hyperplasia.
Right: Higher magnification shows that the lining epithelial cells resemble foveolar cells.

When high-grade dysplasia is present in papillary adenomas of intestinal type the distinction from a papillary carcinoma may become problematic. However, the extent of cytologic atypia and the number of mitotic figures is greater in carcinomas than in adenomas. In addition, most papillary carcinomas contain no Paneth cells or when present are fewer in number than in papillary adenomas. Finally, the stromal desmoplasia and intramural invasion, seen in many carcinomas, do not occur in papillary adenomas.

Papillary adenomas of the biliary type should be distinguished from primary and secondary papillary hyperplasia. The latter two lesions lack circumscription and do not develop papillary structures with fibrovascular stalks. They are composed of either hyperplastic mucosal folds lined by cells similar to those found in normal gallbladder epithelium or by columnar cells with interspersed goblet and Paneth cells. Since papillary adenomas of the biliary type reveal minimal cytologic atypia, the distinction from papillary carcinoma is not difficult.

Molecular Pathology

The molecular pathology of adenomas of the gallbladder differs from that of carcinomas. Of 16 adenomas, 14 pyloric and 2 intestinal, analyzed genetically, none showed p53 and p16 Ink4/CDKN2a gene mutations which are the most common and sometimes the only molecular abnormalities detected in carcinomas (19a,23a). Four adenomas (25 percent) had K-ras mutations (two in codon 12 and two in codon 61), which are considered rare and late events in the pathogenesis of carcinomas of the gallbladder. Only one adenoma of intestinal type showed loss of heterozygosity at 5q22 (19a).

CYSTADENOMA

Definition and General Features. Cystadenomas are multiloculated neoplasms lined by columnar epithelium reminiscent of bile duct or foveolar gastric epithelium. The cellular subepithelial stroma resembles ovarian stroma and shows fibrosis of variable extent. More common in the extrahepatic bile ducts than in the gallbladder, cystadenomas are larger than non-cystic adenomas and invariably cause symptoms (25–29,34). The only three patients reported with cystadenomas of the gallbladder were adult females (27,28,30). Some of these tumors may measure 20 cm and lead to obstructive jaundice or chronic cholecystitis-like symptoms (27,30). Elevated serum levels of the tumor-associated antigen CA19-9 have recently been reported in patients with these tumors (32).

Grossly, the tumors are cystic and multiloculated. The thickness of the cyst wall varies from 0.3 to 3 cm. The locules contain mucinous fluid and the inner surface is finely granular or trabeculated. Small polypoid structures project into the lumen.

Pathologic Findings. Although mucinous cystic neoplasms of the pancreas, liver, and extrahepatic biliary tract share gross features, an ovarian-like stroma, and a minor endocrine component, biliary cystadenomas have a more homogenous epithelial cell population (24,27). Characteristically, the cyst wall has three layers: an inner layer of cuboidal or columnar biliary type epithelium that contains mucin, a cellular mesenchymal stroma, and an outer layer of hyalinized fibrous tissue (figs. 3-23, 3-24). In a few tumors, clusters of goblet cells and serotonin-containing (EC) cells are admixed with the cuboidal or columnar cells, indicating intestinal metaplasia. Focal dysplastic changes are found in approximately 13 percent of the tumors suggesting that progression to cystadenocarcinoma may occur.

The columnar or cuboidal epithelial cells are cytokeratin, epithelial membrane antigen, and carcinoembryonic antigen positive. They also show strong cytoplasmic positivity for CA19-9 by immunocytochemistry (32). The spindle stromal cells are diffusely immunoreactive for vimentin and focally reactive for muscle-specific actin, indicating focal myofibroblastic differentiation. Estrogen and progesterone receptors are positive in the mesenchymal stromal cells but not in the lining epithelium (33).

By electron microscopy, three cell types have been described in the stroma: undifferentiated mesenchymal cells, fibroblasts, and myofibroblasts. The stroma closely resembles ovarian stroma. This impression is further substantiated by the close similarity of the well-demarcated hyalinized areas to corpus albicans. However, ectopic ovarian tissue has never been reported in cystadenomas of the extrahepatic biliary tree. Chronic inflammatory cells, edema, hemorrhage,

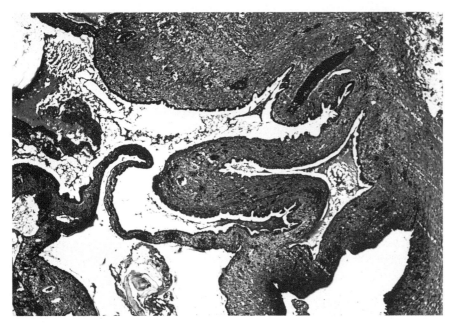

Figure 3-23
CYSTADENOMA OF
THE GALLBLADDER
Low-power view of a multi-
loculated biliary cystadenoma of
the gallbladder.

and extensive fibrosis may distort or even efface the three-layer architecture.

It has recently been suggested that biliary cystadenomas arise from displaced embryonic tissue destined to form the gallbladder (31). However, this hypothesis is unlikely because similar tumors are found in the retroperitoneum unattached to any organ, and the primitive mesenchymal stroma is shared by mucinous cystic tumors of the pancreas. Moreover, estrogen receptors have been demonstrated in the mesenchymal stromal cells of both pancreatic and biliary cystadenomas (33) while estrogen receptors are lacking in the stroma of the fetal gallbladder. Finally, this hypothesis fails to explain the almost exclusive occurrence of biliary cystadenomas among adult women (28).

Biliary cystadenomas may recur following incomplete excision. A single example of biliary cystadenocarcinoma has been reported in the gallbladder (28). However, it is not clear whether this tumor resulted from malignant transformation of a cystadenoma or arose de novo.

THE ADENOMA-CARCINOMA SEQUENCE

In recent years, the role played by adenomas of the gallbladder as possible precursors of invasive cancer has been investigated. Some authors have claimed that the adenoma-carcinoma sequence is the usual route for the development of

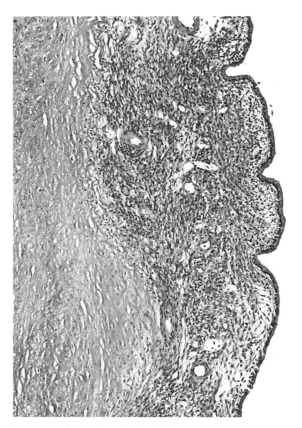

Figure 3-24
BILIARY CYSTADENOMA
Higher magnification of biliary cystadenoma shown in figure 3-23. The biliary epithelium, the cellular mesenchymal stroma, and the dense fibrous tissue are clearly seen.

invasive carcinoma of the gallbladder. For example, in one study remnants of an adenoma were found in 15 of 79 (19 percent) invasive carcinomas (37). Another study, based on 35 cases of early carcinoma (larger than 5 mm) and 16 microcarcinomas (equal to or less than 5 mm) of the gallbladder, revealed that 7 (13.7 percent) arose in adenomas (36). In some of these cases, however, the carcinomatous changes were limited to the adenomas, and therefore, could be regarded as in situ carcinomas within adenomas. In our series of 32 adenomas, only 2 progressed to invasive carcinoma (35).

There is data against the hypothesis that adenomas are the usual pathway in the development of most invasive carcinomas. In a review of more than 600 invasive carcinomas of the gallbladder, we found remnants of a tubular or papillary adenoma in less than 5 percent of the cases. Carcinomas of the gallbladder may show a spectrum of cytologic abnormalities that ranges from minimal nuclear atypia to overt malignant changes. Areas with minimal atypia may easily be interpreted as the remnants of an adenoma. Also, the hyperplasia of metaplastic pyloric type glands that is often seen in the vicinity of carcinomas, has been confused with adenomas. The prevalence of adenoma is not high in geographic areas in which cholelithiasis and carcinoma are endemic. The association of adenoma with lithiasis is not as common as the association of carcinoma with lithiasis. Even in areas in which gallbladder cancer is sporadic, adenomas are less common than malignant epithelial tumors. Finally, adenomas have molecular abnormalities that differ from those found in carcinomas (38). We therefore believe that adenomas play a minor role in the pathogenesis of invasive carcinoma of the gallbladder.

REFERENCES

Adenomas

1. Albores-Saavedra J, Henson DE. Tumors of the gallbladder and extrahepatic bile ducts. Atlas of Tumor Pathology, 2nd Series, Fascicle 22. Washington, D.C.: Armed Forces Institute of Pathology, 1986.
2. Albores-Saavedra J, Henson DE, Sobin LE. Histological typing of tumours of the gallbladder and extrahepatic bile ducts. World Health Organization. Berlin: Springer-Verlag, 1991.
3. Albores-Saavedra J, Vardaman C, Vuitch F. Non-neoplastic polypoid lesions and adenomas of the gallbladder. Pathol Ann 1993;28:145–77.
4. Christensen AH, Ishak KG. Benign tumors and pseudotumors of the gallbladder. Report of 180 cases. Arch Pathol 1970;90:423–32.
5. Foster DR, Foster DB. Gallbladder polyps in Peutz-Jeghers syndrome. Postgrad Med J 1980;56:373–6.
6. Kijima H, Watanabe H, Iwafuchi M, Ishihara N. Histogenesis of gallbladder carcinoma from investigation of early carcinoma and microcarcinoma. Acta Pathol Jpn 1989;39:235–44.
7. Kosuka S, Tsubone M, Yasui A, Hachisuka K. Relation of adenoma to carcinoma in the gallbladder. Cancer 1982;50:2226–34.
8. Kushima R, Remmele W, Stolte M, Borchard F. Pyloric gland type adenoma of the gallbladder with squamoid spindle cell metaplasia. Pathol Res Pract 1996;192:963–9
9. Lauwers GY, Wahl SJ, Scott GV, DeRoux SJ. Papillary mucinous adenoma arising in adenomyomatous hyperplasia of the gallbladder. J Clin Pathol 1995;48:965–7.
10. Lin G, Hägerstrand I. Multiple adenomas of the gallbladder. Acta Path Microbiol Immunol Scand [A] 1983;91:475–6.
11. Miyazaki K, Date K, Imamura S, Ogawa Y, Nakayam F. Familial occurrence of anomalous pancreaticobiliary duct union associated with gallbladder neoplasms. Am J Gastroenterol 1989;84:176–81.
12. Mogilner JG, Dharan M, Siplovich L. Adenoma of the gallbladder in childhood. J Pediatr Surg 1991;26:223–4.
13. Molina LM, DeDiego JA, Diez M, et al. Obstruction of the bile duct by a papillary adenoma of the gallbladder. Hepatogastroenterology 1988;35:91–3.
14. Nakajo S, Yamamoto M, Tahara E. Morphometric analysis of gallbladder adenoma and adenocarcinoma: with reference to histogenesis and adenoma-carcinoma sequence. Virchows Arch [A] 1990;417:49–56.
15. Nishihara K, Yamaguchi K, Hashimoto H, Enjoji M. Tubular adenoma of the gallbladder with squamoid spindle cell metaplasia. Report of 3 cases with immunohistochemical study. Acta Pathol Jpn 1991;41:41–5.
16. Sato H, Mizushima M, Ito J, Doi K. Sessile adenoma of the gallbladder. Reappraisal of its importance as a precancerous lesion. Arch Pathol Lab Med 1985;109:65–9.
17. Tantachamrun T, Borvonsombat S, Theetranont C. Gardner's syndrome associated with adenomatous polyp of the gallbladder. J Med Assoc Thai 1979;62:441–7.
18. Wada K, Tanaka M, Yamaguchi K, Wada K. Carcinoma and polyps of the gallbladder associated with Peutz-Jeghers syndrome. Digestive Dis Sci 1987;32:943–6.

19. Walsh N, Qizilbash A, Banerjee R, Waugh GA. Biliary neoplasia in Gardner's syndrome. Arch Pathol Lab Med 1987;111:76–7.

19a. Wistuba I, Miquel AF, Gazdar AF, Albores-Saavedra J. Gallbladder adenomas have molecular abnormalities different from those present in gallbladder carcinomas. Hum Pathol 1999;30:21–5.

20. Yamaguchi K, Enjoji M. Gallbladder polyps: inflammatory, hyperplastic and neoplastic types. Surg Pathol 1988;1:203–13.

21. Yamaguchi K, Maeda S, Kitamura K. Papillary adenoma of the gallbladder associated with regurgitation of pancreatic juice through abnormally shaped union. Acta Chir Scand 1989;155:549–52.

22. Yamamoto M, Murakami H, Ito M, Nakajo S, Tahara E. Ectopic gastric mucosa of the gallbladder: comparison with metaplastic polyp of the gallbladder. Am J Gastroenterol 1989;84:1423–26.

23. Yamamoto M, Nakajo S, Tahara E. Histological classification of epithelial polypoid lesions of the gallbladder. Acta Pathol Jpn 1988;38:181–92.

23a. Yoshida S, Tadoroki T, Ichikawa Y, et al. Mutations of p16Ink4/CDKN2 and p15Ink4B/MTS2 genes in biliary tract cancers. Cancer Res 1995;55:2756–60.

Cystadenomas

24. Albores-Saavedra J, Gould EW, Angeles-Angeles A, Henson DE. Cystic tumors of the pancreas. Pathol Ann 1990;25:19–50.

25. Albores-Saavedra J, Henson DE. Tumors of the gallbladder and extrahepatic bile ducts. Atlas of Tumor Pathology, 2nd Series, Fascicle 22. Washington, D.C.: Armed Forces Institute of Pathology, 1986.

26. Albores-Saavedra J, Henson DE, Sobin LE. Histological typing of tumours of the gallbladder and extrahepatic bile ducts. World Health Organization. Berlin: Springer-Verlag, 1991.

27. Albores-Saavedra J, Vardaman C, Vuitch F. Non-neoplastic polypoid lesions and adenomas of the gallbladder. Pathol Ann 1993;28:145–77.

28. Devaney K, Goodman ZD, Ishak KG. Hepatobiliary cystadenoma and cystadenocarcinoma. A light microscopic and immunohistochemical study of 70 patients. Am J Surg Pathol 1994;18:1078–91.

29. Ishak KG, Willis GW, Cummins SD, Bullock AA. Biliary cystadenoma and cystadenocarcinoma: report of 14 cases and review of the literature. Cancer 1977; 39:322–38.

30. Simmons T, Miller C, Pesigan A, Lewin K. Cystadenoma of the gallbladder. Am J Gastroenterol 1989;84:1427–30.

31. Subramony C, Herrera GA, Turbat-Herrera E. Hepatobiliary cystadenoma. A study of five cases with reference to histogenesis. Arch Path Lab Med 1993;117:1036–42.

32. Thomas JA, Seriven MW, Puntis MC, Jasani B, Williams GT. Elevated CA19-9 levels in hepatobiliary cystadenoma with mesenchymal stroma. Two case reports with immunohistochemical confirmation. Cancer 1992;70:1841–6.

33. Vuitch F, Battifora H, Albores-Saavedra J. Demonstration of steroid hormone receptors in pancreato-biliary mucinous cystic neoplasms. Lab Invest 1993;68:114A.

34. Wheeler DA, Edmondson HA. Cystadenoma with mesenchymal stroma (CMS) in the liver and bile ducts. A clinicopathologic study of 17 cases, 4 with malignant change. Cancer 1985;56:1434–45.

Adenoma-Carcinoma Sequence

35. Albores-Saavedra J, Vardaman C, Vuitch F. Non-neoplastic polypoid lesions and adenomas of the gallbladder. Pathol Ann Part I, 1993;28:145–77.

36. Kijima H, Watanabe H, Iwafuchi M, Ishihara N. Histogenesis of gallbladder carcinoma from investigation of early carcinoma and microcarcinoma. Acta Pathol Jpn 1989;39:235–44.

37. Kosuka S, Tsubone M, Yasui A, Hachisuka K. Relation of adenoma to carcinoma in the gallbladder. Cancer 1982;50:2226–34.

38. Wistuba I, Miquel AF, Gazdar AF, Albores-Saavedra J. Gallbladder adenomas have molecular abnormalities different from those present in gallbladder carcinomas. Hum Pathol 1999;30:21–5.

39. Yoshida S, Tadoroki T, Ichikawa Y, et al. Mutations of p16Ink4/CDKN2 and p15Ink4B/MTS2 genes in biliary tract cancers. Cancer Res 1995;55:2756–60.

✧✧✧

4

GALLBLADDER CANCER: EPIDEMIOLOGY, ETIOLOGY, CLINICAL MANIFESTATIONS, AND LABORATORY STUDIES

EPIDEMIOLOGY

The distribution of gallbladder cancer is unique among malignant neoplasms. Its incidence not only varies in different parts of the world, but it also varies in different ethnic groups within the same country. In the United States, for example, carcinoma of the gallbladder is more common in Native Americans than in whites or blacks. Similar high rates are also found in some areas of Latin America, especially in Chile, Mexico, and Bolivia (8). In other countries, such as Japan, the incidence is intermediate between that of the American Indians and whites (12).

Incidence

Cancer of the gallbladder is not a common disease. In the United States for the years 1982 to 1991, the age-adjusted rate for histologically proven invasive cancer of the gallbladder was 0.72 cases per 100,000 males and 1.36 cases per 100,000 females, accounting for 0.17 percent of all cancers in males and 0.49 percent in females (5). In general, females with carcinoma of the gallbladder outnumber males 2 to 1, although this ratio varies in different parts of the world.

In Native Americans the rates are much higher. In New Mexico, for example, the rates are 5.1 per 100,000 males and 21.1 for females, compared with 0.8 for white males and 1.4 for white females. Spanish descendants living in the same area have intermediate rates, 2.0 for males and 10.5 for females (7). Clinically, cancers of the gallbladder and extrahepatic bile ducts are found in 5.4 percent of all biliary tract operations among Southwestern Native Americans. These cancers are the third most common malignant tumor found in female Native Americans (10).

Some of the lowest rates are seen in blacks in the United States and Africa (2). However, according to the Surveillance, Epidemiology, and End Results Program of the National Cancer Institute, the age-adjusted rates are the same for black and white men (0.78 and 0.75, respec-

tively), but lower in black females than in white females (1.04 and 1.43, respectively).

The high rate of gallbladder cancer found in Mexico, 8.5 per 100,000 women, is also found in Mexican Americans (6). In the Los Angeles area carcinoma of the gallbladder is the third most common type of malignant tumor seen in Mexican American women (11).

Age Distribution

Cancer of the gallbladder is a disease of older age groups. The average age is 72.2 years and the median is 73 years. For males, the average age is 71 years and for females, 72.7 years (5). Carcinoma of the gallbladder was found in an 11-year-old Indian girl, the youngest case on record (9). Figure 4-1 shows the age-specific rates for carcinoma of the gallbladder for males and females. For all age groups, this rate is greater in females. Since cancer of the biliary tract occurs primarily in older age groups, the incidence of carcinoma discovered in patients undergoing surgery for biliary tract disease increases with age. In some referral centers, approximately 10 percent of patients 65 years of age and older who come to surgery for biliary tract disease can be expected to have carcinoma of the gallbladder or extrahepatic bile ducts (3,4). In general, unsuspected carcinoma of the gallbladder is found in approximately 2 percent of cholecystectomy specimens (1).

ETIOLOGY

A number of factors have been associated with the etiology of gallbladder cancer. The three most important are genetic, stones, and a congenitally abnormal choledochopancreatic junction.

Genetic

As discussed under Epidemiology, cancer of the gallbladder is concentrated in certain racial and ethnic groups. Unusually high rates are found among Native Americans and Hispanic Americans,

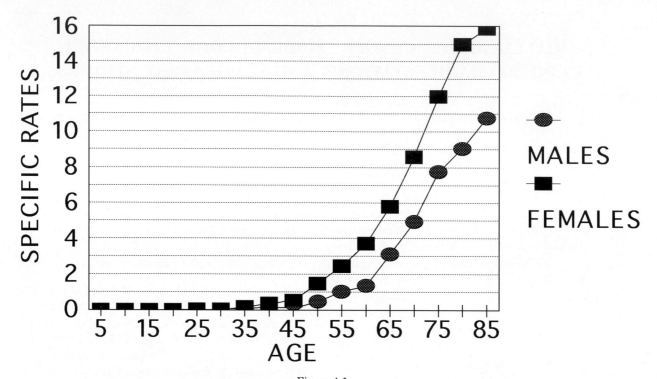

Figure 4-1
AGE-SPECIFIC RATES FOR CANCERS OF THE GALLBLADDER
Data taken from the Surveillance, Epidemiology, and End Results Program, National Cancer Institute, for the years 1981 to 1990. The rates reflect histologically proven invasive cancers only. Data include all histologic types.

especially those living in Arizona and California, and among South and Central American Indians. The Hispanic Americans, it should be recalled, are descendants of the early Spanish settlers and have an ethnic background that is both Native American and Spanish. Familial aggregation of gallbladder cancer has been recorded in the United States and other countries (24,61).

The high incidence of carcinoma of the gallbladder in Hispanic Americans seems to be the result of racial intermixture, since the Iberian Spaniards, the historical source of New Mexico's original settlers, do not have high rates of gallbladder cancer: 2.7 per 100,000 for females and 1.8 for males (24). Studies of Hispanics in Colorado indicate that the Indian contribution to the gene pool is as high as 40 percent. It is possible, therefore, that the high rates observed in some countries in Latin America may also be the result of racial intermixture between the Spanish immigrants and the Native Americans.

The incidence of cancer of the gallbladder in other Hispanic groups, such as in Puerto Ricans and Cubans who have a different ethnic background, is 1.9 per 100,000, the same as that found in the United States. Countries in Latin America that had a large Indian population during the Spanish migration have higher rates of gallbladder cancer than countries that did not. Most likely the genetic tendency is to stone formation. The high incidence of carcinoma can be attributed to the high incidence of cholelithiasis, although other factors may be involved.

Gallstones

The association of carcinoma of the gallbladder with gallstones has been known since 1861. Found in more than 80 percent of cases, this association is cited by many as indicating a causal relationship and is the reason for the view that elective cholecystectomy for cholelithiasis is a preventive measure for carcinoma of the gallbladder (23,57).

Gallstones should be considered a risk factor for carcinoma of the gallbladder. The incidence of gallbladder cancer is higher in patients with gallstones than in patients without stones (35, 36,42). There is a higher incidence of carcinoma in females, who have a higher incidence of stones than males. Gallstones are more common in the gallbladder than the bile ducts, and gallbladder cancer is more common than bile duct cancer. The incidence of gallbladder cancer is higher in ethnic groups, such as Native Americans, who have a higher incidence of stones, and is lower in ethnic groups, such as African Americans, who have a low incidence of stones. While some authors have reported a correlation between gallstone size and the risk of cancer (25,40), others have not found such a correlation (45).

While gallstones are considered a risk factor, the overall incidence of carcinoma of the gallbladder in patients with cholelithiasis is less than 0.2 percent (43). This percentage, however, varies with race, sex, and length of exposure to the stones (39).

Although the relationship of cholelithiasis to carcinoma is not understood, most observers assume that chronic irritation promotes neoplastic transformation, an assumption that has experimental support. Epithelium from lithiferous gallbladders, for example, incorporates tritiated thymidine 23 times greater than normal epithelium (56). Furthermore, biochemical studies have shown that stones from cancer patients are formed through standard mechanisms of cholesterol precipitation and not secondary to stasis or infection, which would be the case if the carcinoma led to stone formation.

Abnormal Choledochopancreatic Junction

Data largely reported from Japan indicate an association between gallbladder cancer and an abnormal junction of the pancreatic and common bile ducts (35,47,66). The abnormal junction is defined as the union of the pancreatic and common bile ducts outside the wall of the duodenum, beyond the influence of the sphincter of Oddi (19). Normally, the main pancreatic duct and the common bile duct unite within the sphincter to form the pancreaticobiliary duct. The pancreaticobiliary duct and the junction are governed by the sphincter, but as a result of the anomaly, the pancreaticobiliary duct is unusually long and no longer under the control of the sphincter. As a result, pancreatic juice can reflux into the common bile duct, since the pressure in the pancreatic duct is usually greater than that in the common duct.

The frequency of these abnormal junctions in patients with diseases of the biliary tree, as assessed by endoscopic retrograde cholangiopancreatography, has varied from 1.5 to 3.2 percent in different reports (35). These abnormal junctions are often associated with choledochal cysts (14,15,35,67). Patients who develop carcinoma of the gallbladder in association with an abnormal junction are usually 10 years younger than those with a normal junction who develop carcinoma, and usually do not have gallstones (35, 66). In addition, there are no sex differences in the incidence in contrast to gallbladder cancer associated with calculi. In Japan, 16.7 percent of gallbladder cancers are associated with an abnormal pancreaticobiliary junction, whereas gallbladder carcinoma occurs in 24.6 percent of patients with an abnormal junction in comparison with a 1.9 percent incidence of this carcinoma among patients with a normal ductal union (35). It should be noted that studies relating gallbladder cancer and this anomaly have not been carried out in many countries, including the United States.

It has been postulated that reflux of pancreatic juice into the common bile duct may lead to the development of acquired choledochal cysts as a result of recurrent inflammation and increased intraluminal pressure (14). Similarly, reflux into the gallbladder or into an established choledochal cyst may eventually lead to the development of cancer (35,47). Pancreatic juice contains an enzyme phospholipase, A2, which converts lecithin to lysolecithin, a substance known to damage cell membranes (49). Cancer is likely to develop in the gallbladder or in choledochal cysts where stasis tends to occur. Metaplastic and hyperplastic changes are frequently seen in gallbladders associated with abnormal junctions (65). High levels of pancreatic amylase have been found in choledochal cysts (22,37).

Carcinomas of the gallbladder occurring in association with an abnormal choledochopancreatic junction have a high incidence of ras mutations,

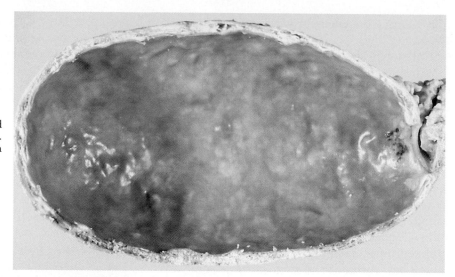

Figure 4-2
PORCELAIN GALLBLADDER
The wall of this large distended gallbladder is rigid and calcified. A stone found in the neck had been previously removed.

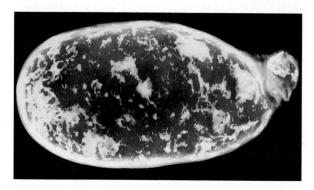

Figure 4-3
PORCELAIN GALLBLADDER
This is a radiograph of the gallbladder shown in figure 4-2. The wall of the gallbladder is diffusely calcified, characteristic of porcelain gallbladder.

which is in contrast to the carcinomas not associated with this anomaly (30). This observation supports the concept that there is more than one pathogenetic mechanism for the development of this carcinoma. Carcinoma of the gallbladder has been associated with choledochal cysts in patients with an anomalous pancreaticobiliary junction (52). Synchronous primary cancers of the gallbladder and common bile duct have also been associated with an abnormal junction (32,34,48,51). These examples of multicentric tumors clearly point to a common etiology.

When carcinoma of the gallbladder is found in the absence of gallstones, the pathologist should recommend evaluation of the choledochopancreatic junction.

Bile Composition

In considering the etiology of carcinoma of the gallbladder, we should note that the composition of bile and gallstones is not uniform in all parts of the world. In La Paz, Bolivia, for example, a city with a five-fold increase in the incidence of carcinoma of the gallbladder compared to that of the United States, only cholesterol stones were found in 138 patients who were studied (59). This is in contrast to Philadelphia, an area with a low incidence of gallbladder cancer, where 27 percent of patients undergoing cholecystectomy had pigment gallstones (62). The stones from Bolivian patients contain a much higher proportion of cholesterol, and therefore much less calcium bilirubinate, calcium carbonate, and other noncholesterol components compared to stones from patients in Philadelphia. Also, in Bolivia, Caucasians, Mestizos, and Indians all have a uniform stone composition, with the cholesterol content greater than 90 percent. This also includes patients with carcinoma of the gallbladder.

Calcification

Another condition predisposing to carcinoma is diffuse calcification, or porcelain gallbladder, which has a characteristic plaque-like appearance on plain radiographs of the abdomen (figs. 4-2–4-4) (33). Occurring in less than 0.1 percent of cholecystectomy specimens, diffuse calcification is associated with carcinoma in 10 to 25

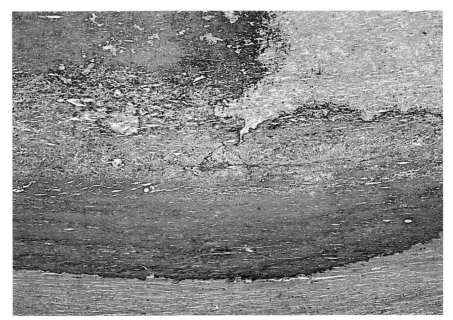

Figure 4-4
PORCELAIN GALLBLADDER
The wall shows extensive calcification involving predominantly the muscular layer.

percent of cases (16). The calcification is considered by many to be the end stage of a longstanding inflammatory process (55). It has also been suggested that calcium salts precipitate in the mucosa following obstruction of the cystic duct, usually by a stone, and exclusion of bile from the gallbladder (53). Ninety-five percent of patients with porcelain gallbladders have gallstones. Histologically, the calcifications appear as broad bands involving the muscle layer, the mucosa, or both (33). Porcelain gallbladders are also found in children (17). They should be removed when discovered and evaluated carefully for carcinoma.

The reason for the increased incidence of cancer in this condition is unknown. We suggest, however, that it may be related to the phenomenon of scar cancer, since there is usually fibrosis in addition to the calcification. For the most part, the tumors are infiltrating adenocarcinomas, although mucinous and squamous cell carcinomas have also been reported.

Ulcerative Colitis

Carcinoma of the gallbladder occasionally occurs in association with ulcerative colitis (27,46,54,63), although this association is less common than the association of ulcerative colitis with carcinomas of the extrahepatic bile ducts. It has been suggested that a cholecystectomy should be considered in those patients with ulcerative colitis who require a colectomy.

Familial Polyposis

A small number of patients with familial adenomatous polyposis coli develop carcinoma of the gallbladder. In support of this association, 26 percent of patients with familial polyposis show gallbladder dysplasia (50), which is considered the most common precursor for gallbladder cancer.

Infections

Reports indicate that chronic carriers of *Salmonella typhi* have a higher incidence of hepatobiliary cancer (18,44,64). From this observation, it was suggested that salmonella surviving in the gallbladder change the bile salts into carcinogenic agents. In one case, carcinoma of the gallbladder developed 67 years after the diagnosis of typhoid cholecystitis (13). It should be noted, however, that chronic carriers of salmonella often have gallstones. Salmonella may also be involved in the etiology of extrahepatic bile duct cancer (see page 183).

When careful culture technique is used, bile from patients with normal gallbladders is consistently sterile (21). In patients with chronic cholecystitis associated with cholesterol or pigment stones, the incidence of positive cultures is less than 33 percent and approaches 10 percent in studies done in the United States (20,29,38). In patients with acute cholecystitis, the incidence of infection increases to 60 percent. Bacteria have been found in bile in 80 percent of patients with carcinoma of the gallbladder (20), although this figure may be related in part to age, since the incidence of positive cultures increases with age. It remains uncertain whether bacteria are involved in the etiology of gallbladder cancer, especially in patients with cholelithiasis.

Bacteria can be recovered from bile, stones, and the wall of the gallbladder. These bacteria are usually mixtures of intestinal flora and include aerobic and anaerobic species (28,58). Anaerobic infection does not occur in the absence of aerobic organisms. Because of their labyrinthine interstices, gallstones once infected are unlikely to be sterilized by systemic antibiotics, even though some of these drugs are concentrated in bile.

In the Orient, infection with *Escherichia coli* is the rule among patients with calcium bilirubinate stones (41). These stones, which contain calcium salts of bilirubin and fatty acids, are thought to form following bacteria deconjugation of bilirubin diglucuronide to bilirubin and bacterial lysis of phospholipid lecithin to lysolecithin and free fatty acids. These patients are subject to recurrent stone formation and to chronic pyogenic cholangitis and cholangiohepatitis, but they do not have an increased incidence of extrahepatic biliary cancer.

Occupation

Cancer of the biliary tract has been associated with exposure to chemicals used in the rubber industry (42). An excess risk has also been found for workers in the nonelectrical machinery and primary metal industries (31). In a remarkable case, asbestos bodies were found within a squamous cell carcinoma that developed in the cystic duct of a patient with an occupational exposure to asbestos (60).

CLINICAL MANIFESTATIONS

Cancer of the gallbladder usually presents late in its course, after the tumor has invaded the liver or caused bile duct obstruction. The signs and symptoms are usually delayed because the tumor develops in a small organ with a blind end and does not interfere with the flow of bile or cause immediate obstruction. Furthermore, the signs and symptoms of a preexisting cholecystitis, which are found in 50 to 90 percent of patients, may mislead the physician and cause a delay in diagnosis.

The signs and symptoms of gallbladder cancer are not specific, often resembling those of chronic cholecystitis (70). Pain, usually the initial complaint, occurs in 75 percent of cases. It may be intermittent or persistent, severe, and, for the most part, localized in the right upper quadrant. There is often a palpable mass, hepatomegaly, and eventually jaundice, nausea, vomiting, anorexia, and weight loss (77). Pruritus usually occurs with jaundice.

Thirty to 60 percent of patients develop jaundice, usually as a result of obstruction from tumor extending to the common duct, or less often caused by extension to the liver. Jaundice is a poor prognostic sign, since 85 percent of patients with jaundice have nonresectable tumors at the time of diagnosis (76). In addition to patients with jaundice, resection is usually not possible in patients with an enlarged liver, palpable abdominal masses, or ascites. About 20 percent of patients present with ascites and 10 percent with duodenal obstruction (83).

Occasionally, a malignant tumor is found incidentally in specimens removed for cholelithiasis. In these cases, the tumor is either in the in situ stage or has invaded but not penetrated the wall of the gallbladder. These patients have the best opportunity of being cured.

The first signs of local recurrence include right upper quadrant pain, a palpable mass, an enlarged liver, back pain, jaundice, and occasionally, ascites.

Systemic Manifestations

In addition to the common signs and symptoms of gallbladder cancer, a very small number of patients present with remote or systemic signs and symptoms.

Carcinoma of the gallbladder has been associated with Cushing s syndrome, the result of ectopic hormone production by the tumor. In our series of 29 patients with small cell carcinoma (68a), one had Cushing's syndrome. Another patient with the syndrome was reported to have an

APUDoma which was probably a small cell carcinoma (86). Carcinoma of the gallbladder has been associated with acanthosis nigricans (69,95) and with bullous-type pemphigoid skin lesions (84).

Carcinoma of the gallbladder has also been associated with the Leser-Trelat sign (rapid growth of multiple seborrheic keratoses) (81). In a unique case, a 31-year-old man with an occupational exposure to aromatic hydrocarbons and carcinoma of the gallbladder presented with Trousseau's sign (26,74). Rarely, hypercalcemia can accompany carcinoma of the gallbladder (92,94) as it does cancers arising in other sites.

Laboratory Findings

Laboratory findings are not diagnostic. Jaundice indicates intrahepatic or extrahepatic obstruction and is manifested by hyperbilirubinemia, bilirubinuria, and elevated levels of serum alkaline phosphatase, 5 nucleotidase, and leucine aminopeptidase. These changes are not specific for carcinoma, but are associated with hepatic obstruction from any cause

In patients who are not jaundiced but complain of pain, nausea, or other symptoms, laboratory findings are either normal or show nonspecific changes. Serum levels of alanine aminotransferase and lactic acid dehydrogenase may be elevated, especially with liver involvement or cholestasis. Normal values do not preclude metastatic lesions in the liver.

Circulating Tumor Markers

A number of circulating tumor markers have been found in patients with carcinoma of the gallbladder. These markers, however, are not diagnostic. They are not present in all patients with cancer and are often elevated in the presence of cholestasis from any cause. Some markers such as CA19-9 can be used to follow the course of the disease. Markers are not useful for early detection because of low sensitivity and specificity.

Carcinoembryonic Antigen. Since carcinomas of the biliary tree produce carcinoembryonic antigen (CEA), it is not surprising that bile and serum levels increase (87,90). However, serum levels may also increase as a result of bile duct obstruction from any cause; therefore, a rise does not necessarily indicate cancer (89,90). Serum levels of CEA may temporarily increase in cases of cholelithiasis.

CA19-9. Elevated levels of the carbohydrate antigen CA19-9 are found in a high proportion of patients with carcinoma of the gallbladder or extrahepatic bile ducts (82). Although the antigen lacks specificity, it may be useful for discriminating patients with gallbladder cancer from those with gallstones and no cancer (87). Serum levels are also associated with a high proliferation index as measured by flow cytometry, although levels in bile are not so associated (86). CA19-9 can be used to follow patients for recurrence. Serum levels may also be elevated in patients with pancreatitis, cholangitis, or cholelithiasis.

Alpha-Fetoprotein. Carcinomas of the gallbladder, especially those of the clear cell type, have been associated with elevated levels of serum alpha-fetoprotein (AFP) (71,78,89,93). Immunohistochemical studies have shown that the tumor cells produce AFP (78,91). Histologically, AFP-producing tumors may show focal hepatoid differentiation (91). Even though AFP-producing tumors of the gallbladder are uncommon, they should be considered in the differential diagnosis of patients with elevated levels of serum AFP, especially in patients with biliary tract disease.

Radiographic Findings

Ultrasonography is usually the initial diagnostic procedure in biliary tract disease. However, differentiation of carcinoma from cholecystitis, adenomyomatous hyperplasia, or adenomas by this method may be extremely difficult (72,73,79,95a). Focal or diffuse thickening of the gallbladder wall, a mass in the gallbladder fossa, or an intraluminal mass are the most common findings (fig. 4-5) (85). Intraoperative ultrasound is especially useful for diagnosis and for evaluating the depth of tumor invasion into the wall of the gallbladder. Computed tomography has also been used in the recognition and staging of gallbladder cancer (80), although it seems less helpful than ultrasound (fig. 4-6). Diagnosis can also be made by angiography which depends on the demonstration of neovascularization (68). Conventional methods for visualizing the gallbladder, such as oral cholecystography, are usually not useful for detecting carcinoma.

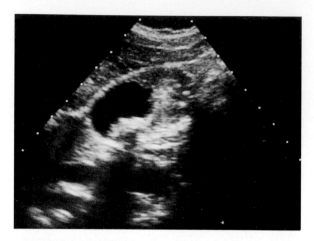
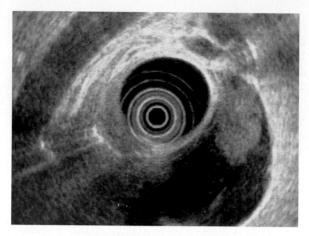

Figure 4-5
CARCINOMAS

Left: Adenocarcinoma. Several stones as well as an irregular infiltrating gallbladder mass are seen in this sonogram.
Right: Adenosquamous carcinoma. Endoscopic ultrasonography reveals a large polypoid infiltrating mass in the gallbladder.

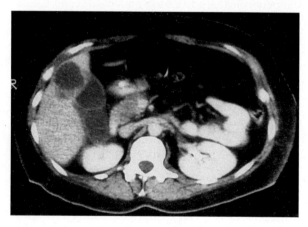

Figure 4-6
ADENOCARCINOMA
Computed tomography shows a large distended gallbladder with a mass infiltrating into the liver.

Most carcinomas are found during exploratory laparotomy, during surgery for cholelithiasis, or during surgery for an obstructive lesion in the biliary tract. Not infrequently, an unsuspected gallbladder cancer is found during abdominal computed tomography for nonspecific complaints (75).

BILE CYTOLOGY

Percutaneous fine needle aspiration (PFNA) under computerized tomographic guidance has occasionally been employed for the diagnosis of malignant gallbladder neoplasms with good results (96,98). Although in one small series PFNA had a sensitivity of 88 percent (96), we would like to emphasize that experience with this procedure is still very limited and its false-positive rate and complications are unknown. Bile for cytologic examination has been obtained preoperatively by endoscopic retrograde cholangiopancreatography or by percutaneous transhepatic cholangiography. The diagnostic sensitivity of these procedures has been around 50 percent, with an unsatisfactory rate of 25 percent and an average false-positive rate of 6 percent (96). Improper collection, handling, and processing of bile may explain the poor results.

Bile for cytology can be collected by gallbladder puncture during peritoneoscopic examination. In a series of 110 punctures, only one patient developed peritonitis, which resolved under conservative treatment indicating that the procedure is safe (100). Bile can also be obtained by puncturing the gallbladder during cholecystectomy or immediately after cholecystectomy after clamping the neck of the gallbladder with forceps (97,99,101). Although these procedures are not used as a diagnostic tool in many countries, including the United States, pathologists can use them to become familiar with the cytology of dysplasia, carcinoma in situ, and

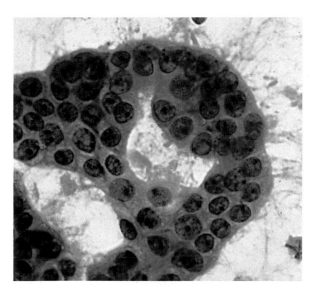

Figure 4-7
SLIGHT DYSPLASIA
Sheets of dysplastic cells show some enlargement of nuclei and loss of normal nuclear cytoplasmic ratio. The nuclei are round, and have finely granular chromatin and small nucleoli.

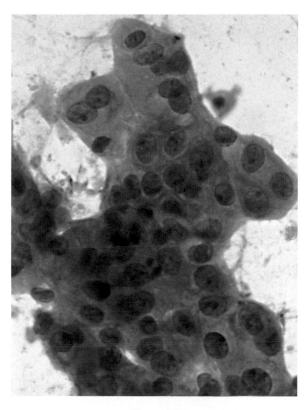

Figure 4-8
MODERATE DYSPLASIA
Clusters of dysplastic epithelial cells, some of which contain prominent nucleoli, are seen.

invasive carcinoma of the gallbladder. To insure good cell preservation smears should be prepared immediately with the aspirated saline irrigated bile. In our experience, this technique allows identification of dysplasia, carcinoma in situ, and invasive carcinoma (97). It has some advantage in those cases in which an invasive carcinoma is not suspected grossly and therefore may easily be missed because of inadequate sampling. If malignant cells are present in the bile smears, but the histologic sections show only inflammatory changes, additional sections must be submitted for diagnostic confirmation.

Dysplasia

Dysplastic cells desquamate in sheets, are less cohesive than normal epithelial cells, and exhibit some variation in size and shape. The nuclei are large, round, or ovoid, with well-defined and uniformly stained nuclear membranes. The chromatin appears finely granular, and nucleoli are more conspicuous than in normal cells. As a consequence of an increase in nuclear volume, there is a moderate increase in the nuclear-cytoplasmic ratio (figs. 4-7, 4-8). Goblet cells often show moderate nuclear atypia.

Carcinoma in Situ

Cell aggregates tend to form sheets. Individual cells show great variation in size and shape and are less cohesive than in dysplasia. There is also considerable variation in the size and shape of the nuclei. Their membranes are reinforced and do not stain uniformly. The chromatin becomes coarsely granular and irregularly distributed. The nucleoli are usually large, pleomorphic, multiple, and more prominent than in dysplasia (fig. 4-9).

Invasive Carcinoma

A tumor diathesis usually occurs in cases of invasive adenocarcinoma. Malignant cells desquamate either singly or in small clusters. Their cytologic features vary according to the type of tumor. Well-differentiated adenocarcinomas show cells with round or ovoid nuclei and prominent nucleoli. These nuclei are vesicular or

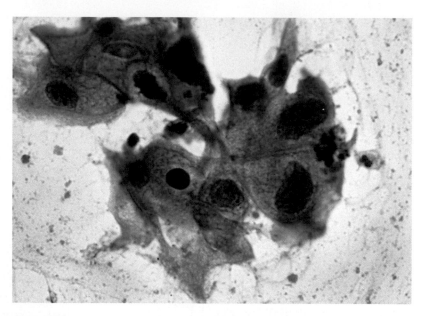

Figure 4-9
CARCINOMA IN SITU
There is great variation in size and shape of the cells. The chromatin is coarsely granular and unevenly distributed. Nucleoli are multiple and prominent.

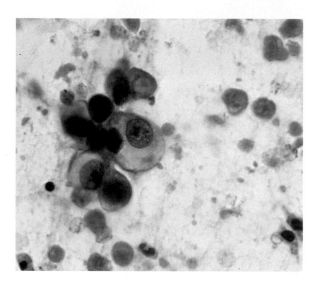

Figure 4-10
WELL-DIFFERENTIATED ADENOCARCINOMA
The malignant epithelial cells have round nuclei, prominent nucleoli, and coalescent cytoplasmic mucin vacuoles.

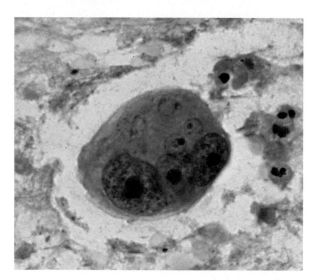

Figure 4-11
UNDIFFERENTIATED GIANT CELL CARCINOMA
A single Reed-Sternberg-like cell with several nuclei and macronucleoli is present.

hyperchromatic. The cytoplasm is usually vacuolated (fig. 4-10). Neoplastic cells arranged around fibrovascular cores is highly suggestive of papillary carcinoma. In giant cell carcinoma, cellular pleomorphism is more pronounced than in other types. Giant neoplastic cells with one or several bizarre nuclei and prominent macro-

nucleoli are seen (fig. 4-11). The cells from small cell carcinoma have large hyperchromatic nuclei with fine chromatin granules and no nucleoli. When nucleoli are present they are inconspicuous. The cytoplasm may not be seen or may appear as a small perinuclear rim.

REFERENCES

Epidemiology

1. Bosmans E, Onsea J, Verboven H. Gallbladder cancer as unexpected finding at cholecystectomy for benign disease. Acta Chir Belg 1990;90:207–12.
2. Fraumini JF Jr. Cancers of the pancreas and biliary tract: epidemiological considerations. Cancer Res 1975;35:3437–46.
3. Glenn F, Hays DM. The scope of radical surgery in the treatment of malignant tumors of the extrahepatic biliary tract. Surg Gynecol Obstet 1954;99:529–41.
4. Glenn F, Hill MR Jr. Extrahepatic biliary-tract cancer. Cancer 1955;8:1218–25.
5. Henson DE, Albores-Saavedra J, Corle D. Carcinoma of the gallbladder. Histologic types, stage of disease, and survival rates. Cancer 1992;70:1493–7.
6. Menck HR, Henderson BE, Pike MD, Mack T, Martin SP, SooHoo J. Cancer incidence in the Mexican-American. JNCI 1975;55:531–6.
7. Morris DL, Buechley RW, Key CR, Morgan MV. Gallbladder disease and gallbladder cancer among American Indians in tricultural New Mexico. Cancer 1978;42:2472–7.
8. Rios-Dalenz J, Takabayashi A, Henson DE, Strom BL, Soloway RD. The epidemiology of cancer of the extrahepatic biliary tract in Bolivia. Int J Epidemiol 1983;12:156–60.
9. Rudolph R, Cohen JJ. Cancer of the gallbladder in an 11-year-old Navajo girl. J Pediat Surg 1972;7:66–7.
10. Rudolph R, Cohen JJ, Gascoigne RH. Biliary cancer among southwestern American Indians. Ariz Med 1970;27:1–4.
11. Steiner PE. Cancer: race and geography. William and Wilkins, Baltimore, 1954.
12. Tominaga S, Kuroishi T, Ogawa H, Shimizu H. Epidemiologic aspects of biliary tract cancer in Japan. NCI Monogr 1979;53:25–34.

Etiology

13. Axelrod L, Munster AM, O Brian TF. Typhoid cholecystitis and gallbladder carcinoma after interval of 67 years. JAMA 1971;217:83.
14. Babbitt DP. Congenital choledochal cysts: new etiological concept based on anomalous relationships of the common bile duct and pancreatic bulb. Ann Radiologie 1969;12:231–40.
15. Babbitt DP, Starshak RJ, Clemett AR. Choledochal cyst: a concept of etiology. Am J Roentgenol 1973;119:17–62.
16. Berk RN, Armbuster TG, Saltzstein SL. Carcinoma in the porcelain gallbladder. Radiology 1973;106:29–31.
17. Casteel HB, Williamson SL, Golladay ES, Fiedorek SC. Porcelain gallbladder in a child: a case report and review. J Pediat Surg 1990;25:1302–3.
18. Caygill CP, Hill MJ, Braddick M, Sharp JC. Cancer mortality in chronic typhoid and paratyphoid carriers. Lancet 1994;343:83–4.
19. Chijiiwa K, Tanaka M, Nakayama F. Adenocarcinoma of the gallbladder associated with anomalous pancreaticobiliary ductal junction. Am Surg 1993;59:430–4.
20. Csendes A, Becerra M, Burdiles P, Demian I, Bancalari K, Csendes P. Bacteriological studies of bile from the gallbladder in patients with carcinoma of the gallbladder, cholelithiasis, common bile duct stones and no gallstones disease. Eur J Surg 1994;160:363–7.
21. Csendes A, Fernandez M, Uribe P. Bacteriology of the gallbladder bile in normal subjects. Am J Surg 1975;129:629–31.
22. Davenport M, Stringer MD, Howard ER. Biliary amylase and congenital choledochal dilatation. J Pedr Surg 1995;30:474–7.
23. De Aretxabala X, Riedeman P, Burgos L, et al. Gallbladder cancer. A case-control study. Revista Med Chile 1995;123:581–6.
24. Devor EJ, Buechley RW. Gallbladder cancer in Hispanic New Mexicans II. Familial occurrence in two northern New Mexico kindreds. Can J Genet Cytol 1979;1:139–45.
25. Diehl AK. Gallstone size and the risk of gallbladder cancer. JAMA 1983;250:2323–6.
26. Diggory P, Jacyna MR, Booth JC, Cook HT, Thomas HC. Gallbladder cancer presenting with Trousseau's sign in a 31-year-old man with occupational exposure to aromatic hydrocarbons. J R Soc Med 1989;82:631–2.
27. Dorudi S, Chapman RW, Kettlewell MG. Carcinoma of the gallbladder in ulcerative colitis and primary sclerosing cholangitis. Report of two cases. Dis Colon Rectum 1991;34:827–8.
28. England DM, Rosenblatt JE. Anaerobes in human biliary tracts. J Clin Microbiol 1977;6:494–8.
29. Goodhart GL, Levison ME, Trotman BW, Soloway RD. Pigment vs cholesterol cholelithiasis: bacteriology of gallbladder stone, bile, and tissue correlated with biliary lipid analysis. Am J Dig Dis 1978;23:877–82.
30. Hanada K, Itoh M, Fujü K, et al. K-ras and p53 mutations in stage I gallbladder carcinoma with an anomalous junction of the pancreaticobiliary duct. Cancer (in press)
31. Houten L, Sonnesso G. Occupational exposure and cancer of the liver. Arch Environ Health 1980;35:51–3.
32. Ikoma A, Nakamura N, Miyazaki T, Maeda M. Double cancer of the gallbladder and common bile duct associated with anomalous junction of pancreaticobiliary ductal system. Surgery 1992;111:595–600.
33. Kane RA, Jacobs R, Katz J, Costello P. Porcelain gallbladder: ultrasound and CT appearance. Radiology 1984;152:137–41.
34. Khan TF. Synchronous carcinoma of the gallbladder in patients with bile duct carcinoma. Aust N Z J Surg 1994;64:275.
35. Kimura K, Ohto M, Saisho H, et al. Association of gallbladder carcinoma and anomalous pancreaticobiliary ductal union. Gastroenterology 1985;89:1258–65.

36. Kimura W, Shimada H, Kuroda A, Morioka Y. Carcinoma of the gallbladder and extrahepatic bile ducts in autopsy cases of the aged, with special reference to its relationship to gallstones. Am J Gastroenterol 1989;84:386–90.

37. Kinoshita H, Nagata E, Hirohashi K, Kobayashi Y. Carcinoma of the gallbladder with an anomalous connection between the choledochus and the pancreatic duct. Report of 10 cases and review of the literature in Japan. Cancer 1984;54:762–9.

38. Lou MA, Mandal AK, Alexander JL, Thadepalli H. Bacteriology of the human biliary tract and the duodenum. Arch Surg 1977;112:965–7.

39. Lowenfels AB, Lindstrom CG, Conway MJ, Hastings PR. Gallstones and risk of gallbladder cancer. JNCI 1985;75:77–80.

40. Lowenfels AB, Walker AM, Althaus DP, Townsend G, Domellof L. Gallstone growth, size, and risk of gallbladder cancer: an interracial study. Int J Epidemiol 1989;18:50–4.

41. Maki T. Pathogenesis of calcium bilirubinate gallstone: role of E coli beta-glucuronidase and coagulation by inorganic ions. Ann Surg 1966;164:90–100.

42. Mancuso TF, Brennan MJ. Epidemiological considerations of cancer of the gallbladder, bile ducts and salivary glands in the rubber industry. J Occup Med 1970;12:333–41.

43. Maringhini A, Moreau JA, Melton J III, Hench VS, Zinsmeister AR, DiMagno EP. Gallstones, gallbladder cancer, and other gastrointestinal malignancies. An epidemiologic study in Rochester, Minnesota. Ann Intern Med 1987;107:30–5.

44. Mellemgaard A, Gaarslev K. Risk of hepatobiliary cancer in carriers of Salmonella typhi [Letter]. JNCI 1988;80:288.

45. Moerman CJ, Lagerwaard FJ, Bueno de Mesquita HB, Van Dalen A, Van Leeuwen MS. Schrover PA. Gallstone size and the risk of gallbladder cancer. Scand J Gastroenterol 1993;28:482–6.

46. Morowitz DA, Glagov S, Dordal E, Kirsner JB. Carcinoma of the biliary tract complicating chronic ulcerative colitis. Cancer 1971;27:356–61.

47. Nagata E, Sakai K, Kinoshita H, Kobayashi Y. The relation between carcinoma of the gallbladder and an anomalous connection between the choledochus and the pancreatic duct. Ann Surg 1985;202:182–90.

48. Nakao A, Sakagami K, Uda M, Mitsuoka S. Double cancers of the gallbladder and bile duct associated with anomalous choledochopancreatic duct junction. J Gastroenterol 1997;32:110–3.

49. Neiderhiser DH, Morningstar WA, Roth HP. Absorption of lecithin and lysolecithin by the gallbladder. J Lab Clin Med 1973;82:891–7.

50. Nugent KP, Spigelman AD, Talbot IC, Phillips RK. Gallbladder dysplasia in patients with familial adenomatosis polyposis. Br J Surg 1994;81:291–2.

51. Ohtani T, Shirai Y, Tsukada K, Hatakeyama K, Muto T. The association between extrahepatic biliary carcinoma and the junction of the cystic duct and the biliary tree. Eur J Surg 1994;160:37–40.

52. Ozmen V, Martin PC, Igci A, Cevikbas U, Webb WR. Adenocarcinoma of the gallbladder associated with congenital choledochal cyst and anomalous pancreaticobiliary ductal junction. Eur J Surg 1991;157:549–51.

53. Phemister DB, Rewbridge AG, Rudisill H Jr. Calcium carbonate gallstones and calcification of the gallbladder following cystic-duct obstruction. Ann Surg 1931;94:493–516.

54. Piehler JM, Crichlow RW. Primary carcinoma of the gallbladder. Surg Gynecol Obstet 1978;147:929–42.

55. Polk HC Jr. Carcinoma and the calcified gallbladder. Gastroenterology 1966;50:582–5.

56. Putz P, Willems G. Proliferative changes in the epithelium of the human lithiasic gallbladder. JNCI 1978;60:283–7.

57. Rothenberg RE, LaRaja RD, McCoy RE, Pryce EH. Elective cholecystectomy and carcinoma of the gallbladder. Am Surg 1991;57:306–8.

58. Shimada K, Inamatsu T, Yamashiro M. Anaerobic bacteria in biliary disease in elderly patients. J Infect Dis 1977;135:850–4.

59. Soloway RD, Takabayashi A, Rios-Dalenz J, et al. Geographic differences in the operative incidence and type of pigment gallstones and in the non-cholesterol components of cholesterol gallstones. Hepatol Rapid Lit Rev 1981;11:1637–8.

60. Szendroi M, Nemeth L, Vajta G. Asbestos bodies in a bile duct cancer after occupational exposure. Environ Res 1983;30:270–80.

61. Trajber HJ, Szego T, Amancio de Camargo HS Jr, et al. Adenocarcinoma of the gallbladder in two siblings. Cancer 1982;50:1200–3.

62. Trotman BW, Soloway RD. Pigment vs cholesterol cholelithiasis: clinical and epidemiological aspects. Am J Dig Dis 1975;20:735–40.

63. Warren KW, Hardy KJ, O'Rourke MG. Primary neoplasia of the gallbladder. Surg Gynec Obstet 1968;126:1036–40.

64. Welton JC, Marr JS, Friedman SM. Association between hepatobiliary cancer and typhoid carrier state. Lancet 1979;1:791–4.

65. Yamamoto M, Nakajo S, Tahara E, et al. Mucosal changes of the gallbladder in anomalous union with the pancreatico-biliary duct system. Pathol Res Pract 1991;187:241–6.

66. Yamauchi S, Koga A, Matsumoto S, Tanaka M, Nakayama F. Anomalous junction of pancreaticobiliary duct without congenital choledochal cyst: a possible risk factor for gallbladder cancer. Am J Gastroenterol 1987;82:20–4.

67. Young WT, Thomas GV, Blethyn AJ, Lawrie BW. Choledochal cyst and congenital anomalies of the pancreatico-biliary junction: the clinical findings, radiology and outcome in nine cases. Br J Radiol 1992;65:33–8.

Clinical Manifestations

68. Abrams RM, Meng CH, Firooznia H, Beranbaum ER, Epstein HY. Angiographic demonstration of carcinoma of the gallbladder. Radiology 1970;94:277–82.

68a. Albores-Saavedra J, Molberg K, Henson DE. Unusual malignant epithelial tumor of the gallbladder. Sem Diag Pathol 1996;13:326–38.

69. Arora A, Choudhuri G, Tandon RK. Acanthosis nigricans associated with adenocarcinoma of the gallbladder. Am J Gastroenterol 1985;80:896–7.

70. Bismuth H, Malt RA. Carcinoma of the biliary tract. N Engl J Med 1979;301:704–6.

71. Brown JA, Roberts CS. Elevated serum alpha-fetoprotein levels in primary gallbladder carcinoma without hepatic involvement. Cancer 1992;70:1838–40.

72. Crade M, Taylor KJ, Rosenfield AT, de Graaff CS, Minihan P. Surgical and pathologic correlation of cholecystosonography and cholecystography. Am J Radiol 1978;131:227–9.

73. Dalla Palma L, Rizzatto G, Possi-Mucelli RS, Bazzocchi M. Grey-scale ultrasonography in the evaluation of carcinoma of the gallbladder. Br J Radiol 1980;53:662–7.

74. Diggory P, Jacyna MR, Booth JC, Cook HT, Thomas HC. Gallbladder cancer presenting with Trousseau's sign in a 31-year-old man with occupational exposure to aromatic hydrocarbons. J R Soc Med 1989;82:631–2.

75. Gale ME, Robbins AH. Computed tomography of the gallbladder: unusual diseases. J Comp Assist Tomograph 1985;9:439–43.

76. Gradisar IA, Kelly TR. Primary carcinoma of the gallbladder. Arch Surg 1970;100:232–5.

77. Hamrick RE Jr, Liner FJ, Hastings PR, Cohn I Jr. Primary carcinoma of the gallbladder. Ann Surg 1982;195:270–3.

78. Haruta J, Kanayama K, Tachino F, et al. A clinicopathological evaluation of AFP-positive gallbladder cancer with special reference to two autopsy cases investigated by an immunological method. Gan No Rinsho 1987;33:1389–45.

79. Hederström E, Forsberg L. Ultrasonography in carcinoma of the gallbladder. Diagnostic difficulties and pitfalls. Acta Radiol 1987;28:715–8.

80. Itai Y. Computed tomographic evaluation of gallbladder disease. Crit Rev Diagn Imaging 1987;27:113–52.

81. Jacobs MI, Rigel DS. Acanthosis nigricans and the sign of Leser-Trelat associated with adenocarcinoma of the gallbladder. Cancer 1981;48:325–8.

82. Ker CG, Chen JS, Lee KT, Sheen PC, Wu CC. Assessment of serum and bile levels of CA19-9 and CA125 in cholangitis and bile duct carcinoma. J Gastroenterol Hepatol 1991;6:505–8.

83. Pemberton LB, Diffenbaugh WF, Strohl EL. The surgical significance of carcinoma of the gallbladder. Am J Surg 1971;122:381–3.

84. Post B, Wilhelmi F, Janner M. Bulloses pemphigoid asl cutanes paraneoplastiches syndrom bei einem galledblasencarcinom. Hautarzt 1973;24:193–7.

85. Rooholamini SA, Tehrani NS, Razavi MK, et al. Imaging of gallbladder carcinoma. Radiographics 1994;14:291–306.

86. Spence RW, Burns-Cox CJ. ACTH-secreting apudoma of gallbladder. Gut 1975;16:473–6.

87. Strom BL, Iliopoulis D, Atkinson B, et al. Pathophysiology of tumor progression in human gallbladder: flow cytometry, CEA, and CA19-9 levels in bile and serum in different stages of gallbladder disease. JNCI 1989;81:1571–80.

88. Strom BL, Maislin G, West SL, Atkinson B, et al. Serum CEA and CA19-9: potential future diagnostic or screening test for gallbladder cancer? Int J Cancer 1990;45:821–4.

89. Sugaya Y, Sugaya H, Kuronuma Y, Hisauchi T, Harada T. A case of gallbladder carcinoma producing both alpha-fetoprotein (AFP) and carcinoembryonic antigen (CEA). Gastroenterol Jpn 1989;24:325–31.

90. Tatsuta M, Yamamura H, Yamamoto R, Morii T, Okuda S, Tamura H. Carcinoembryonic antigen in the bile in patients with pancreatic and biliary cancer. Correlation with cytology and percutaneous transhepatic cholangiography. Cancer 1982;50:2903–9.

91. Vardaman C, Albores-Saavedra J. Clear cell carcinoma of the gallbladder and extrahepatic bile ducts. Am J Surg Pathol 1995;19:91–9.

92. Villabona CM, Esteve M, Vidaller A, et al. Hypercalcemic crisis in gallbladder cancer. Acta Gastroenterol Belg 1986;49:532–5.

93. Watanabe M, Hori Y, Nojima T, et al. Alpha-fetoprotein-producing carcinoma of the gallbladder. Dig Dis Sci 1993;38:561–4.

94. Watanabe Y, Ogino Y, Ubukata E, Sakamoto Y, Matsuzaki O, Shimizu N. A case of a gallbladder cancer with marked hypercalcemia and leukocytosis. Jpn J Med 1989;28:722–6.

95. Werko L. Acanthosis nigricans associated with carcinoma of gallbladder and plantar hyperkeratosis. Acta Derm Venereol 1945;26:70–83.

95a. Wibbenmeyer LA, Sharafuddin MJ, Walverson MK, Heiberg EV, Wade TP, Shields JB. Sonographic diagnosis of unsuspected gallbladder cancer. AJR Am J Roentgenol 1995;165:1169–74.

Bile Cytology

96. Akosa AB, Barker F, Desa L, et al. Cytologic diagnosis in the management of gallbladder carcinoma. Acta Cytol 1995;39:494–8.

97. Alonso-DeRuiz P, Albores-Saavedra J, Henson DE, Monroy MN. Cytopathology of the precursor lesions of invasive carcinoma of the gallbladder. Acta Cytol 1982;26:144–52.

98. Dodd LG, Moffatt J, Hudson ER, Layfield LJ. Fine needle aspiration of primary gallbladder carcinoma. Diagn Cytopathol 1996;15:151–6.

99. Ishikawa O, Ohhigashi H, Sasaki Y, et al. The usefulness of saline irrigated bile for the intraoperative cytologic diagnosis of tumors and tumor-like lesions of the gallbladder. Acta Cytol 1988;32:475–81.

100. Ropertz, S, Wagner K. Puncture of the gallbladder during peritoneoscopy—technique and diagnostic relevance. Leber Megen Darm 1976;6:19–24.

101. Verma K, Bhargava DK. Cytologic examinations as an adjunct to laparoscopy and guided biopsy in the diagnosis of hepatic and gallbladder neoplasia. Acta Cytol 1982;26:311–6.

5
DYSPLASIA AND CARCINOMA IN SITU OF GALLBLADDER

INTRODUCTION

Many studies have shown that invasive carcinoma of the gallbladder is preceded by dysplasia and carcinoma in situ (1–14,16). However, the incidence of these precursors varies in different parts of the world. In Australia, for example, the incidence of dysplasia was 3.3 percent and the incidence of carcinoma in situ was 1.6 percent in gallbladders with lithiasis (14). In Finland, the incidence of mild dysplasia was 24 percent, of moderate dysplasia 8.5 percent, and of severe dysplasia 1.4 percent in gallbladders containing stones (11). In Mexico and Chile, where carcinoma of the gallbladder is considered to be endemic, the incidence of dysplasia has varied from 13.5 to 16.0 percent and that of carcinoma in situ between 3.5 to 2.5 percent (1,10). This variation in incidence is attributable to several factors: 1) *Method of sampling.* If only one or two random sections are taken from the gallbladder, as is customary in most pathology laboratories, the probability of finding these lesions decreases; 2) *Study design.* Prospective studies usually show a higher incidence of dysplasia and carcinoma in situ than retrospective studies (9); 3) *The country in which the study is performed.* Carcinoma of the gallbladder is sporadic in many countries and endemic in others (2,6). The rate of dysplasia and carcinoma in situ is a reflection of the rate of gallbladder carcinoma in those countries; and 4) *Histologic criteria.* Reactive atypia is often seen in acute and chronic cholecystitis (3). If it is misinterpreted as dysplasia or carcinoma in situ the incidence of these two lesions will increase. Morphologic criteria for distinguishing mild dysplasia from intestinal metaplasia are subtle and variable among pathologists.

Since these precursor lesions represent a morphologic continuum from hyperplasia to carcinoma in situ, some variability in interpretation by pathologists is inevitable. This problem is enhanced by the lack of markers that can separate atypical reactive cells from dysplastic cells and the latter from neoplastic cells. Genetic analysis has shown similar molecular abnormalities in metaplastic, dysplastic, and carcinoma cells, making their separation impossible even at the molecular level (16). As a result, pathologists must rely on conventional histologic sections to classify these lesions, a morphologic exercise which is largely subjective. With these limitations in mind, we shall proceed to describe these lesions.

Dysplasia and carcinoma in situ are usually not visible macroscopically, but are invariably discovered during histologic examination. However, the papillary form of dysplasia and carcinoma in situ may appear as small cauliflower-like excrescences that are visible grossly above the mucosal surface. These lesions are usually focal and may be multiple. However, they can involve wide areas of the mucosa and even extend into the cystic duct.

According to their growth pattern, two types of dysplasia and carcinoma in situ are recognized: papillary and flat, the latter being more common. The papillary type is characterized by short fibrovascular stalks that are covered by dysplastic or neoplastic cells.

Since dysplasia and carcinoma in situ are often seen in association with cholelithiasis, they usually arise in an abnormal mucosa showing pyloric gland or intestinal metaplasia (3,6,17, 19). Dysplasia and carcinoma in situ have also been described in patients with familial adenomatous polyposis coli (7,13). The lesions usually begin on the surface and subsequently extend laterally and downward into the Rokitansky-Aschoff sinuses and into metaplastic pyloric glands located in the lamina propria (20). This extension should not be mistaken for stromal invasion. Rarely, dysplasia and carcinoma in situ may arise from the Rokitansky-Aschoff sinuses or from metaplastic glands.

Dysplasia is characterized by columnar, cuboidal, or elongated cells showing variable degrees of pseudostratification, nuclear atypia, loss of polarity, and mitotic figures (figs. 5-1–5-3). Atypical goblet cells are also found in some cases. Dysplasia is graded as mild, moderate, or severe, or classified as low or high grade based on the extent of cytologic atypia and loss of polarity.

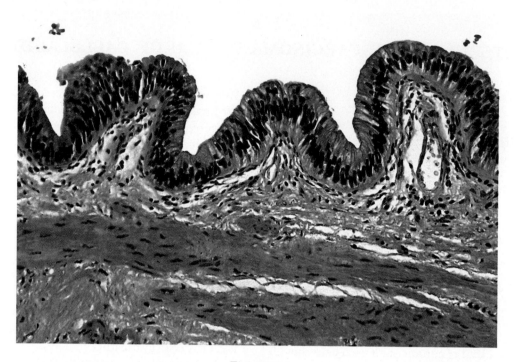

Figure 5-1
MILD (LOW-GRADE) DYSPLASIA
The enlarged, hyperchromatic nuclei are pseudostratified and some are not basally located.

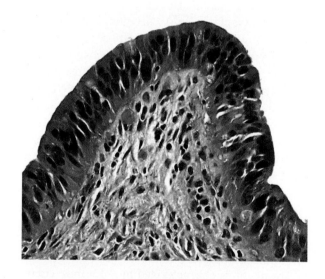

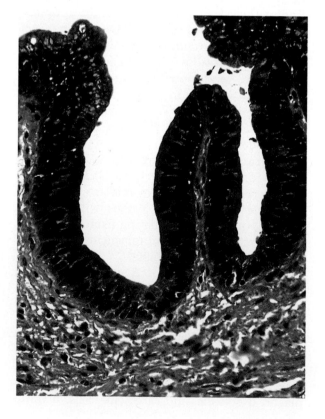

Figure 5-2
SEVERE (HIGH-GRADE) DYSPLASIA
Above: The enlarged nuclei are vesicular and contain prominent nucleoli.
Right: The columnar cells show elongated, hyperchromatic, and pseudostratified nuclei.

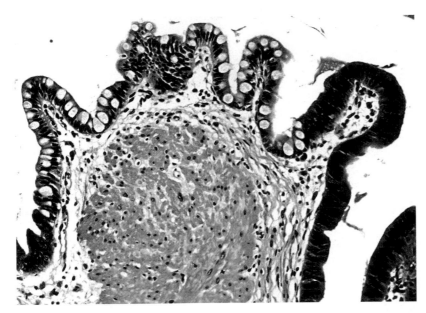

Figure 5-3
HIGH-GRADE DYSPLASIA
ADJACENT TO
INTESTINAL METAPLASIA
The surface epithelium shows hyperchromatism and nuclear enlargement adjacent to mature or slightly dysplastic goblet cells.

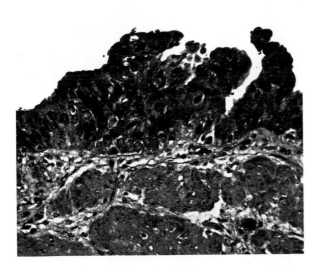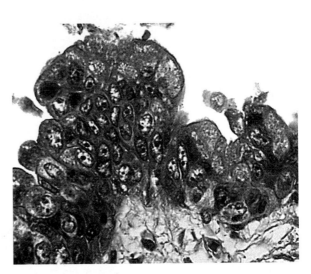

Figure 5-4
CARCINOMA IN SITU
Left: The epithelial lining is highly atypical. The cells are pseudostratified and have large, bizarre, hyperchromatic nuclei.
Right: In this carcinoma in situ the cells contain prominent nucleoli.

Carcinoma in situ is defined as epithelium with the histologic features of carcinoma but without evidence of stromal invasion. The cellular overgrowth expands upward and laterally within the confines of the epithelium (fig. 5-4). True stratification occurs in some cases (figs. 5-4–5-8). The histologic features vary only in degree when compared to those of dysplasia: the nuclei of carcinoma in situ are larger and contain a coarse granular chromatin, while the nucleoli are more prominent and usually increased in number. Giant cells with large hyperchromatic nuclei are observed in some in situ carcinomas. Mitotic figures are relatively common. We should emphasize, however, that the histologic differences between severe dysplasia and carcinoma in situ are often arbitrary and separation of the two lesions is not always possible. This is not important because the two lesions are closely related biologically.

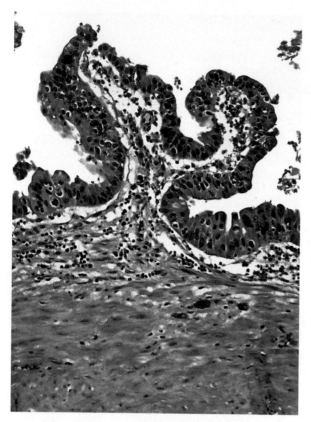

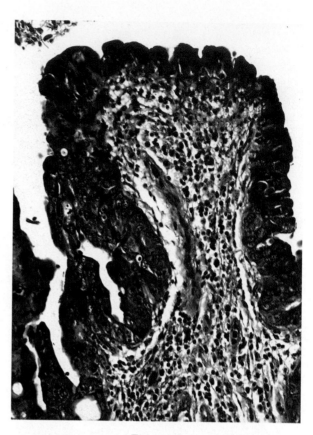

Figure 5-5
CARCINOMA IN SITU
A mucosal fold is lined by pleomorphic epithelial cells that are pseudostratified and show mitotic activity.

Figure 5-6
CARCINOMA IN SITU
A mucosal fold is lined by neoplastic epithelial cells with vesicular nuclei and prominent nucleoli.

Figure 5-7
PAPILLARY CARCINOMA
IN SITU
Papillary structures are lined by neoplastic cells with vesicular nuclei and prominent nucleoli.

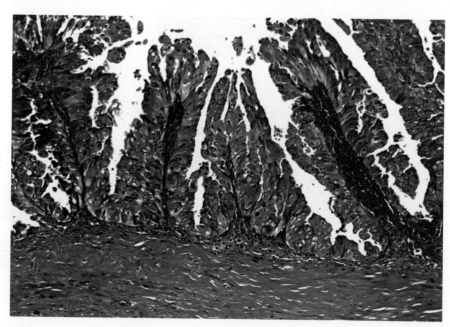

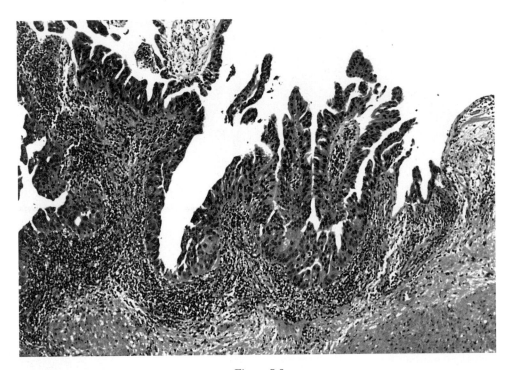

Figure 5-8
CARCINOMA IN SITU
This in situ papillary carcinoma shows a dense lymphocytic infiltrate in the lamina propria.

However, differentiation of dysplasia or carcinoma in situ from the epithelial atypia of repair is of great clinical significance because the latter does not progress to carcinoma. Atypia of repair consists of a heterogeneous cell population in which columnar mucus-secreting cells, low cuboidal cells, atrophic-appearing epithelium, and penciloid cells are present. In addition, reactive atypia shows a gradual transition of the cellular abnormalities, in contrast to the abrupt transition seen in dysplasia and carcinoma in situ (3), and the extent of nuclear atypia is less pronounced.

Nuclear DNA ploidy studies by flow cytometry in paraffin-embedded material do not allow separation of reactive atypia from dysplasia and carcinoma in situ. Some cases of atypia secondary to repair are aneuploid as are most in situ carcinomas (Vardaman C, Albores-Saavedra J. Unpublished observations, 1991). On the other hand, morphometric analysis appears to be useful in differentiating atypia of repair and dysplasia from invasive carcinoma (12). This technique, however, does not allow distinction between atypia of repair and true dysplasia or carcinoma in situ.

IMMUNOHISTOCHEMISTRY AND MOLECULAR PATHOLOGY

By immunohistochemical methods it has been shown that dysplasia and carcinoma in situ are immunoreactive for polyclonal and monoclonal carcinoembryonic antigen (CEA) (5) and for the carbohydrate antigen CA19-9 (21). The reactivity is usually focal and in a linear pattern along the apical cytoplasmic border. However, faint cytoplasmic staining is also seen, mainly with CEA. This oncofetal antigen can be detected as well in both the bile and serum, but an elevated CEA level is not diagnostic of dysplasia or carcinoma because extrahepatic bile duct obstruction from any cause leads to a rise. The lack of specificity of CEA limits its use in the diagnosis of early carcinoma of the gallbladder.

Recent studies have shown a crucial role of p53 gene mutations in the early pathogenesis of gallbladder carcinoma (14a). By immunohistochemistry, p53 nuclear staining was found in 32 percent of dysplasias and 44 percent of in situ carcinomas (fig. 5-9) (15). Genetic analysis has shown a high incidence of loss of heterozygosity

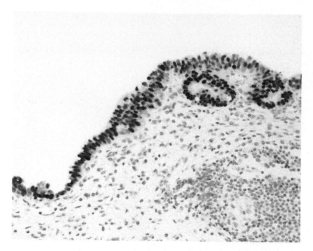

Figure 5-9
IMMUNOHISTOCHEMICAL OVEREXPRESSION
OF P53 PROTEIN BY DYSPLASTIC CELLS

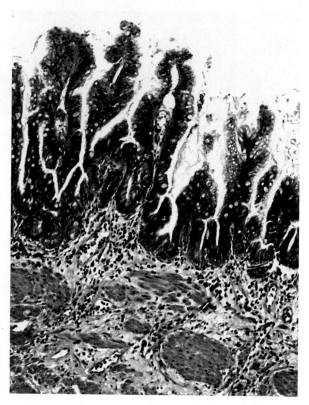

Figure 5-10
INTESTINAL TYPE CARCINOMA IN SITU
This papillary in situ carcinoma is composed of columnar cells, goblet cells, and Paneth cells, the latter of which are difficult to recognize at low power. Endocrine cells were demonstrated with silver stains.

at the p53 gene in both dysplasia (58 percent) and carcinoma in situ (85 percent). Other molecular abnormalities include loss of heterozygosity at 9p and 8p loci and the 18q gene. These molecular abnormalities are early events and most likely contributing factors in the pathogenesis of gallbladder carcinoma (16). K-*ras* mutations were not detected in either lesion (16).

HISTOLOGIC SUBTYPES OF CARCINOMA IN SITU

Rarely, in situ carcinomas may contain numerous goblet cells, Paneth cells, and endocrine cells. Consequently, these lesions are considered to be the preinvasive phase of the intestinal type of adenocarcinoma (fig. 5-10).

We have seen two examples of signet ring cell carcinoma confined to the surface epithelium and the epithelial invaginations of the gallbladder (fig. 5-11) (4). The signet ring cells were reactive for cytokeratin and CEA (fig. 5-12). Despite multiple sections, stromal invasion was not found. These in situ signet ring cell carcinomas represented incidental findings in cholecystectomy specimens and are cytologically similar to those reported in the stomach. This unusual form of carcinoma in situ should be distinguished from epithelial cells which acquire signet ring cell morphology when desquamated within the lumen of dilated metaplastic pyloric glands in cases of chronic cholecystitis. The

CEA-negative cells are often poorly preserved, lack nuclear atypia, and appear to "float" with other degenerating epithelial and inflammatory cells. Likewise, mucin-containing histiocytes (muciphages) that are occasionally seen in mucoceles of the gallbladder may simulate signet ring cell carcinoma in situ. These muciphages, however, are cytokeratin and CEA negative.

Squamous cell dysplasia and squamous cell carcinoma in situ are often seen in the vicinity of invasive squamous cell carcinoma (fig. 5-13). This suggests that these pathologic changes are the intermediate steps in the development of invasive squamous cell carcinoma.

The morphologic type of in situ carcinoma does not always correspond with that of the invasive carcinoma. For example, we have seen conventional adenocarcinoma in situ in the mucosa adjacent to invasive squamous cell carcinoma,

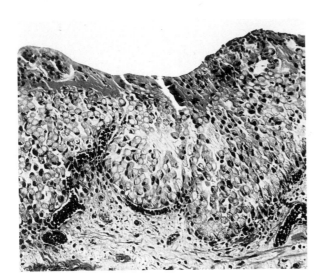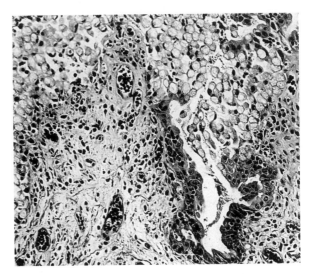

Figure 5-11
SIGNET RING CELL CARCINOMA IN SITU
Left: The neoplastic cells are confined to the mucosa.
Right: Detail of neoplastic signet ring cells, some of which extend along an epithelial invagination.

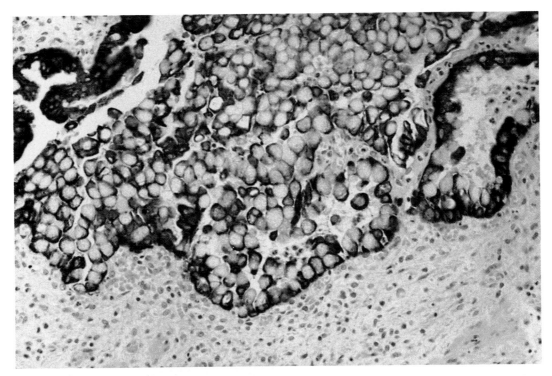

Figure 5-12
SIGNET RING CELL CARCINOMA IN SITU
Neoplastic signet ring cells show cytokeratin reactivity. Similar reactivity was obtained with CEA.

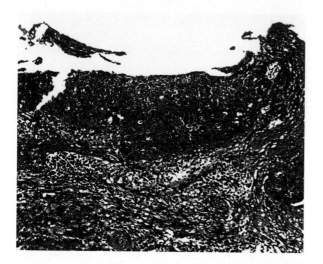 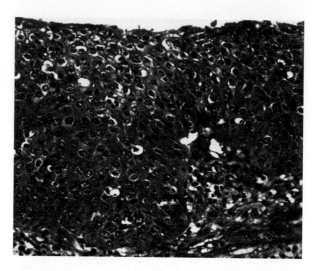

Figure 5-13
SQUAMOUS CELL CARCINOMA IN SITU
Left: The surface epithelium of the gallbladder is replaced by neoplastic squamous cells.
Right: Detail of squamous cells showing nuclear enlargement and loss of polarity.

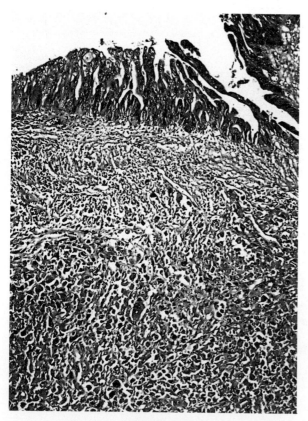

Figure 5-14
CARCINOMA IN SITU
This carcinoma in situ with micropapillary features overlies a spindle and giant cell carcinoma.

small cell carcinoma, and undifferentiated carcinoma, spindle and giant cell types (fig. 5-14).

Little is known about the natural history of dysplasia and carcinoma in situ of the gallbladder. Most of these lesions are diagnosed after cholecystectomy and the entire lesion removed. This is a limiting factor in the study of their rate of progression. Similarly, the proportion of invasive carcinomas that pass through the sequence of dysplasia and carcinoma in situ is unknown. However, there is evidence that progression from in situ to infiltrating carcinoma does occur. For instance, when in situ carcinomas were studied by subserial sections, foci of microinvasion were found in the lamina propria continuous with the overlying carcinoma in situ (3). Dysplasia and carcinoma in situ are seen in the areas of intact mucosa that are found adjacent to nearly all invasive carcinomas (3,18–22). These two changes do not represent lateral neoplastic growth because normal or metaplastic epithelium is often seen between the invasive and the in situ carcinomas. Dysplasia and carcinoma in situ are most often found in the fundus and body, the areas of the gallbladder from which most invasive carcinomas arise. Finally, patients with dysplasia on average are 5 years younger than those with carcinoma in situ and patients with carcinoma in situ are on average 10 years younger than those with invasive carcinoma (1).

When dysplasia or carcinoma in situ is found in the gallbladder, multiple sections should be examined to exclude invasion. We would like to emphasize that extension of carcinoma in situ along Rokitansky-Aschoff sinuses should not be confused with stromal invasion. These structures are epithelial invaginations lined by non-neoplastic biliary epithelium with an intact basal lamina (fig. 5-15). Likewise, extension of carcinoma in situ into metaplastic pyloric glands may simulate invasion. If no invasive carcinoma is found, no further treatment is recommended. Patients with invasive carcinoma extending into the lamina propria or superficial portion of the muscle layer are at risk for metastatic disease (3). Of 101 patients with carcinoma in situ of the gallbladder collected by the Surveillance, Epidemiology, and End Results (SEER) Program of the National Cancer Institute, 100 percent survived 5 years (fig. 5-16). However, 33 percent died of tumor at 10 years, suggesting that either an invasive component was missed or patients developed a second primary that was not recorded.

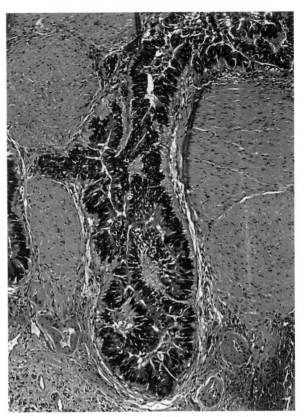

Figure 5-15
CARCINOMA IN SITU EXTENDING ALONG
A ROKITANSKY-ASCHOFF SINUS
The tumor cells are sharply demarcated from the muscle layer and serosa.

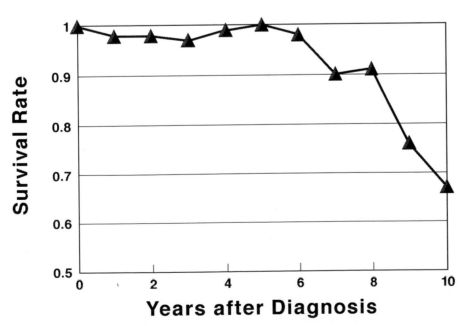

Figure 5-16
TEN-YEAR RELATIVE
SURVIVAL RATE FOR
101 PATIENTS WITH
IN SITU CARCINOMA
OF THE GALLBLADDER
Data taken from the Surveillance, Epidemiology, and End Results Program of the National Cancer Institute for the years 1981–1990.

REFERENCES

1. Albores-Saavedra J, Alcantra-Vazquez A, Cruz-Ortiz H, Herrera-Goepfert R. The precursor lesions of invasive gallbladder carcinoma. Cancer 1980;45:919–27.

2. Albores-Saavedra J, Henson DE. Gallbladder and extrahepatic bile ducts. In: Henson DE, Albores-Saavedra, eds. Pathology of incipient neoplasia, 2nd ed. Philadelphia: WB Saunders, 1993:167–81.

3. Albores-Saavedra J, Manrique JJ, Angeles-Angeles A, Henson DE. Carcinoma in situ of the gallbladder. A clinicopathologic study of 18 cases. Am J Surg Pathol 1984;8:323–33.

4. Albores-Saavedra J, Molberg K, Henson DE. Unusual malignant epithelial tumors of the gallbladder. Sem Diagn Pathol 1996;13:326–38.

5. Albores-Saavedra J, Nadji M, Morales AR, Henson DE. Carcinoembryonic antigen in normal, preneoplastic and neoplastic gallbladder epithelium. Cancer 1983; 52:1069–72.

6. Black WC. The morphogenesis of gallbladder carcinoma. In: Fenoglio CM, Wolff M, eds. Progress in surgical pathology, Vol. II. New York: Masson Publishing, 1980:207–23.

7. Bombi JA, Rives A, Astudillo E, Pera C, Cardesa A. Polyposis coli associated with adenocarcinoma of the gallbladder. Report of a case. Cancer 1984;53:2561–3.

8. Dowling GP, Kelly JK. The histogenesis of adenocarcinoma of the gallbladder. Cancer 1986;58:1702–8.

9. Chang KW. Review of 253 cases of significant pathology in 7,910 cholecystectomies in Hong Kong. Pathology 1988;20:20–3.

10. Duarte I, Llanos O, Domke H, Harz C, Valdivieso V. Metaplasia and precursor lesions of gallbladder carcinoma. Frequency, distribution and probability of detection in routine histologic samples. Cancer 1993;72:1878–84.

11. Laitio M. Histogenesis of epithelial neoplasms of human gallbladder. I. Dysplasia. Pathol Res Pract 1983;178:51–6.

12. Nakajo S, Yamamoto M, Tahara E. Morphometric analysis of gallbladder adenocarcinoma: discrimination between carcinoma and dysplasia. Virchows Arch [A] 1989;416:133–40.

13. Nugent KP, Spigelman AD, Talbot IC, Phillips RK. Gallbladder dysplasia in patients with familial adenomatous polyposis. Br J Surg 1994;81:291–2.

14. Ojeda VJ, Shilkin KB, Walters MN. Premalignant epithelial lesions of the gallbladder. A prospective study of 120 cholecystectomy specimens. Pathology 1985;17:451–4.

14a. Wistuba I, Albores-Saavedra J. Genetic abnormalities involved in the pathogenesis of gallbladder carcinoma. J Hepatobiliary Pancreat Surg 1999;6:237–44.

15. Wistuba II, Gazdar AF, Roa I, Albores-Saavedra J. P53 protein over–expression in gallbladder carcinoma and its precursor lesions: an immunohistochemical study. Hum Pathol 1996;27:360–5.

16. Wistuba II, Sugio K, Hung J, et al. Allele-specific mutations involved in the pathogenesis of endemic gallbladder carcinoma in Chile. Cancer Res 1995;55:2511–5.

17. Yamagiwa H. Dysplasia of gallbladder. Its pathological significance. Acta Pathol Jpn 1987;37:747–54.

18. Yamagiwa H. Mucosal dysplasia of gallbladder: isolated and adjacent lesions to carcinoma. Jpn J Cancer Res 1989;80:238–43.

19. Yamagiwa H, Tomiyama H. Intestinal metaplasia-dysplasia-carcinoma sequence of the gallbladder. Acta Pathol Jpn 1986;36:989–97.

20. Yamaguchi A, Hachisuka K, Isogai M, et al. Carcinoma in situ of the gallbladder with superficial extension into the Rokitansky-Aschoff sinuses and mucous glands. Gastroenterol Jpn 1992;27:765–72.

21. Yamaguchi K, Enjoji M. Carcinoma of the gallbladder. A clinicopathology of 103 patients and a new proposed staging. Cancer 1988;62:1425–32.

22. Yamamoto M, Nakajo S, Tahara E. Dysplasia of the gallbladder. Its histogenesis and correlation to gallbladder adenocarcinoma. Pathol Res Pract 1989;185:454–60.

✧✧✧

6

PATHOLOGY OF INVASIVE CARCINOMA OF GALLBLADDER

Although the gallbladder has a relatively simple histologic structure, it gives rise to a wide variety of malignant tumors. More than 98 percent of such tumors are carcinomas, most of which result, in our experience, from the neoplastic transformation of the lining epithelium.

Carcinomas of the gallbladder are not likely to cause diagnostic problems. Most are well- or moderately differentiated adenocarcinomas that are cytologically heterogeneous. Most carcinomas consist of a mixture of cell types. Many of these cells resemble those of biliary epithelium while others show an intestinal phenotype. A small proportion of tumors contain, in addition, cells similar to those of gastric foveolar epithelium. Moreover, carcinomas of the gallbladder exhibit different growth patterns and varying degrees of differentiation. Undifferentiated carcinomas usually coexist with foci of well-differentiated adenocarcinoma. A significant proportion of small cell carcinomas have a glandular component. Clear cell carcinomas often contain elements of a well- or moderately differentiated adenocarcinoma and may even show focal areas of hepatoid differentiation.

In tumors with more than one histologic pattern, the trend has been to classify them according to the predominant pattern. However, since knowledge of the natural history of these tumors is incomplete and the response of the different histologic types to therapy not well known, we recommend that pathologists record all patterns in the final diagnosis.

Recording the histologic type is clinically important, since patients with some types have a better prognosis. For example, the relative 5-year survival rate for patients with papillary carcinoma is 36 percent, while the 5-year relative survival rate for those with adenocarcinoma is 13 percent (2). Because small cell carcinomas can cause endocrine manifestations, such as Cushing's syndrome, they should be correctly reported. Perhaps a more important reason for separation is that the chemotherapeutic approach to small cell carcinomas differs from that for adenocarcinomas.

GROSS FEATURES

Small infiltrating carcinomas may appear as a focal thickening of the gallbladder wall, a raised mucosal plaque, a bulging submucosal nodule, a polypoid structure protruding into the lumen, or a combination of these features. At an early stage, a small tumor may be confused with chronic cholecystitis and not recognized grossly (fig. 6-1). As carcinomas enlarge, some cause

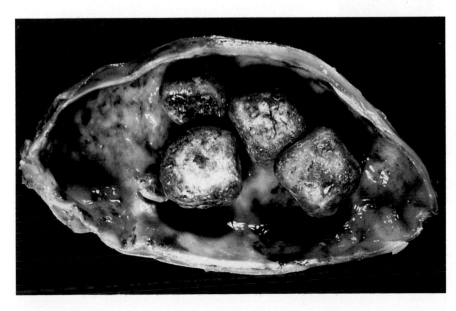

Figure 6-1
ADENOCARCINOMA
Gallbladder excised for cholelithiasis. A small infiltrating carcinoma, not grossly visible, was found in a thickened area of the fundus. This early gross change is difficult to recognize and is usually mistaken for chronic cholecystitis.

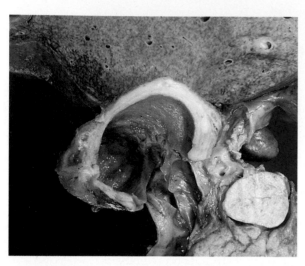

Figure 6-2
INTRAMURAL INFILTRATION
Diffuse intramural infiltration of a well-differentiated adenocarcinoma that had also metastasized to a peripancreatic lymph node. In cases of diffuse infiltration the site of origin of the tumor is not possible to identify.

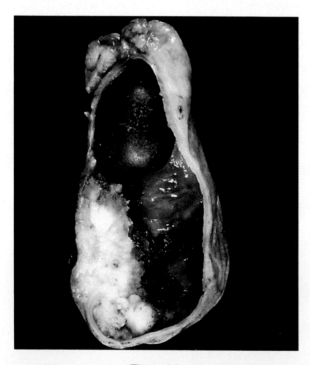

Figure 6-3
ADENOCARCINOMA
The usual gross features of a well-differentiated adenocarcinoma are shown. The fungating tumor which is associated with stones involves the body and the fundus, and has invaded the full thickness of the wall.

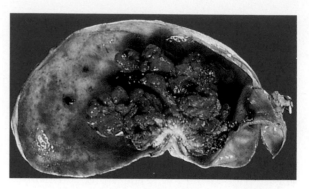

Figure 6-4
PAPILLARY ADENOCARCINOMA
This papillary adenocarcinoma arose from the body of the gallbladder. It has a cauliflower-like appearance and protrudes into the lumen. Despite its large size, limited invasion into the wall was demonstrated microscopically. (Pl. IB from Fascicle 22, 2nd Series.)

diffuse thickening and induration of the entire gallbladder wall (fig. 6-2). Most carcinomas, however, grow as an infiltrating, gray-white mass that can be recognized without much difficulty as a malignant neoplasm, and their site of origin can be located with some degree of certainty (fig. 6-3). The gallbladder may be distended by the tumor, contracted, or collapsed due to obstruction of the neck or cystic duct. It can also assume an hourglass deformity when the tumor arises in the body and constricts the lateral walls.

Papillary carcinomas are usually sessile and exhibit a polypoid or cauliflower-like appearance (fig. 6-4). Mucinous and signet ring cell carcinomas have a mucoid or gelatinous cut surface (fig. 6-5). Although any type of gallbladder cancer may show necrosis, undifferentiated giant cell and small cell carcinomas are usually the most necrotic (figs. 6-6, 6-7). Submucosal growth is an important feature of signet ring and small cell carcinomas.

Carcinomas arising in the neck of the gallbladder not only lead to obstruction, which may result in hydrops, but commonly infiltrate the wall of the bile ducts including the mucosa, so that in some cases it is not possible to specify whether the tumor originated in the neck or in the cystic duct.

When extension to the liver takes place, the tumor often surrounds the gallbladder. The result is a thick neoplastic wall in which the gallbladder becomes encased (fig. 6-8).

Approximately 60 percent of carcinomas originate in the fundus, 30 percent in the body, and 10 percent in the neck. In some cases, the tumor

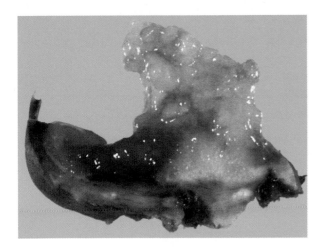

Figure 6-5
MUCINOUS CARCINOMA
A polypoid and infiltrating mass with a gelatinous appearance as shown here is characteristic of mucinous carcinomas.

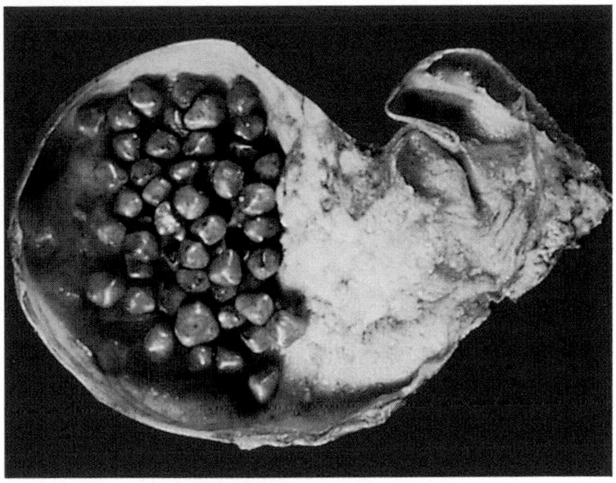

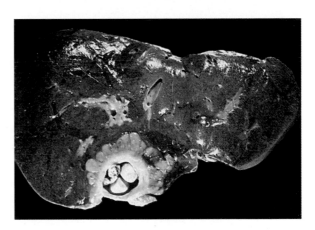

Figure 6-7
SMALL CELL CARCINOMA
This small cell carcinoma which arose in the body shows extensive necrosis. It is associated with stones. (Pl. ID from Fascicle 22, 2nd Series.)

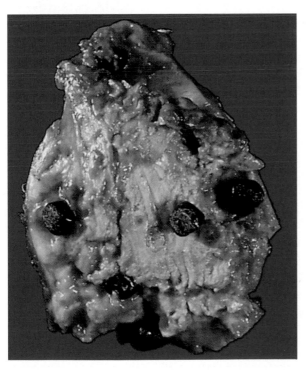

Figure 6-6
UNDIFFERENTIATED CARCINOMA,
SPINDLE AND GIANT CELL TYPE
The tumor which is largely necrotic and associated with stones has filled most of the lumen of the gallbladder. (Pl. IC from Fascicle 22, 2nd Series.)

Figure 6-8
A NEOPLASTIC WALL
A thick neoplastic wall encases the gallbladder, which contains several stones. Histologically, this tumor was a signet ring cell carcinoma.

gin impossible to ascertain. Carcinoma can develop in a gallbladder stump years after a partial cholecystectomy (1,3).

HISTOLOGIC TYPES

Table 6-1 shows the distribution of the different histologic types of gallbladder cancer recorded in the Surveillance, Epidemiology, and End Results (SEER) Program of the National Cancer Institute. The table includes all cases of

may involve the entire gallbladder, apparently from diffuse intramural infiltration, and its ori-

Table 6-1

HISTOLOGIC DISTRIBUTION FOR CANCERS OF THE GALLBLADDER, 1982–1991*

Histologic Types	Number of Patients	Percent of Total	Males	Percent of Total	Females	Percent of Total
Carcinoma in situ	126	4.36	31	3.99	95	4.49
Adenocarcinoma, NOS	2211	76.43	589	75.8	1622	76.65
Papillary adenocarcinoma	127	4.39	35	4.5	92	4.35
Adenocarcinoma, intestinal type	1	0.03	0	0	1	0.05
Mucinous adenocarcinoma	150	5.18	47	6.05	103	4.87
Clear cell carcinoma	2	0.07	1	0.13	1	0.05
Signet ring cell carcinoma	18	0.62	9	1.16	9	0.43
Adenosquamous carcinoma	94	3.25	24	3.09	70	3.31
Squamous cell carcinoma	48	1.66	13	1.67	35	1.65
Small cell carcinoma	12	0.41	6	0.77	6	0.28
Adenocarcinoma in villous adenoma	10	0.35	3	0.39	7	0.33
Cholangiocarcinoma	6	0.21	0	0	6	0.28
Infiltrating duct carcinoma	12	0.41	1	0.13	11	0.52
Undifferentiated carcinoma	30	1.04	6	0.77	24	1.13
TOTAL	2847	98.41	765	98.46	2082	98.39
Carcinoid tumors	5	0.17	2	0.26	3	0.14
Mixed carcinoid-adenocarcinoma	0	0	0	0	0	0
TOTAL	5	0.17	2	0.26	3	0.14
Sarcoma, NOS	3	0.1	1	0.13	2	0.09
Rhabdomyosarcoma	0	0	0	0	0	0
Kaposi's sarcoma	0	0	0	0	0	0
Leiomyosarcoma	1	0.03	0	0	1	0.05
Malignant fibrous histiocytoma	0	0	0	0	0	0
Angiosarcoma	0	0	0	0	0	0
TOTAL	4	0.14	1	0.13	3	0.14
Carcinosarcoma	11	0.38	3	0.39	8	0.38
Malignant melanoma	0	0	0	0	0	0
Malignant lymphoma	2	0.07	1	0.13	1	0.04
Others, NOS	24	0.83	5	0.64	19	0.9
TOTAL INVASIVE	2767	95.64	746	96.01	2021	95.51
TOTAL INVASIVE and IN SITU	2893	100	777	100	2161	100

*Data from the Surveillance, Epidemiology, and End Results Program, National Cancer Institute.

histologically proven malignant tumors of the gallbladder occurring in 10 percent of the population for the years 1982–1991. Adenocarcinoma is the most common histologic type. Table 6-2, which can be compared to Table 6-1, shows the different histologic types in our series of 386 cases collected over a 20-year period. The cases listed in Table 6-1 were diagnosed by many contributing pathologists. The differences in the histologic distribution in Tables 6-1 and 6-2 probably reflect a variation in histologic criteria and use of different terminology.

Table 6-2

DISTRIBUTION OF HISTOLOGIC TYPES IN 386 PATIENTS WITH MALIGNANT TUMORS OF THE GALLBLADDER

Histologic Type	Number of Patients (%)	Sex Distribution	
		Males	Females
Adenocarcinoma, well to moderately differentiated	186 (48.2)	31	155
Undifferentiated spindle and giant cell carcinoma	51 (13.2)	14	37
Adenosquamous carcinoma	37 (9.58)	2	35
Poorly differentiated adenocarcinoma, small cell type	25 (6.48)	3	22
Small cell carcinoma	18 (4.66)	2	16
Papillary adenocarcinoma	17 (4.40)	1	16
Mucinous carcinoma	16 (4.14)	5	11
Carcinoma in situ	14 (3.63)	1	13
Signet ring cell carcinoma	10 (2.59)	3	7
Squamous cell carcinoma	4 (1.04)	1	3
Intestinal type adenocarcinoma	4 (1.04)	1	3
Adenocarcinoma with choriocarcinoma-like areas	1 (0.26)	0	1
Carcinosarcoma	1 (0.26)	0	1
Carcinoid tumor	1 (0.26)	1	0
Malignant fibrous histiocytoma	1 (0.26)	0	1
TOTAL	386	65	321

Adenocarcinoma

Well-differentiated adenocarcinoma, the most common type of invasive carcinoma of the gallbladder, is characterized by a proliferation of different sized glands which tend to branch and divide (fig. 6-9). Small tubular glands, medium-sized glands, and large or cystically dilated glands may all be present in the same tumor (figs. 6-10, 6-11). The glandular epithelium is characteristically tall columnar, less frequently cuboidal, or rarely, flat and then superficially resembles endothelium (fig. 6-12). The round, oval, or elongated basal or centrally located nuclei are often vesicular with marginal chromatin, although coarsely granular, diffusely distributed chromatin often results in nuclear hyperchromatism (figs. 6-13, 6-14). The cytoplasm is eosinophilic or slightly granular, but also can be pale or clear. Scattered goblet cells located between the columnar or cuboidal cells are occasionally present.

Both the columnar and goblet cells are immunoreactive for cytokeratin and epithelial membrane antigen. Approximately one third of well-differentiated adenocarcinomas contain a population of argyrophil and argentaffin cells, most of which are immunoreactive for serotonin and less frequently for peptide hormones including somatostatin, gastrin, and pancreatic polypeptide (fig. 6-15) (6,7). Presumably, serotonin and peptide hormones pass into the circulation, however, their clinical significance is unknown. Occasionally isolated Paneth cells are found. The presence of goblet cells, serotonin immunoreactive cells, and Paneth cells reflects focal intestinal differentiation and in our experience has no relationship to prognosis.

The number of mitotic figures varies considerably: in some tumors they are numerous, while in others they are relatively rare. In addition to glands, the neoplastic cells may form sheets or

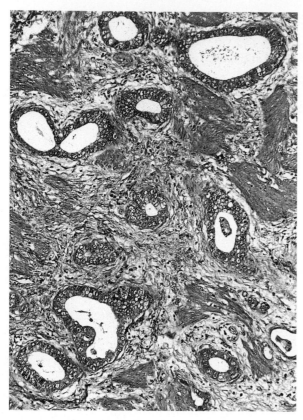

Figure 6-9
WELL-DIFFERENTIATED ADENOCARCINOMA
A well-differentiated adenocarcinoma is composed of variable sized glands that infiltrate the muscular wall of the gallbladder.

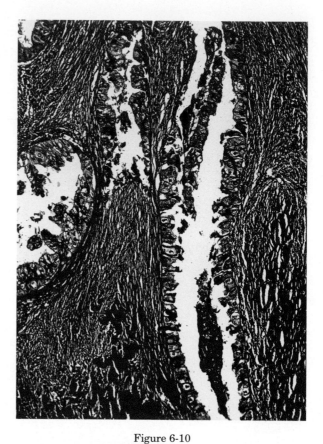

Figure 6-10
WELL-DIFFERENTIATED ADENOCARCINOMA
This adenocarcinoma is composed of long tubular glands separated by dense fibrous bands.

Figure 6-11
WELL-DIFFERENTIATED
ADENOCARCINOMA
Well-differentiated adenocarcinoma composed of small and medium sized glands with minimal intervening stroma.

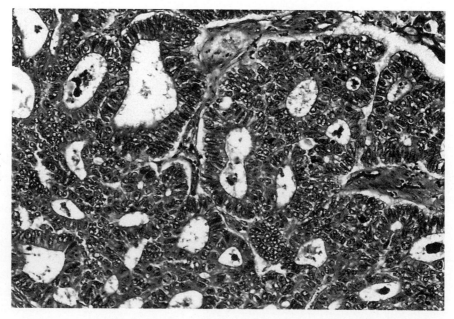

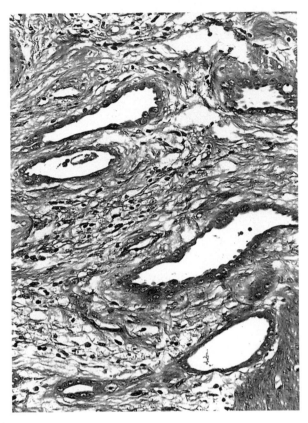

Figure 6-12
WELL-DIFFERENTIATED ADENOCARCINOMA
This well-differentiated adenocarcinoma contains glands lined by low cuboidal or flat epithelium superficially resembling endothelium.

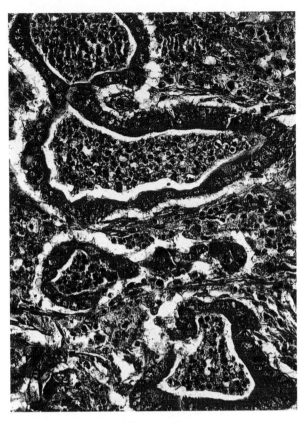

Figure 6-13
WELL-DIFFERENTIATED ADENOCARCINOMA
In this well-differentiated adenocarcinoma, the glands are filled with polymorphonuclear leukocytes.

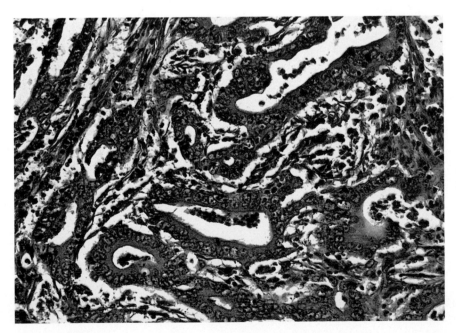

Figure 6-14
WELL-DIFFERENTIATED
ADENOCARCINOMA
The vesicular nuclei of this well-differentiated adenocarcinoma contain prominent nucleoli.

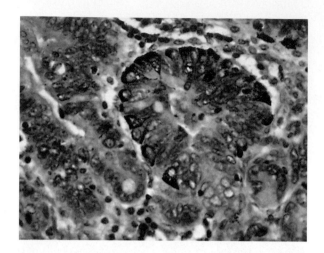 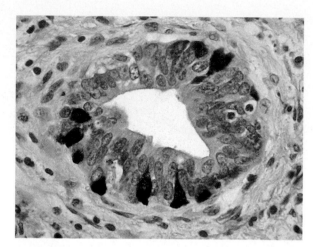

Figure 6-15
WELL-DIFFERENTIATED ADENOCARCINOMA
Left: Grimelius-positive cells in a well-differentiated adenocarcinoma.
Right: Serotonin containing cells in a well-differentiated adenocarcinoma of the gallbladder.

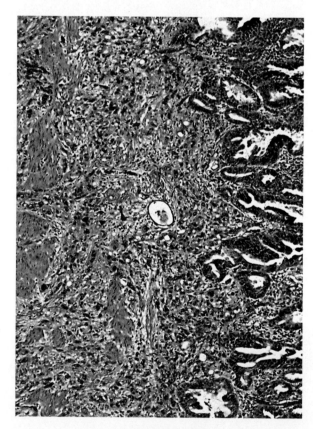

Figure 6-16
MODERATELY DIFFERENTIATED
ADENOCARCINOMA
The well-defined glandular component is seen in the superficial portion of the tumor whereas the cord-like arrangement is present in the deep portion.

cords. The diagnosis of well-differentiated adenocarcinoma requires that 95 percent of the tumor contains glands; for moderately differentiated adenocarcinoma, 40 to 94 percent of the tumor should be composed of glands; and for poorly differentiated adenocarcinoma, 5 to 39 percent of the tumor should contain glands (figs. 6-16, 6-17). More than 95 percent of undifferentiated carcinomas consist of cord or solid growth patterns.

The poorly differentiated component of adenocarcinoma may be accompanied by a prominent acute and chronic inflammatory response. The neoplastic epithelial cells are mixed with the inflammatory cells often mimicking a malignant fibrous histiocytoma (fig. 6-18). Immunostains for cytokeratin highlight the epithelial cells and clarify the diagnosis.

With the periodic acid–Schiff (PAS), Alcian blue, and colloidal iron stains, mucin can be detected in some cells and in the lumen of the neoplastic glands (fig. 6-19). The amount of intracellular and extracellular mucin, however, is variable even in different areas of the same tumor. This substance is predominantly a nonsulfated acid and neutral mucin. Occasionally, the PAS and Alcian blue stains are positive only along the apical border or luminal surface of the cell. Most adenocarcinomas of the gallbladder are immunoreactive for carcinoembryonic antigen and for the tumor-associated antigen, CA19-9 (7,24,35).

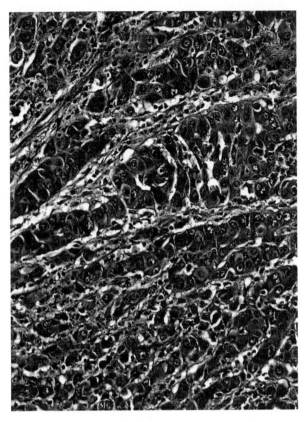

Figure 6-17
POORLY DIFFERENTIATED ADENOCARCINOMA
Most of the tumor displays a cord-like architecture. A single neoplastic gland is visible in the right upper corner.

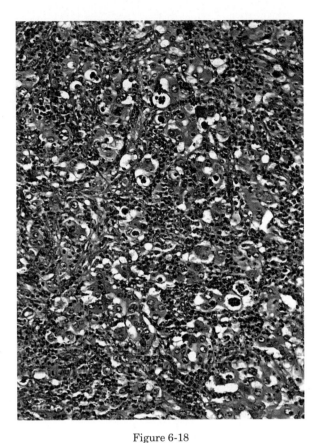

Figure 6-18
POORLY DIFFERENTIATED ADENOCARCINOMA
Small clusters of epithelial cells are intimately mixed with inflammatory cells. The pattern is reminiscent of a malignant fibrous histiocytoma.

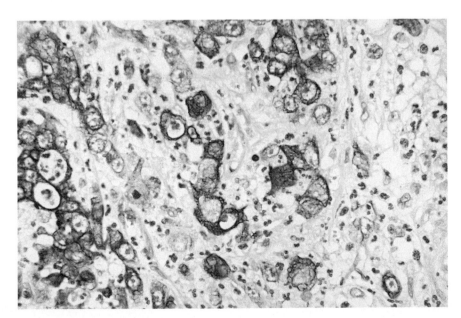

Figure 6-19
POORLY DIFFERENTIATED
ADENOCARCINOMA
The immunostain for cytokeratin highlights the epithelial cells.

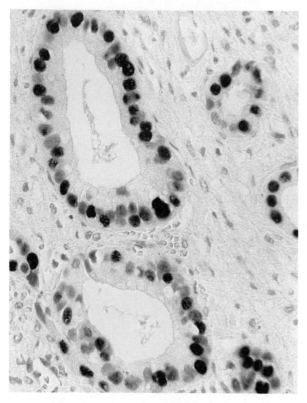

Figure 6-20
WELL-DIFFERENTIATED ADENOCARCINOMA
Nuclear staining for p53 protein is strong in this well-differentiated adenocarcinoma of the gallbladder. The p53 immunoreactivity is confined to the nucleus.

However, these nonspecific immunohistochemical markers have little diagnostic value.

The wall of the gallbladder shows variable degrees of fibrosis as well as an acute or chronic inflammatory cell infiltrate that may also be present within the lumen of the neoplastic glands. The fibrous tissue may widely separate these glands, especially in tumors with excessive desmoplasia. In tumors arising in porcelain gallbladders the fibrotic wall is extensively calcified. Occasionally, carcinomas in early stages (microcarcinomas) invade the lamina propria and muscle layer without provoking a fibroblastic reaction. Neoplastic growth along Rokitansky-Aschoff sinuses is common.

Immunohistochemical Findings. In addition to the focal enteroendocrine cell phenotype, and reactivity for carcinoembryonic antigen and the tumor associated antigen, CA19-9, immunohistochemistry shows further evidence of divergent differentiation in adenocarcinomas of the gallbladder. Pepsinogens I and II, normally found in the pyloric mucosa, have been detected immunohistochemically in most adenocarcinomas (30). Likewise, immunoreactivity for the p53 protein is found in 65 to 70 percent of cases (fig. 6-20) (31,33,34). No correlation, however, has been found between p53 immunoreactivity and the histologic type, grade, or level of invasion (34).

The search for antimetastatic activity has led to the discovery of a new family of genes, *nm23*, which was first described in murine melanoma cell lines. The human *nm23-H1* gene encodes a 17-kD nuclear and cytoplasmic protein which has been shown to be reduced in a variety of human carcinomas. Immunohistochemical expression of the nm23-H1 protein has been investigated in carcinomas of the gallbladder with conflicting results. In one study, absent or weak nm23-H1 protein immunoreactivity was found in most poorly differentiated adenocarcinomas and in 50 percent of the cases of moderately differentiated adenocarcinomas (29). In another study, however, 72 percent of 107 carcinomas expressed nm23 protein regardless of histologic type, depth of invasion, or stage of disease. Moreover, nm23 protein was detected in 60 percent and 74 percent of cases with and without lymph node metastases, respectively, suggesting that in gallbladder carcinomas decreased expression of nm23 protein does not have implications for metastasis (14).

Epidermal growth factor receptors (EGFR) contribute to cell transformation and may facilitate cellular proliferation (32). Immunohistochemical staining has shown overexpression of EGFR in nearly all adenocarcinomas of the gallbladder, regardless of the histologic grade (20).

Estrogen receptor (ER) immunoreactivity was found in 26 of 114 (22.8 percent) cases of gallbladder adenocarcinoma (36); there was no sex difference in the incidence of reactivity. Likewise, no differences in survival were seen in patients with ER-positive or ER-negative tumors.

Electron Microscopic Findings. The ultrastructure of well- to moderately differentiated adenocarcinomas of the gallbladder resembles, to some degree, normal gallbladder epithelium (19). Thus, two of the three epithelial cell types found in the normal human gallbladder, the predominant ordinary columnar cell and the rare penciloid cell (fig. 6-21), are present in most

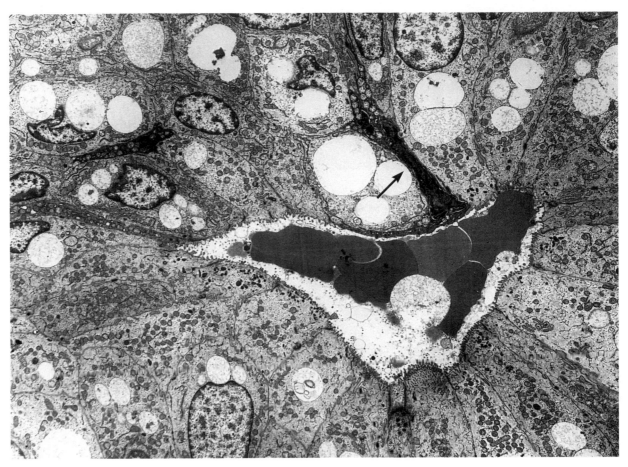

Figure 6-21
ADENOCARCINOMA: ULTRASTRUCTURE
Neoplastic columnar and penciloid cells are seen in a well-differentiated adenocarcinoma. The columnar cells contain mucin droplets and are covered by microvilli. The penciloid cells are darker and appear compressed by adjacent columnar cells (arrow). (Courtesy of Dr. Carlos Manivel, Minneapolis, MN.)

tumors. The third cell type, the basal cell, has not been identified in any of the tumors that we have examined, nor was it mentioned in the two other published ultrastructural studies on gallbladder adenocarcinoma (17,19,21). The columnar cells are oriented around gland lumens and rest on a basal lamina, which may be thickened or even duplicated. The apical portions of the lateral walls of adjacent tumor cells are connected by junctional complexes. These walls, which may show complex infoldings, are separated by intercellular spaces which in normal cells are considered important for fluid transport.

The predominant neoplastic cell, the ordinary light columnar cell, has a large central or basal nucleus which may be round, ovoid, irregular, or elongated. The nuclei, which occasionally show multiple indentations, contain coarse marginal chromatin and one or two nucleoli. Cytoplasmic organelles include a moderate number of mitochondria, and a well-developed rough endoplasmic reticulum and Golgi apparatus. Lysosomes are also present in the apical portion of the cytoplasm. These cells usually secrete excessive mucin. They contain either multiple small mucin droplets of variable electron density or large coalescent vacuoles that occupy most of the cytoplasm. Intracytoplasmic lumen formation is occasionally seen. Microvilli emerge from the apical surface and project into the gland lumen (fig. 6-22). Their number, height, and morphology vary: most are short and blunt, while others are tall and slender.

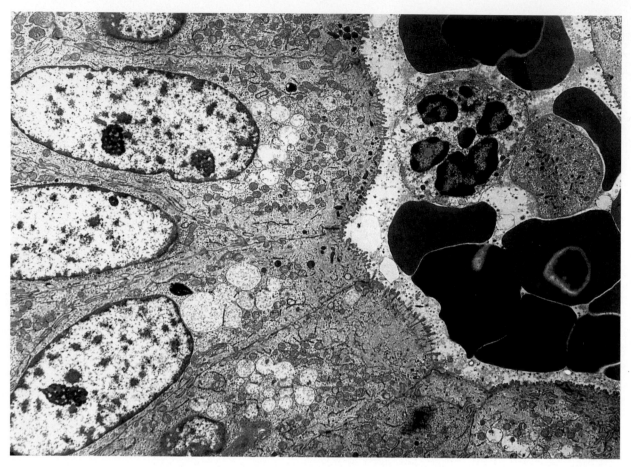

Figure 6-22
ADENOCARCINOMA: ULTRASTRUCTURE
Neoplastic columnar cells are oriented around a gland lumen. They have large nuclei, prominent nucleoli, and numerous mucin vacuoles. (Courtesy of Dr. Carlos Manivel, Minneapolis, MN.)

Approximately one third of well- to moderately differentiated adenocarcinomas show focal intestinal metaplasia characterized by the presence of goblet cells, Paneth cells, and endocrine cells. The latter cells contain round and pleomorphic dense core secretory granules. The endocrine cells have a suprabasal location and are similar to the enterochromaffin and enterochromaffin-like cells described in association with the intestinal metaplasia found in chronic cholecystitis. Their clinical significance in adenocarcinomas is unknown. The columnar cells have a well-defined brush border produced by uniform slender and closely spaced microvilli. These microvilli contain microfilament bundles which are continuous with those of the adjacent cytoplasm, the so called microvillous core rootlets (21). Part of these microvilli are covered with a filamentous glycocalyx. Round or oval, membrane-bound structures known as glycocaliceal bodies are seen above and between the microvilli, especially those with core rootlets (fig. 6-23). These glycocaliceal bodies have a focal or diffuse distribution and a diameter less than 25 percent of an individual microvillus. Unfortunately, these two distinct microvilli-related structures (microvillous core rootlets and glycocaliceal bodies) are not specific, since they are identical to those found in some adenocarcinomas of the stomach, intestine, pancreas, lung, ovary, and cervix (15). As a consequence their diagnostic value is limited.

Penciloid cells are rarely seen. Located between columnar cells, they extend from the basal lamina to the lumen, although sometimes they do not reach the lumen or even the basal lamina. Their dark appearance, narrow profile, well-developed,

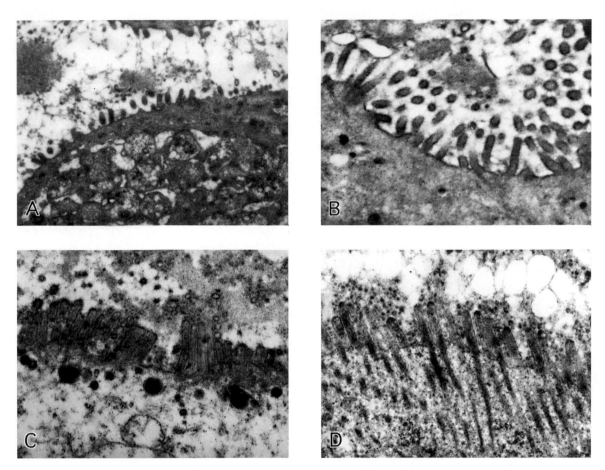

Figure 6-23
ADENOCARCINOMA: ULTRASTRUCTURE
Four different types of microvilli found in a well-differentiated adenocarcinoma are illustrated. The top panels reveal small and poorly developed microvilli, while the lower panels show well-developed intestinal type microvilli. In addition, dark electron dense cytoplasmic bodies are present in the left lower panel. Closely spaced microvilli with core rootlets and glycocaliceal bodies above and between the microvilli are seen in the right lower panel. (Fig. 97 from Fascicle 22, 2nd Series.)

supranuclear, rough surface endoplasmic reticulum, and minimal mucin content allow easy separation from ordinary columnar cells. The apical surface contains short and scattered microvilli while the opposite end becomes attenuated, resulting in a slender cytoplasmic process which penetrates between columnar cells. Cytoplasmic projections extending to the basal lamina are not seen, a feature usually found in normal penciloid cells.

Although the penciloid cell is considered a modified columnar cell, its function in normal and pathologic conditions remains to be determined. Its extensive supranuclear, granular endoplasmic reticulum and its presence in malignant tumors do not support the hypothesis that it is a degenerate or inactive cell (13).

Flow Cytometric Findings. There have been few investigations of flow cytometry on gallbladder adenocarcinomas (11,12,37). Two studies (11,37) showed that most gallbladder cancers are aneuploid (89 percent). However, no significant correlation was found between DNA ploidy, stage of disease, and outcome (11). In one study, the rate of aneuploidy was 46 percent (37).

Unusual Histologic Types of Adenocarcinoma

Rarely, adenocarcinomas grow in solid nodules or broad trabeculae which contain uniform, punched-out spaces producing a cribriform pattern. This growth pattern is often focal, but may be seen throughout the tumor, resembling cribriform

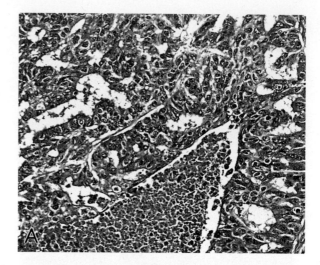

Figure 6-24
ADENOCARCINOMA, CRIBRIFORM TYPE
A: Adenocarcinoma displaying a focal cribriform pattern with necrosis.
B: This tumor has a predominant cribriform pattern of growth and is similar to cribriform carcinoma of the breast.
C: Higher magnification of B showing cell detail in a cribriform area.

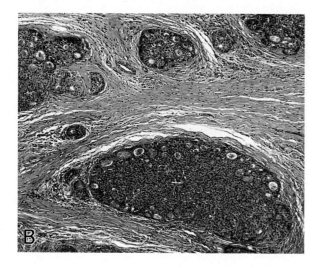

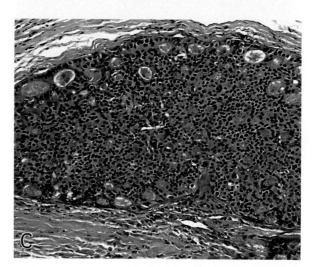

carcinoma of the breast (fig. 6-24). We have seen three such cases in females with cholelithiasis and no clinical evidence of breast carcinoma (8).

Well- to moderately differentiated adenocarcinomas may show anastomosing vascular-like spaces having small papillary projections with hyalinized cores that closely resemble angiosarcoma (figs. 6-25, 6-26). However, the cells that line these pseudovascular structures are cytokeratin positive and do not stain for endothelial markers (8). Pseudovascular carcinomas have been reported in many organs including the breast, lung, and skin (10,23). The mechanism of formation of the pseudovascular space in adenocarcinomas of the gallbladder is unknown.

Occasionally, calcium precipitates in the mucus that accumulates in the lumen of the neoplastic glands (fig. 6-27) (25). This calcium, which is often visible on radiographs, is a diagnostic help to the radiologist. Calcification occurs in less than 1 percent of all gallbladder carcinomas. It is usually found in those tumors that are well differentiated (28). Similar calcium deposits can occur in carcinoma of the stomach or colon.

Adenocarcinoma with Choriocarcinoma-Like Areas. Malignant epithelial neoplasms with choriocarcinoma-like areas have been reported in many sites including the lung (5,26), esophagus (22), stomach (27), urinary bladder (16), and colon (18). We have seen only one gallbladder adenocarcinoma that contained choriocarcinoma-like elements. The glandular component was well differentiated; that is, most glands were well formed and lined by tall, uniform columnar

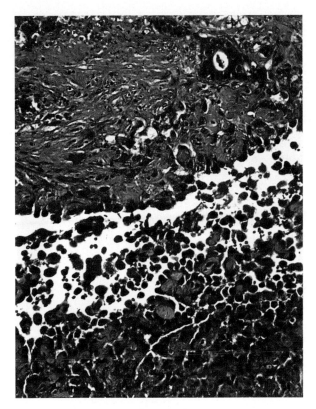

Figure 6-25
ADENOCARCINOMA WITH
ANGIOSARCOMA-LIKE AREAS
A single neoplastic gland is seen in the right upper corner.

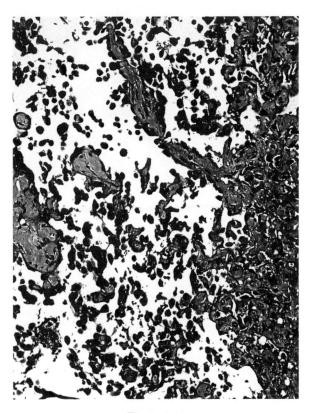

Figure 6-26
ADENOCARCINOMA WITH
ANGIOSARCOMA-LIKE AREAS
In another field of the tumor shown in figure 6-25, the angiosarcoma-like areas predominate.

cells. Some contained multinucleated giant cells in their lumens (fig. 6-28). In addition, solid cords and trabeculae with a central mass of cytotrophoblastic-like neoplastic cells surrounded by syncytiotrophoblastic cells infiltrated the stroma (fig. 6-29). Extensive necrosis was noted, but not of the hemorrhagic type seen in the typical gonadal or uterine choriocarcinoma. Moreover, tumor cells lacked immunoreactivity to human chorionic gonadotropin. The only other case reported as adenocarcinoma with choriocarcinoma of the gallbladder is not convincing microscopically, despite positive immunostaining for the beta subunit of human chorionic gonadotropin (4). Immunohistochemical reactivity for human chorionic gonadotropin in a tumor does not make it a choriocarcinoma. Several types of carcinomas of the gallbladder, including adenosquamous and undifferentiated spindle and giant cell carcinomas, may synthesize human chorionic gonadotropin which can be

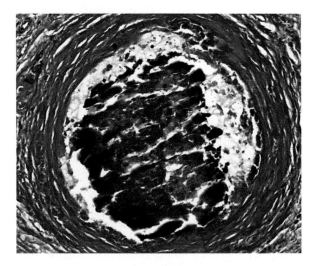

Figure 6-27
CALCIFICATION IN
WELL-DIFFERENTIATED ADENOCARCINOMA
Neoplastic glands in the wall of the gallbladder contain precipitated calcium. The epithelial lining is poorly preserved. A ring of collagen fibers surrounds the gland.

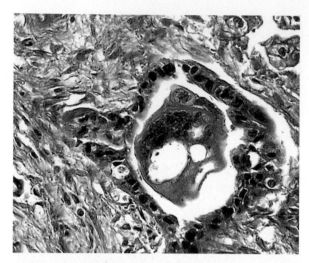

Figure 6-28
ADENOCARCINOMA WITH
CHORIOCARCINOMA-LIKE AREAS
Floating in the gland lumen is a multinucleated giant cell with vacuolated cytoplasm. Another syncytiotrophoblast-like cell is seen in the stroma.

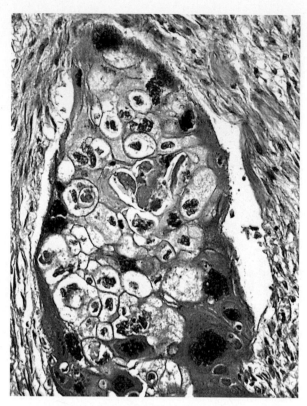

Figure 6-29
ADENOCARCINOMA WITH
CHORIOCARCINOMA-LIKE AREAS
Neoplastic syncytiotrophoblastic-like cells surround cells with cytotrophoblastic-like features. In other areas this tumor showed the pattern of a well-differentiated adenocarcinoma.

detected in the patient's serum or in tumor cells by immunohistochemical methods. The presence of trophoblastic elements in adenocarcinomas of the gallbladder should be viewed within the context of divergent differentiation.

Papillary Adenocarcinoma. Papillary carcinoma is a well-differentiated adenocarcinoma that grows predominantly towards the lumen of the gallbladder (fig. 6-30). The tumor consists of branching fibrovascular stalks of different width and length, lined by cuboidal or columnar cells with basal hyperchromatic nuclei, and a vacuolated cytoplasm containing mucin (figs. 6-31, 6-32). Foci of intestinal metaplasia, consisting of goblet cells, argyrophil and argentaffin cells, as well as a few Paneth cells, are present in some tumors. Most endocrine cells are immunoreactive for serotonin. Less frequently, immunoreactivity for peptide hormones is also expressed. Only rarely are goblet cells the predominant cell type (fig. 6-33). Gastric phenotypic expression, as shown by the immunohistochemical detection of pepsinogens I and II, has been found in most papillary adenocarcinomas (30). The nuclear atypia and number of mitotic figures vary considerably. Cases with slight atypia, few mitoses, and minimal or no invasion are often difficult to distin-

guish from papillary adenomas. As a rule however, the degree of nuclear atypia and the number of mitotic figures seen in carcinomas exceeds those found in papillary adenomas (fig. 6-32, right). Paneth and endocrine cells are more abundant in adenomas than in carcinomas.

These papillary carcinomas may fill the lumen of the gallbladder before invading the wall. For this reason, they are associated with a better prognosis than tumors that infiltrate early. In general, the infiltrating portion of the tumor forms tubular glands rather than papillary structures, but in some areas the papillary pattern is preserved, even in metastatic deposits. Occasionally, papillary carcinomas that have not invaded the wall extend along Rokitansky-Aschoff sinuses and mimic stromal invasion (fig. 6-34).

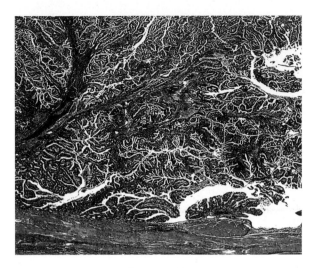

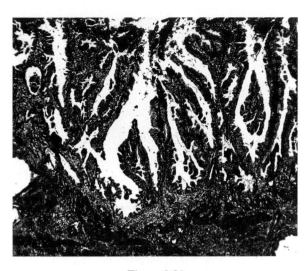

Figure 6-30
PAPILLARY ADENOCARCINOMA
A large papillary adenocarcinoma is growing into the lumen of the gallbladder. The wall of the gallbladder, which is thickened and fibrotic, has not been invaded.

Figure 6-31
PAPILLARY ADENOCARCINOMA
This small papillary adenocarcinoma invades the lamina propria and muscle coat. A neoplastic gland is visible in the wall of the gallbladder.

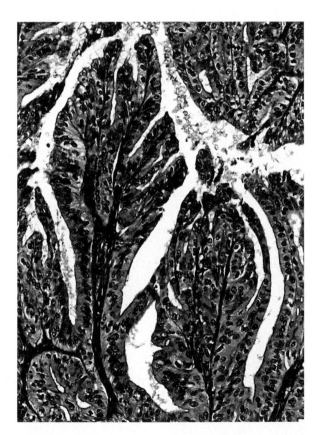

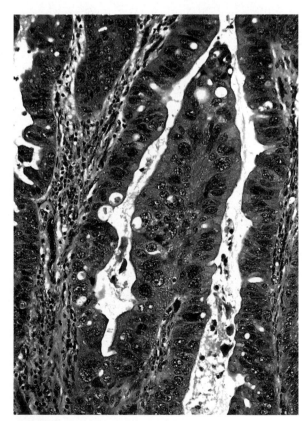

Figure 6-32
PAPILLARY ADENOCARCINOMA
Left: Higher magnification of papillary adenocarcinoma showing a complex papillary growth pattern. The branching papillae project into the lumen of the gallbladder and are lined by columnar biliary type cells.
Right: Marked nuclear atypia is seen in this papillary adenocarcinoma.

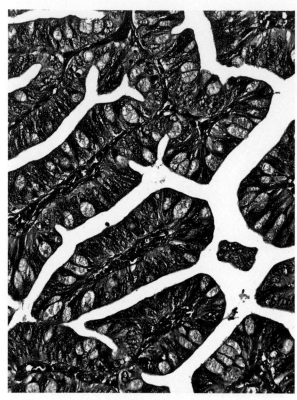

Figure 6-33
PAPILLARY ADENOCARCINOMA
WITH INTESTINAL FEATURES
In this infiltrating papillary carcinoma, the papillary structures are lined by tall columnar and goblet cells.

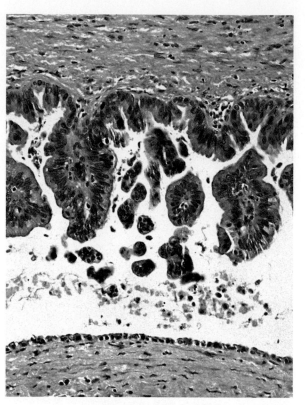

Figure 6-34
NONINVASIVE PAPILLARY CARCINOMA
This noninvasive papillary carcinoma extends into a Rokitansky-Aschoff sinus. Non-neoplastic low cuboidal biliary epithelium is still visible.

Intestinal Type Adenocarcinoma. This type, we believe, is a variant of the well-differentiated adenocarcinoma. However, because it resembles intestinal epithelium, it should be separated from that tumor (9). One type is composed of different sized glands lined chiefly by goblet cells. These cells have basal hyperchromatic nuclei and a cytoplasm distended by single or multiple mucinous vacuoles (fig. 6-35). These distended cells seem to compress adjacent columnar cells, some of which contain no mucous material. A small number of argyrophil and argentaffin cells, identified with the Grimelius or Fontana Masson stain, respectively, are present in approximately one third of the tumors. The endocrine cells are immunoreactive for serotonin and a variety of peptide hormones including somatostatin and pancreatic polypeptide. Paneth cells are found in a smaller number. The glands contain variable amounts of mucous material.

A second type of intestinal adenocarcinoma consists predominantly of glandular structures that resemble those of a colonic adenocarcinoma (fig. 6-36). In some tumors eosinophilic necrotic material is present in the lumen of some glands (fig. 6-37). The epithelium is tall columnar, pseudostratified, and usually with a well-defined brush border. Few goblet cells and a variable number of endocrine cells are interspersed between columnar cells (fig. 6-38). Most endocrine cells are immunoreactive for serotonin. Very often, these tumors are mixed and focally show, in addition, the pattern of an ordinary well-differentiated adenocarcinoma of the gallbladder. The number of mitotic figures varies from tumor to tumor, but generally it is low.

Intestinal differentiation can occur as a focal change in other adenocarcinomas, especially the well-differentiated, papillary, and signet ring cell types. However, isolated goblet, endocrine,

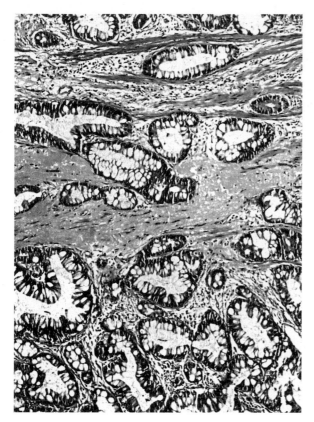

Figure 6-35
INTESTINAL TYPE ADENOCARCINOMA
The neoplastic glands of this intestinal type adenocarci-
noma are lined almost exclusively by goblet cells.

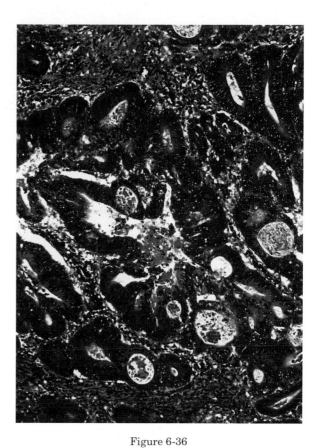

Figure 6-36
INTESTINAL TYPE ADENOCARCINOMA
The glandular structures are similar to those of a well-
differentiated colonic adenocarcinoma. The cytoplasm of
most cells lacks mucin.

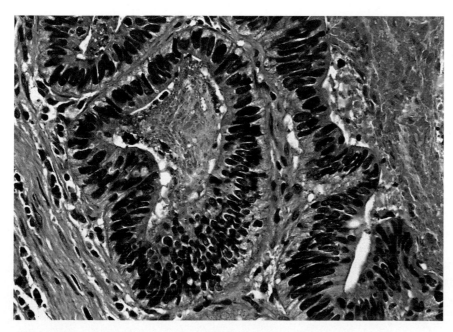

Figure 6-37
INTESTINAL TYPE
ADENOCARCINOMA
Several glands are lined by
pseudostratified columnar cells
with vesicular nuclei and prominent nucleoli. Eosinophilic necrotic
material is present in the lumen of
the glands.

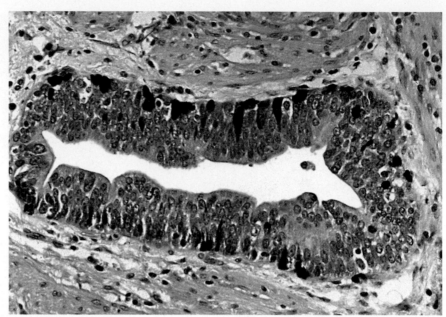

Figure 6-38
INTESTINAL TYPE
ADENOCARCINOMA
Chromogranin-positive cells are mixed with the columnar epithelial cells.

or Paneth cells are more often seen than the fully developed intestinal metaplasia that includes all three cell types.

Clear Cell Adenocarcinoma. Not infrequently, clear cells occur as a focal change in well- to moderately differentiated adenocarcinomas of the gallbladder. However, tumors composed predominantly of clear cells are exceedingly rare and may give rise to diagnostic problems, especially in metastatic deposits (38,44). We reported six examples of this type of tumor and have recently encountered two additional cases (44). All patients but one were females in the fifth or sixth decades of life with coexisting cholelithiasis. Two had elevated serum carcinoembryonic antigen levels and one markedly elevated circulating levels of alpha-fetoprotein and areas of hepatoid differentiation.

The histologic pattern is variable. In addition to the clear cell component all tumors contained foci of conventional adenocarcinoma, usually with mucin production. A single tumor exhibited extensive hepatoid differentiation, which was more prominent in the omental and peritoneal metastatic deposits. The clear cells form glands, solid sheets, cords, trabeculae, and small papillary structures in variable proportions (figs. 6-39–6-41). While the major component of some tumors consists of cords, trabeculae, and papillary structures, in others glandular structures predominate.

The neoplastic cells are uniform in appearance, being cuboidal columnar or polygonal. They have a central or eccentric hyperchromatic nucleus and abundant clear cytoplasm with well-defined borders. Neoplastic cells with subnuclear and supranuclear vacuoles reminiscent of secretory endometrium predominate in some neoplasms (fig. 6-42). Most tumors show mild nuclear pleomorphism and few mitotic figures. Occasionally, however, anaplastic areas containing multinucleated giant cells with bizarre nuclei and numerous mitotic figures are recognized.

The cytoplasm of the clear cells is rich in glycogen as shown by the PAS-positive reaction, which becomes negative after diastase digestion. The mucicarmine, Alcian blue, and colloidal iron stains are usually negative. Rarely, however, the clear cells contain mucin droplets. The conventional adenocarcinomatous component consists predominantly of glands and small papillary structures, both lined by cuboidal or columnar cells, most of which contain cytoplasmic mucin. In some tumors, collections of signet ring cells or extracellular mucin are present. The areas of hepatoid differentiation consist of cells with abundant, eosinophilic cytoplasm and central round nuclei with prominent nucleoli (38,44). These cells exhibit a trabecular growth pattern with acini formation. Focally, the tumor is indistinguishable from a hepatocellular carcinoma. Transitions

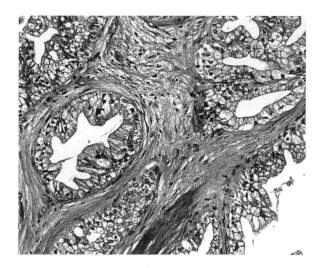

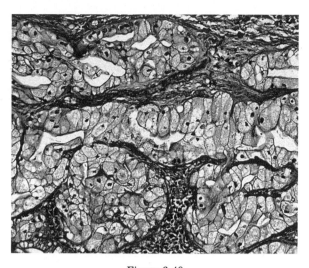

Figure 6-39
ADENOCARCINOMA, CLEAR CELL TYPE
The glands are lined by clear cells and infiltrate the wall of the gallbladder.

Figure 6-40
ADENOCARCINOMA, CLEAR CELL TYPE
Long tubular glands are lined by columnar cells with ample clear cytoplasm and hyperchromatic nuclei.

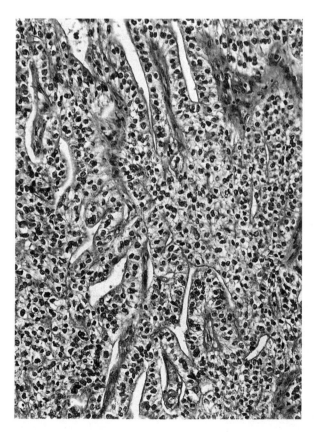

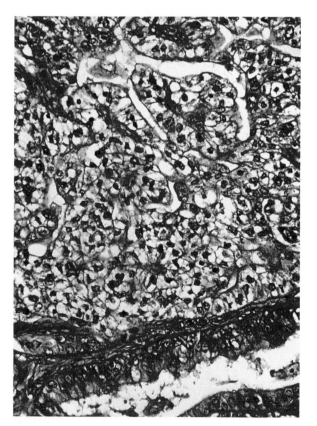

Figure 6-41
CLEAR CELL ADENOCARCINOMA
Left: A sheet-like pattern and small papillary structures are shown.
Right: A neoplastic gland characteristic of conventional adenocarcinoma is seen adjacent to sheets and small papillary structures lined by clear cells.

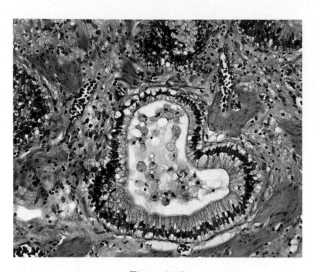

Figure 6-42
CLEAR CELL ADENOCARCINOMA
A neoplastic gland is lined by columnar cells with sub-nuclear and supranuclear vacuoles.

from the clear cells to the hepatoid cells have been noted (fig. 6-43, left). The hepatoid cells are immunoreactive for alpha-fetoprotein by immunohistochemistry (fig. 6-43, right).

Ultrastructurally, the neoplastic cells show apical microvilli, a well-developed rough endoplasmic reticulum, and a moderate number of mitochondria. Abundant glycogen particles are seen in the cytoplasm of some cells. Although there is no bile present, structures closely resembling bile canaliculi are seen with the electron microscope (fig. 6-44).

Hepatoid differentiation is not a specific feature of clear cell carcinomas. We have also seen it in a case of carcinosarcoma of the gallbladder. However, the hepatoid areas of this carcinosarcoma were found adjacent to a minor clear cell component of the tumor. Moreover, some of the conventional gallbladder adenocarcinomas associated with elevated serum levels of alpha-fetoprotein contained a

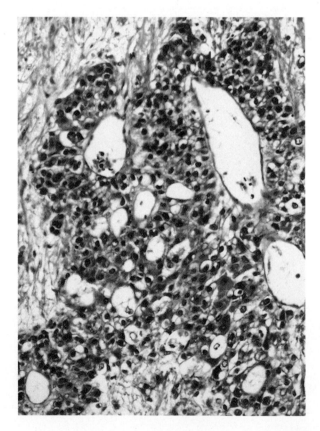

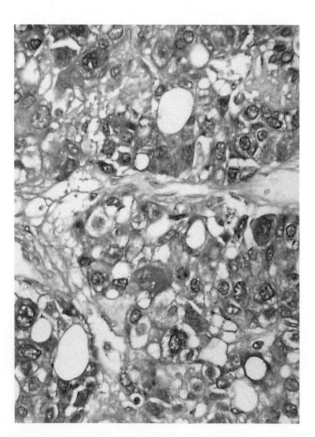

Figure 6-43
HEPATOID AREA IN CLEAR CELL ADENOCARCINOMA
Left: Some of the cells still show a clear cytoplasm.
Right: Some of the cells are immunoreactive for alpha-fetoprotein.

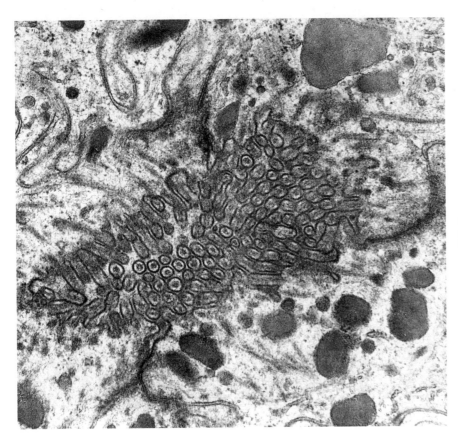

Figure 6-44
CLEAR CELL
ADENOCARCINOMA
A structure similar to a bile canaliculus is in a hepatoid area of clear cell adenocarcinoma. Note the microvilli and the tight junctions.

population of clear cells (41,43,45). This suggests a relationship between clear cells, hepatoid differentiation, and alpha-fetoprotein synthesis.

Due to the similarity of the clear cell component of gallbladder carcinomas to renal cell carcinomas in both histologic structure and antigenic profile, their separation may pose problems for the surgical pathologist. Clear cell adenocarcinomas of the gallbladder can be distinguished from metastatic renal cell carcinomas by identifying areas of conventional adenocarcinoma, most of which show mucin production of variable extent, and carcinoembryonic antigen (CEA) positivity by immunohistochemistry. In a recent study (40), cytokeratin 7 and CEA were found to be useful markers because they were positive in clear cell adenocarcinoma and negative in metastatic renal cell carcinoma. Likewise, the presence of dysplasia or carcinoma in situ in the adjacent mucosa strongly favors a primary carcinoma of the gallbladder. If the gallbladder carcinoma is predominantly glandular, the distinction presents no difficulties. In small biopsy specimens or in metastatic deposits showing only the clear cell

component with a tubuloglandular, nesting, or trabecular pattern, this separation may be extremely difficult because the clear cell component of some adenocarcinomas of the gallbladder is negative for CEA.

Metastases of renal cell carcinoma in the gallbladder and extrahepatic bile ducts are distinctly uncommon, even at autopsy (39,46). The incidence was 0.6 percent in one large series (39) and 0.4 percent in another (46). The few reported cases of symptomatic metastases of renal cell carcinoma fall into two clinical settings: patients with a history of nephrectomy several months or years prior to the appearance of the metastases or patients with coexisting renal cell carcinoma (42). However, we have recently seen a single polypoid gallbladder metastasis as the first manifestation of a renal cell carcinoma in a kidney transplant recipient.

Mucinous Carcinoma

This tumor, which is uncommon, represents 4 percent of all gallbladder carcinomas in our material. There are two histologic variants. The

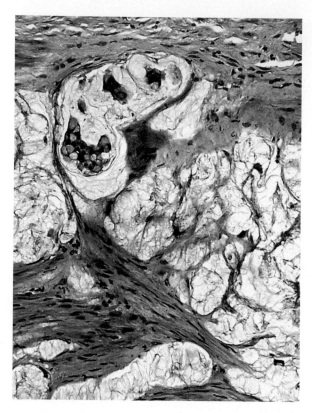
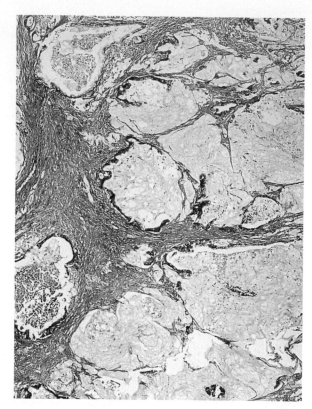

Figure 6-45
MUCINOUS CARCINOMA
Left: Small nests of neoplastic epithelial cells lie in pools of basophilic mucin.
Right: Cystically dilated glands filled with mucin and pools of acellular mucin are evident.

first and most common is similar to that found in the breast and other sites and is characterized by small clusters of malignant epithelial cells surrounded by large deposits of extracellular mucin (greater than 50 percent of the tumor) (fig. 6-45, left). The mucin, which dominates the histologic picture, usually stains basophilic. Very often, the mucous pools, especially the larger ones, are surrounded by fibrous septa. In general, there are a few glandular elements. The malignant cells either show no mucin or have compressed peripheral nuclei and a cytoplasm engorged with mucin. Large pools of acellular mucin are present. In some tumors, multiple sections are needed to demonstrate the clusters of neoplastic cells.

The second morphologic variant of mucinous carcinoma is characterized by cystically dilated glands filled with mucin and lined by mucin-producing columnar cells with mild to moderate nuclear atypia (fig. 6-45, right). Smaller glands and pools of acellular mucin are also seen.

It should be kept in mind that conventional well-to moderately differentiated adenocarcinomas and clear cell carcinomas of the gallbladder may have a focal mucinous component. Therefore, the diagnosis of pure mucinous carcinoma, as in the colon, requires that more than 50 percent of the tumor be composed of extracellular mucin containing few neoplastic cellular elements.

A diagnosis of mucinous carcinoma should be suspected from gross examination when a nodular or polypoid, infiltrating, gelatinous mass having a smooth and glistening surface is found in the wall of the gallbladder.

Because mucinous carcinomas are uncommon, we have not been able to compare their clinical behavior or modes of spread with other types of carcinoma of the gallbladder. It has been reported that these tumors are more apt to spread to the peritoneum than other histologic types, a metastatic pattern we have had the opportunity to confirm in three cases.

Mucinous carcinoma should be distinguished from a benign mucocele. The abundant extracellular mucin present in this lesion can penetrate the full thickness of the wall and may be seen in the serosa. Although the mucin lacks neoplastic cells it may induce a histiocytic response. The histiocytes may phagocytize mucin and be confused with signet ring cells. Immunohistochemical stains for cytokeratin and CEA solve the problem: they are positive in mucinous carcinoma and negative in the muciphages.

Signet Ring Cell Carcinoma

As the name indicates, signet ring cells are the predominant, or even the exclusive, element in these tumors which constitute 3 percent of all malignant tumors of the gallbladder. Rarely, they contain small clusters of argyrophil cells that are chromogranin positive and immunoreactive for serotonin and peptide hormones. Occasionally, scattered Paneth cells are seen. If the neoplastic signet ring cells are confined to the surface epithelium or extend into the epithelial invaginations, but show no stromal invasion, the tumor should be regarded as signet ring cell carcinoma in situ. We have had the opportunity to study two such cases which were incidental findings in cholecystectomy specimens and were recognized on microscopic examination. When neoplastic cells infiltrate the wall they grow either in cords, nests, and sheets, or form incomplete glandular structures which usually lie in a mucoid stroma (figs. 6-46, 6-47). The diffusely infiltrating linear pattern, resembling linitis plastica of the stomach, is observed in some cases. Rarely, the neoplastic signet ring cells are admixed with and obscured by inflammatory cells (fig. 6-48). Submucosal growth is prominent in some tumors, especially those in which a mucosal ulceration is not apparent. Some signet ring cell tumors are not pure and contain foci of well-differentiated neoplastic glands. If a tumor predominantly consists of well-differentiated neoplastic glands with a few foci of signet ring cells, it should be classified as an adenocarcinoma.

The neoplastic signet ring cells are positive with Mayer's mucicarmine, Alcian blue, and PAS stains (figs. 6-49, 6-50). They are also immunoreactive for cytokeratin and CEA, whereas, the endocrine cells, in addition to cytokeratin, have

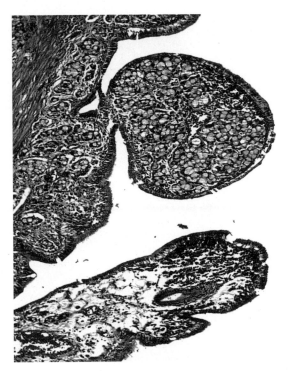

Figure 6-46
SIGNET RING CELL CARCINOMA
Tumor cells infiltrate the lamina propria and muscle coat, leaving the overlying epithelium intact. This type of growth pattern is often seen in signet ring cell carcinoma of the gallbladder.

shown immunoreactivity for chromogranin, serotonin, somatostatin, pancreatic polypeptide, and gastrin. Tumors that contain endocrine cells can be confused with signet ring or goblet cell carcinoid. However, this tumor is seen almost exclusively in the appendix, ovary, and rarely, ampulla of Vater. It is composed of nests or tubular structures lined by columnar and goblet cells, with minimal cytologic atypia. Often the mucin material is intracellular or confined to the lumen of the tubules. Immunoreactivity for chromogranin is more extensive in goblet cell carcinoids than in signet ring cell carcinomas.

Florid pyloric gland metaplasia can occur in association with signet ring cell carcinomas.

Electron microscopy reveals that the cytoplasm of the neoplastic cells is occupied by abundant mucin which displaces the nucleus toward the periphery (fig. 6-51). Intracytoplasmic lumina lined by short microvilli are also filled and distended with mucin (fig. 6-52). Consequently, there is room for few cytoplasmic organelles

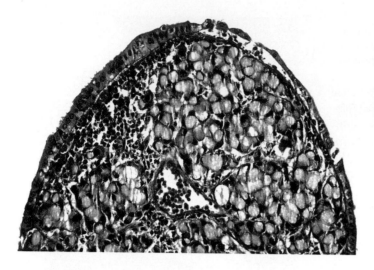

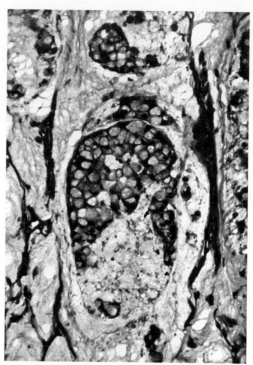

Figure 6-47
SIGNET RING CELL CARCINOMA
Above: Detail of neoplastic signet ring cells in the lamina propria.
Right: Small groups of neoplastic signet ring cells lie in a mucoid stroma.

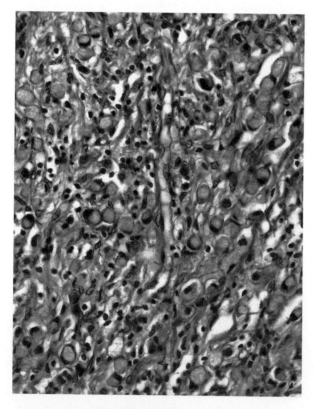

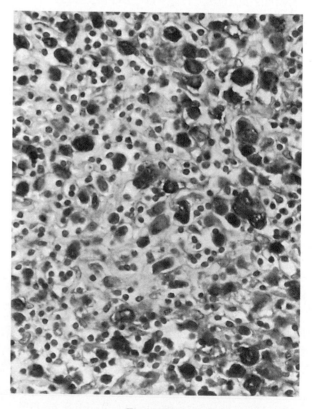

Figure 6-48
SIGNET RING CELL CARCINOMA
Small groups and isolated neoplastic signet ring cells are mixed with inflammatory cells.

Figure 6-49
SIGNET RING CELL CARCINOMA
The mucicarmine stain highlights the neoplastic signet ring cells, which are admixed with lymphocytes.

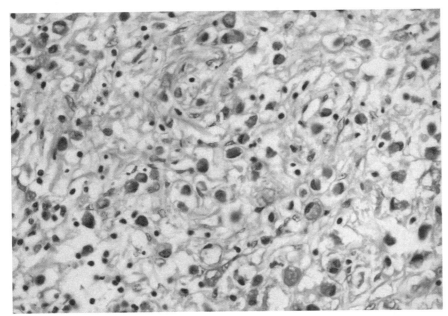

Figure 6-50
SIGNET RING
CELL CARCINOMA
The signet ring cells are Alcian
blue positive.

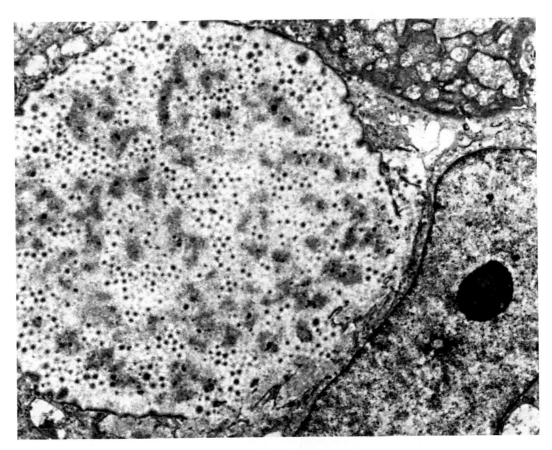

Figure 6-51
SIGNET RING CELL CARCINOMA: ULTRASTRUCTURE
A large intracytoplasmic lumen containing mucus has compressed the nucleus (lower right) and cytoplasmic structures.
(Fig. 98 from Fascicle 22, 2nd Series.)

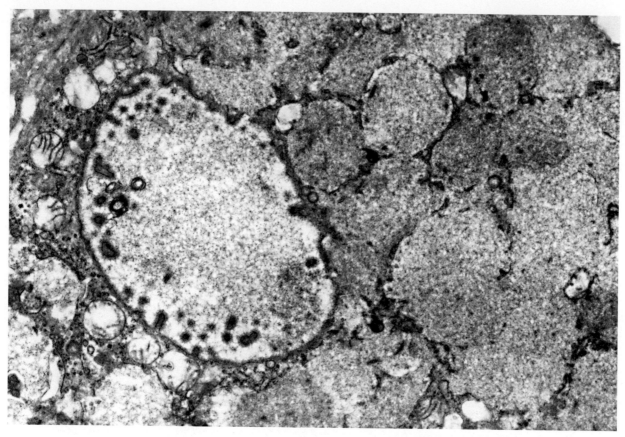

Figure 6-52
SIGNET RING CELL CARCINOMA: ULTRASTRUCTURE
A small intracytoplasmic lumen containing microvilli and mucus is visible. In the remainder of the cytoplasm, there is abundant mucus and scattered mitochondria. (Fig. 99 from Fascicle 22, 2nd Series.)

including small mitochondria, rough endoplasmic reticulum, and Golgi apparatus. The nuclei are large and ovoid or reniform, and usually contain a single prominent nucleolus. The endocrine cells show membrane-bound, dense core, round or pleomorphic neurosecretory granules. Some of these granules are associated with the Golgi apparatus. Cells containing both cytoplasmic mucin and neurosecretory granules have not been reported.

Adenosquamous Carcinoma

According to different series, adenosquamous carcinoma accounts for 7 to 9 percent of all gallbladder carcinomas (47,50). It consists of a variable mixture of two malignant but different epithelial components, one glandular and the other squamous (fig. 6-53). The glands are similar to those seen in well- to moderately differen-

tiated adenocarcinomas. A unique example of adenosquamous carcinoma showing gastric foveolar type epithelium has recently been reported (51). A superficial papillary growth pattern is noted in some adenosquamous carcinomas. The squamous component may be scattered, focal, or occupy large areas of the tumor. It may be mixed with glandular epithelium or appear independent from the glands and separated by fibrous stroma.

The degree of differentiation of the squamous elements varies from tumor to tumor, but, in general, tumors tend to be moderately differentiated. Whorls, keratohyaline, or keratin pearls are often present. Only a few tumors show poorly differentiated or anaplastic features in both components. Occasionally, spindle cells, which are usually cytokeratin positive, predominate in the squamous component (53). Reactive osteoclast-like

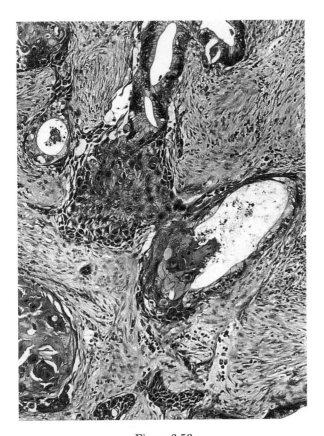

Figure 6-53
ADENOSQUAMOUS CARCINOMA
Well-differentiated malignant squamous cells fill the lumen of a neoplastic gland lined by cuboidal and columnar cells.

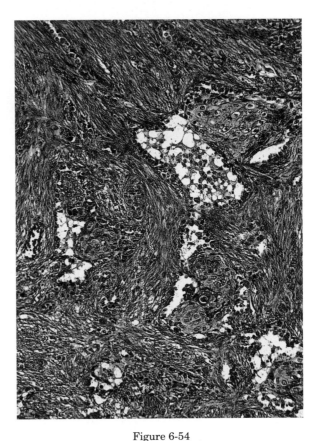

Figure 6-54
ADENOSQUAMOUS CARCINOMA
A cellular fibroblastic stroma surrounds glands filled with neoplastic squamous cells. The glands are lined by low cuboidal epithelial cells.

giant cells have rarely been observed in the stroma (49). In our experience, approximately 20 percent of adenosquamous carcinomas contain scattered endocrine cells admixed with the neoplastic columnar and squamous cells (48). Although lacking trophoblastic differentiation, immunoreactivity for human chorionic gonadotropin has been detected in 42 percent of adenosquamous carcinomas (50). The lack of anaplastic giant cells in tumors with a spindle cell–rich component excludes the diagnosis of undifferentiated spindle and giant cell carcinoma. An occasional tumor shows a reactive cellular fibroblastic stroma with mitotic activity, a feature that may lead to confusion with carcinosarcoma or undifferentiated carcinoma (fig. 6-54). However, the lack of cytologic atypia in the fibroblasts allows correct identification of the pseudosarcomatous stromal response. Both the glandular and squamous components are cytokeratin positive and contain CEA.

Adenosquamous carcinomas are not a mixture of two cell lines, each with a separate phenotype that is squamous or glandular, but result from the instability of differentiation of a single cell line; the neoplastic cells are able to express both phenotypes (52). Flow cytometric studies have shown DNA heterogeneity of the two phenotypes, providing additional support for the hypothesis of genetic instability of the original tumor cell clone (50).

By electron microscopy, adenosquamous carcinomas are composed of variable proportions of three cell types: one purely glandular which is columnar with cytoplasmic lumina, mucin droplets, and apical microvilli; another purely squamous; and a third with dual differentiation with tonofilament bundles, mucin droplets, intracytoplasmic lumina, and microvilli. Cells of the first type and those with dual differentiation form glandular structures

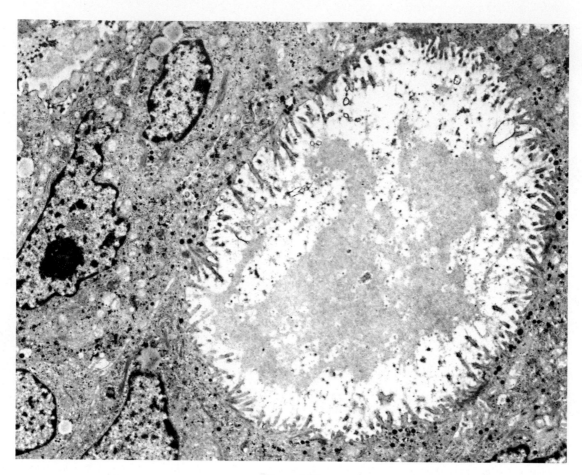

Figure 6-55
ADENOSQUAMOUS CARCINOMA: ULTRASTRUCTURE
A glandular structure contains mucus and is lined by epithelial cells with long microvilli, one of which exhibits dense core rootlets. In addition to the mucin, the cytoplasm of the neoplastic cells contains tonofilament bundles. This dual cellular differentiation is a characteristic feature of adenosquamous carcinomas (Uranyl acetate and lead citrate). (Fig. 100 from Fascicle 22, 2nd Series.)

which are surrounded by the basement membrane (fig. 6-55). These cells are joined by junctional complexes located at the apical ends and show prominent interdigitations that become more complicated near the cell base. The cells with purely squamous features are arranged in nests or cords, but do not form glandular structures. When present, endocrine cells contain membrane-bound, round or pleomorphic electron dense granules. These cells are seen admixed with the columnar glandular cells.

Squamous Cell Carcinoma

Squamous cell carcinoma, which constitutes 1 percent of all malignant tumors of the gallbladder, probably arises in areas of squamous metaplasia of the surface epithelium. In three of seven cases we have examined, we were able to demonstrate squamous metaplasia, dysplasia, and carcinoma in situ in the mucosa adjacent to the invasive cancer (fig. 6-56). Foci of conventional adenocarcinoma in situ were also found in one of these three cases. As with squamous cell carcinomas in other sites, the tumor consists of cords, islands, or sheets of malignant squamous cells separated by a dense fibrous stroma (figs. 6-57, 6-58). The extent of differentiation of the squamous cells varies from the anaplastic to the mature keratinizing type. One of the squamous cell carcinomas in our series was composed predominantly of large glycogen-rich clear cells displaying a trabecular growth pattern (fig. 6-59). CEA is present in the neoplastic squamous cells.

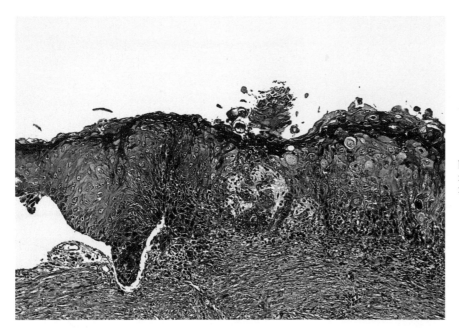

Figure 6-56
SQUAMOUS DYSPLASIA
The surface epithelium has been replaced by mature squamous epithelium which shows focal dysplastic changes.

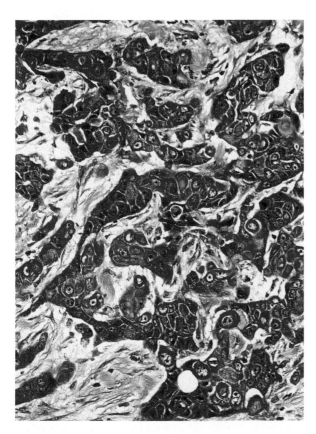

Figure 6-57
SQUAMOUS CELL CARCINOMA
Cords of malignant squamous cells are growing beneath the gallbladder epithelium (not shown in the photomicrograph).

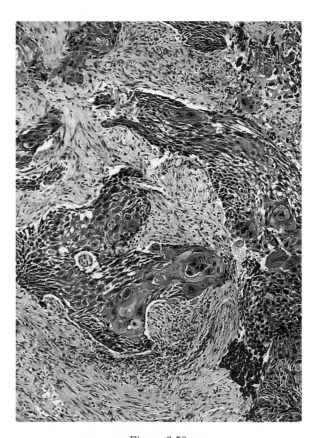

Figure 6-58
SQUAMOUS CELL CARCINOMA
Nests of well-differentiated, neoplastic, keratinizing squamous cells infiltrate the wall of the gallbladder and are surrounded by dense fibrous tissue.

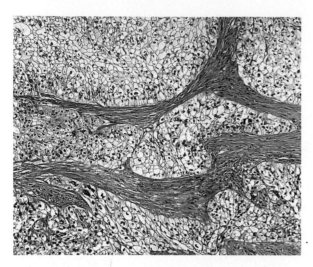

Figure 6-59
CLEAR CELL SQUAMOUS CARCINOMA
The neoplastic clear cells are arranged in trabecular structures. In other areas (not shown) the tumor exhibited squamous differentiation.

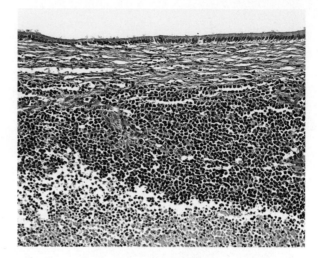

Figure 6-60
SMALL CELL CARCINOMA
Tumor cells are small, round, and hyperchromatic. The tumor exhibits submucosal growth, which is characteristic of small cell carcinomas. Extensive necrosis has occurred.

The spindle cell variant of squamous carcinoma also occurs in the gallbladder. When the tumor is composed entirely of spindle cells its separation from undifferentiated carcinoma or even malignant fibrous histiocytoma is difficult based on hematoxylin and eosin–stained sections alone. The presence of epithelial markers, such as keratin and epithelial membrane antigen in the spindle cells, is useful and the best way to establish the squamous nature of the tumor. We must caution, however, that before a diagnosis of pure squamous cell carcinoma is issued, multiple sections must be examined because some adenosquamous carcinomas have a minor glandular component that represents 5 to 10 percent of the tumor.

Ultrastructurally, squamous cell carcinomas of the gallbladder do not differ from those in other anatomic locations. Tumor cells are joined by well-developed desmosomes in which bundles of tonofilaments are inserted. These tonofilaments extend into the cytoplasm, which may contain a few mucin droplets. Electron microscopy may help identify the spindle cell variant of squamous carcinoma of the gallbladder.

Small Cell Carcinoma

Small cell carcinoma is a rare but distinctive neoplasm that accounts for 4 percent of all primary gallbladder carcinomas. Since first de-scribed in 1981 (54), approximately 50 cases have been reported (55–64). We have recently updated our observations based on 29 cases (55). Because of its characteristic morphologic features, highly aggressive clinical behavior, occasional association with endocrine manifestations, and sensitivity to chemotherapy it should be separated from undifferentiated carcinoma (55,64). Combined forms showing glandular or squamous differentiation have also been recognized (54,55,61,61a,62). Regardless of the extent of these two components, these forms should not be included in the adenocarcinoma or squamous cell carcinoma category because, in our experience, they behave as small cell carcinomas.

The histologic appearance of small cell carcinoma of the gallbladder is comparable to that of the corresponding lung and gastrointestinal tumors (55–57,66). Small round cells, usually mixed with spindle cells, predominate (figs. 6-60–6-62). Multinucleated giant cells are uncommon, occurring in less than 5 percent of the cases. Both the round and spindle cells have hyperchromatic nuclei, finely dispersed chromatin, and inconspicuous nucleoli. The cytoplasm is sparse, eosinophilic, and of imprecise limits. Although these cells usually grow in a diffuse manner, a focal nesting, trabecular, or festoon pattern is often seen. Tubular structures and pseudorosettes are

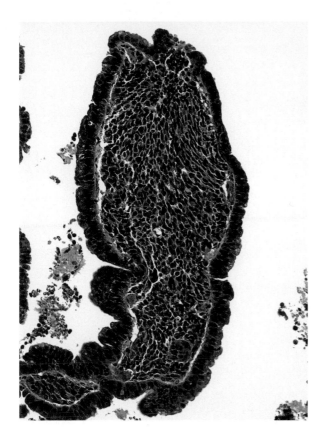

Figure 6-61
SMALL CELL CARCINOMA
The lamina propria of this mucosal fold is expanded by a
small cell carcinoma. The overlying epithelium is dysplastic.

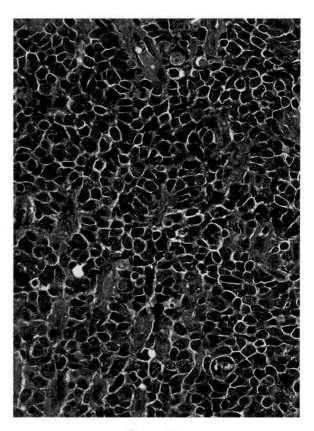

Figure 6-62
SMALL CELL CARCINOMA
A rosette-like structure is shown in this small cell carci-
noma of the gallbladder.

uncommon (fig. 6-62). Central necrosis of the trabeculae often results in a comedocarcinoma-like pattern. In areas of extensive necrosis, which are present in almost every tumor, the only viable-appearing tumor cells are those surrounding blood vessels (fig. 6-63). The walls of the vessels rarely exhibit the deep basophilic staining which is the result of DNA deposition. In two of our patients, the gallbladder epithelium overlying the tumor showed dysplastic changes and carcinoma in situ, but cells from these lesions did not resemble those of the infiltrating small cell carcinoma. Furthermore, foci of squamous differentiation and areas of well-differentiated neoplastic glands are found in 6 and 30 percent of the tumors, respectively (figs. 6-64, 6-65). The neoplastic glands are usually confined to a few areas, but rarely they may be a major component. This divergent differentiation has been documented in small cell carcinomas arising in

other anatomic sites including the gastrointestinal tract (57). In our experience, the incidence of divergent differentiation is related to sampling. Tumors studied by multiple sections often show foci of neoplastic glands whereas small biopsy specimens usually lack this component. We have also seen a carcinosarcoma in which the carcinomatous component was of the small cell type.

Unexpectedly the Grimelius stain reveals fine argyrophil granules in 15 percent of the tumors. In contrast, most small cell carcinomas show endocrine differentiation by immunohistochemistry. In our experience, approximately 75 percent are positive for neuron-specific enolase, about 40 percent are focally immunoreactive for chromogranin, and 50 percent express synaptophysin (figs. 6-66, 6-67). Positivity for Leu-7 is less common (20 percent of cases). Focal serotonin and adrenocorticotropin hormone (ACTH) reactivity have occasionally been detected in

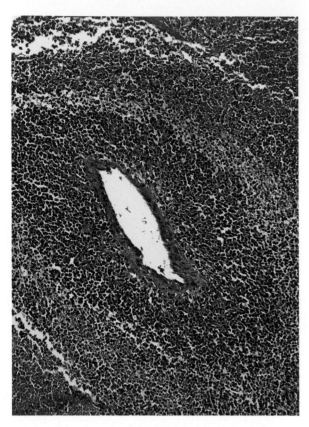

Figure 6-63
SMALL CELL CARCINOMA
Extensive necrosis is seen in this small cell carcinoma. The only viable tumor cells surround a blood vessel.

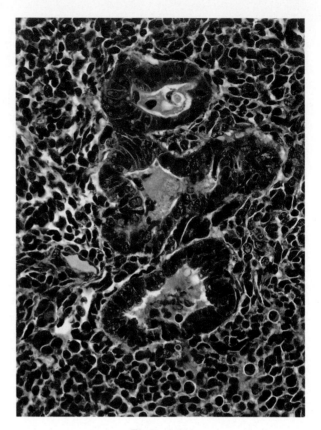

Figure 6-64
COMBINED SMALL CELL AND ADENOCARCINOMA
Neoplastic glands are surrounded by small cells with hyperchromatic nuclei.

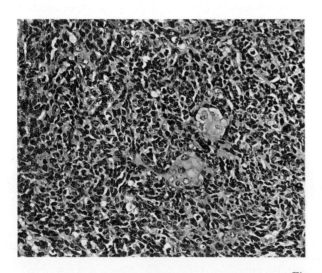

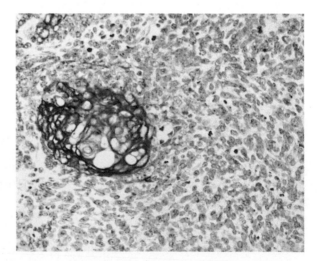

Figure 6-65
SMALL CELL CARCINOMA WITH SQUAMOUS DIFFERENTIATION
Left: Two foci of squamous cells are surrounded by small cell carcinoma.
Right: The focus of squamous cells is strongly cytokeratin positive whereas the small cells are only weakly positive.

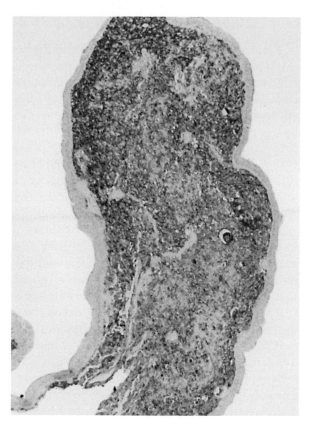

Figure 6-66
SMALL CELL CARCINOMA SHOWING DIFFUSE
NEURON-SPECIFIC ENOLASE REACTIVITY
The overlying dysplastic epithelium is NSE negative.

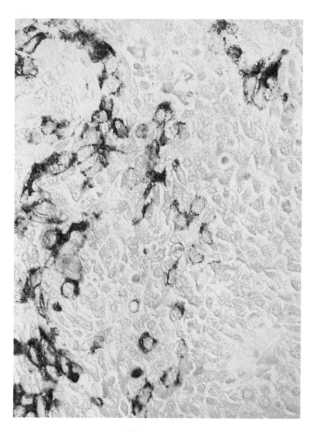

Figure 6-67
SMALL CELL CARCINOMA WITH
FOCAL CHROMOGRANIN POSITIVITY

these tumors by immunohistochemical techniques (63). Endocrine differentiation is absent in the squamous foci but may be present in the glandular component. Most small cell carcinomas are cytokeratin positive and approximately 25 percent are immunoreactive for CEA. These tumors also express p53 protein. Since endocrine differentiation is seen in many carcinomas, including poorly differentiated and undifferentiated carcinomas of the gallbladder, immunohistochemistry has limited diagnostic value for small cell carcinomas. The diagnosis should be based on histologic grounds using conventional stains. By electron microscopy, a few neurosecretory granules are seen in some of the neoplastic cells (fig. 6-68). Flow cytometric studies have shown that 78 percent of the tumors are aneuploid (63).

Small cell carcinomas can be confused with malignant lymphomas. However, the presence of cords, ribbons, festoons, and neoplastic cells that show nuclear molding and dispersed granular chromatin exclude malignant lymphoma. Also, the lymphoma cells are positive for leukocyte common antigen, B- or T-cell markers, do not express cytokeratin or endocrine markers, and lack the neurosecretory granules and cell junctions that characterize small cell carcinomas. Rarely, carcinoid tumors of the gallbladder which are composed predominantly of small round cells can be misinterpreted as small cell carcinoma. This distinction is crucial because carcinoid tumors are much less aggressive than small cell carcinomas. Carcinoid tumors are often small submucosal nodules that histologically show a more organoid pattern, lack necrosis, and exhibit minimal mitotic activity. Neoplastic cells have more open nuclei and more abundant cytoplasm that is usually argyrophilic and diffusely immunoreactive for chromogranin, serotonin, and peptide hormones. Small cell carcinomas should also be distinguished from undifferentiated carcinomas composed predominantly of

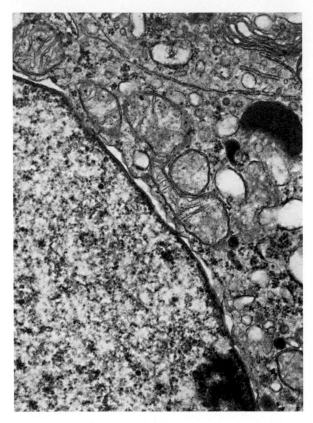

Figure 6-68
SMALL CELL CARCINOMA: ULTRASTRUCTURE
Portions of two cells, one of which contains three small membrane-bound neurosecretory granules (uranyl acetate and lead citrate). (Fig. 101 from Fascicle 22, 2nd Series.)

small cells. The latter tumors rarely have poorly defined glandular structures, but often contain cytoplasmic mucin. Moreover, cells from these tumors have vesicular nuclei and very prominent nucleoli. In metastatic deposits it is not possible to separate small cell carcinomas of the gallbladder from those originating in other sites.

Small cell carcinomas of the gallbladder are probably under-represented in the medical literature, since these tumors are often reported as undifferentiated or anaplastic carcinomas or as apudomas (65). In our initial series of 386 gallbladder cancers (54a), we found 18 cases (4.7 percent) of small cell carcinoma. They were more common than pure squamous cell carcinoma of the gallbladder. In the SEER program, small cell carcinomas constituted 0.41 percent of all gallbladder cancers (Table 6-1).

Undifferentiated Carcinoma

Four morphologic variants, spindle and giant cell type, small cell type, those with a nodular or lobular growth pattern, and those with osteoclast-like giant cells are included in the undifferentiated category (70). The most common variant is composed predominantly of variable proportions of spindle and giant cells (74). It resembles different types of sarcomas (69,71,81) and is similar to the undifferentiated carcinomas found in other organs such as lung (67,76), thyroid gland (68,73), small and large intestines (72), and pancreas (80). We have now studied 58 examples of this tumor which is the most pleomorphic and anaplastic member of the undifferentiated group. Histologically, variable proportions of spindle and giant cells form sheets or interlacing bundles, often separated by a desmoplastic stroma (fig. 6-69). Although round and polygonal cells are also found they are usually a minor component. Both spindle and giant cells contain large bizarre nuclei with prominent nucleoli (fig. 6-70). The cytoplasm is abundant, deeply eosinophilic, and may contain phagocytized red blood cells, polymorphonuclear leukocytes, lymphocytes, or nuclear debris in various stages of degeneration (figs. 6-71, 6-72). Focal rhabdoid features have rarely been described (79). Approximately 10 percent of the tumors contain anaplastic multinucleated giant cells with distinct PAS-positive hyaline globules, which are also seen in an extracellular location, presumably the result of extrusion from the cells. Focal squamous differentiation has been noted in 8 percent of tumors and clusters of multinucleated osteoclast-like giant cells in 2 percent. If adequately sampled, foci of well- to moderately differentiated neoplastic glands or in situ changes are found in approximately two thirds of the tumors (fig. 6-73). These foci of adenocarcinoma usually represent less than 5 percent of the tumor.

Transitions from the lining glandular epithelium to the anaplastic spindle and giant cell component are occasionally observed. Endocrine cells, which are present in 10 percent of the tumors, are usually found among the columnar cells lining the glands. Mitotic figures are more common in the spindle and giant cells than in the neoplastic glandular cells. Likewise, the proliferative activity, as measured by positivity with the Ki-67

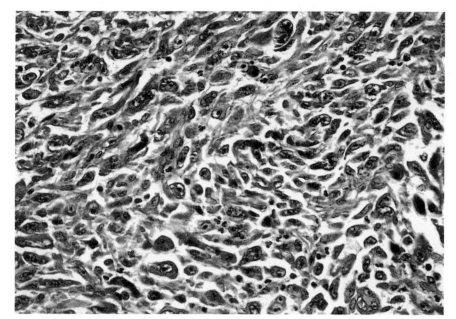

Figure 6-69
UNDIFFERENTIATED
SPINDLE AND
GIANT CELL CARCINOMA
Fascicles of spindle cells predominate in this undifferentiated carcinoma. These areas closely resemble a sarcoma.

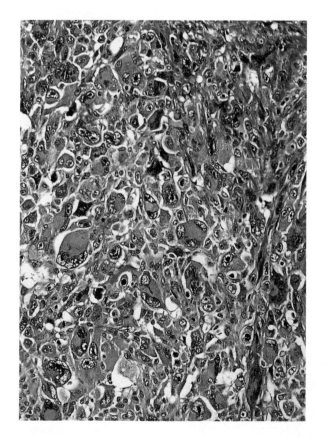 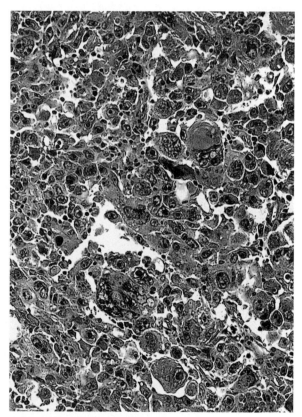

Figure 6-70
UNDIFFERENTIATED SPINDLE AND GIANT CELL CARCINOMA
Pleomorphic spindle and multinucleated giant cells with abundant eosinophilic cytoplasm and prominent nucleoli characterize this tumor.

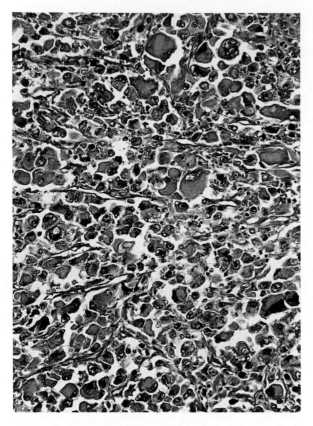

Figure 6-71
UNDIFFERENTIATED SPINDLE
AND GIANT CELL CARCINOMA

Large bizarre cells with abundant eosinophilic cytoplasm form the bulk of this tumor.

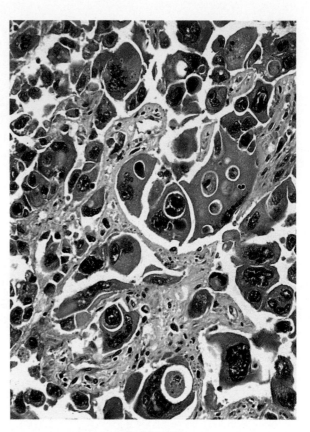

Figure 6-72
UNDIFFERENTIATED SPINDLE
AND GIANT CELL CARCINOMA

Some of the multinucleated giant cells contain phagocytized polymorphonuclear leukocytes and nuclear debris, common features of undifferentiated pleomorphic giant cell adenocarcinomas of the gallbladder.

Figure 6-73
UNDIFFERENTIATED
SPINDLE AND
GIANT CELL CARCINOMA

A single neoplastic gland is highlighted by the cytokeratin stain. The large, pleomorphic, spindle and giant cells around the gland are cytokeratin negative.

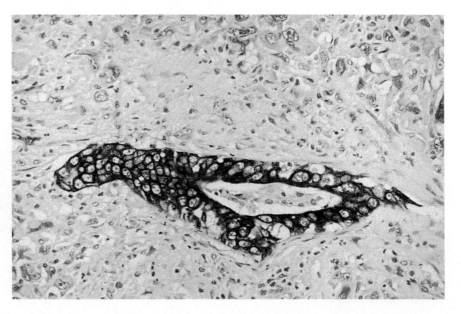

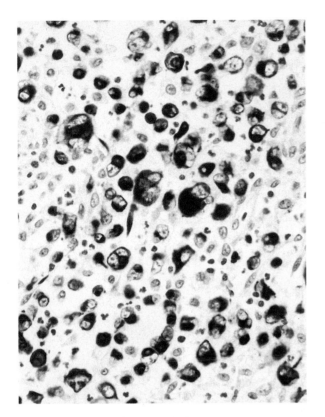

Figure 6-74
UNDIFFERENTIATED SPINDLE
AND GIANT CELL CARCINOMA
Most tumor cells are cytokeratin positive.

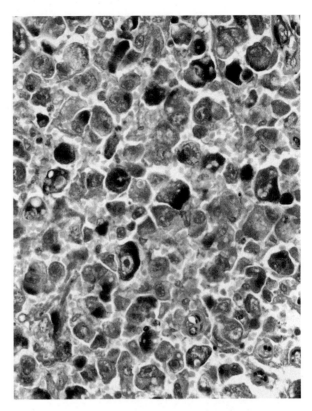

Figure 6-75
UNDIFFERENTIATED SPINDLE
AND GIANT CELL CARCINOMA
Some vimentin-positive cells are seen in this undifferentiated spindle and giant cell carcinoma.

antibody, is higher in the spindle and giant cell component (75). An inflammatory infiltrate rich in polymorphonuclear leukocytes and lymphocytes is often seen in the stroma, admixed with the neoplastic cells. In 70 percent of the tumors at least some of the undifferentiated spindle and giant cells stain for cytokeratin and less frequently (20 percent) for CEA, thus supporting their epithelial derivation (fig. 6-74). Often the reactivity is focal. Likewise, most of these tumors are immunoreactive for vimentin (fig. 6-75). Half of the tumors that have been analyzed by flow cytometry have been aneuploid (78).

The lack of heterologous elements such as cartilage and bone allows distinction from carcinosarcoma. Moreover, the sarcomatous component of these tumors has been cytokeratin negative in the nine cases we have studied by immunohistochemistry.

The two predominant cell types displayed by undifferentiated carcinomas at the light micro-

scopic level are also recognized by electron microscopy. Mononuclear and multinucleated giant cells with large irregular nuclei and prominent nucleoli are joined by desmosomes (fig. 6-76). The cytoplasm, which contains a moderate number of mitochondria and a well-developed endoplasmic reticulum, usually shows no specific line of differentiation. Occasionally, however, a few mucin droplets are present. We did not find tonofilaments or neurosecretory granules in two cases we examined. The spindle cells have large nuclei, prominent nucleoli, a well-developed endoplasmic reticulum, and a moderate number of mitochondria (fig. 6-77). Tonofilament bundles and neurosecretory granules are lacking.

The second most common variant of undifferentiated carcinoma is characterized by the proliferation of small round cells that grow in solid sheets, nodules, cords, or trabeculae (fig. 6-78). Individual cells contain round or ovoid hyperchromatic nuclei,

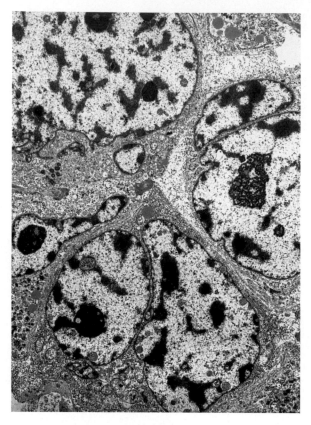

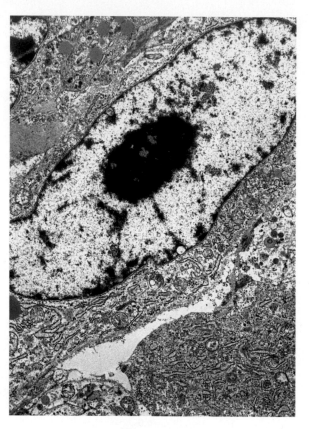

Figure 6-76
UNDIFFERENTIATED SPINDLE
AND GIANT CELL CARCINOMA

Electron micrograph showing large mononuclear and binucleated undifferentiated cells.

Figure 6-77
UNDIFFERENTIATED SPINDLE
AND GIANT CELL CARCINOMA

A neoplastic spindle cell with a large nucleus, a prominent nucleolus, and abundant endoplasmic reticulum is illustrated.

Figure 6-78
UNDIFFERENTIATED
CARCINOMA,
SMALL CELL TYPE

Tumor cells are arranged in long slender cords or single files. Some of the neoplastic cells contain mucin.

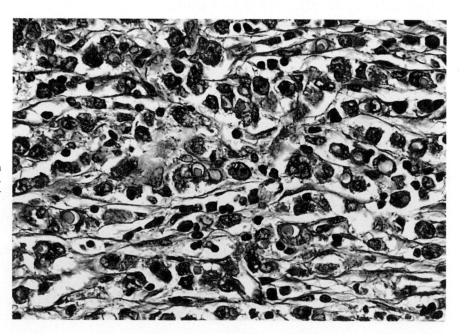

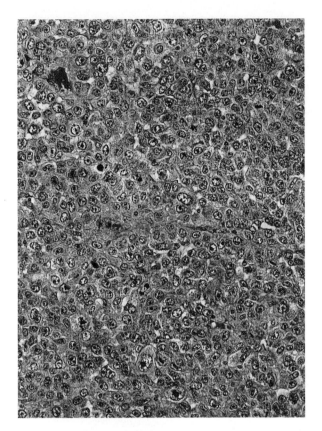

Figure 6-79
UNDIFFERENTIATED CARCINOMA
Sheets of undifferentiated epithelial cells with vesicular nuclei and prominent nucleoli are seen.

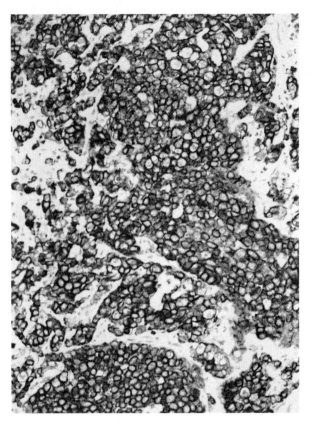

Figure 6-80
UNDIFFERENTIATED CARCINOMA
Nearly all neoplastic cells are cytokeratin positive.

with eosinophilic, often vacuolated cytoplasm (fig. 6-78). A small proportion of tumors contain a population of endocrine cells that are immunoreactive for chromogranin, serotonin, and peptide hormones. A few signet ring cells are also noted in some tumors. When undifferentiated carcinomas are composed predominantly of small cells with vesicular nuclei, prominent nucleoli, and little or no cytoplasmic mucin they can be confused with malignant lymphomas (fig. 6-79). However, the immunohistochemical identification of cytokeratin and CEA excludes lymphoma (fig. 6-80). Minimal gland formation can be detected in some undifferentiated carcinomas, a feature that is also helpful in differentiation from malignant lymphoma. Mitotic figures are numerous, and necrosis and vascular invasion are common.

The absence of ribbons, festoons, and pseudorosettes, as well as a lack of spindle cells and secretory granules, differentiate this variant of undifferentiated carcinoma from small cell carcinoma. Furthermore, the cells of undifferentiated carcinoma, which often have vesicular nuclei and contain mucin, tend to be larger than those of small cell carcinoma.

The third morphologic variant of undifferentiated carcinoma consists of well-defined nodular or lobular structures resembling those seen in lobular carcinoma of the breast (70). The cells are uniform in size, and have round nuclei and inconspicuous nucleoli (figs. 6-81, 6-82). Tubular glands are absent in this third variant.

The most uncommon but distinctive form of undifferentiated carcinoma consists of sheets of round and ovoid cells, and fascicles of spindle cells admixed with numerous osteoclast-like multinucleated giant cells, thereby mimicking giant cell tumor of bone (fig. 6-83) (70). The mononuclear cells, which show varying degrees of nuclear atypia, are immunoreactive for epithelial

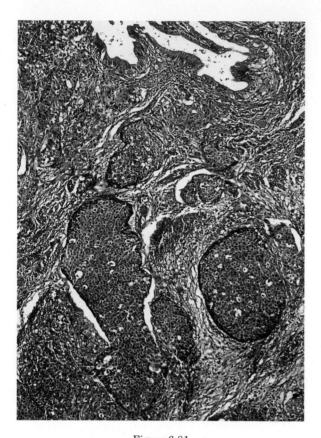

Figure 6-81
UNDIFFERENTIATED CARCINOMA
This tumor displays a well-defined nodular growth pattern, mimicking lobular carcinoma of the breast.

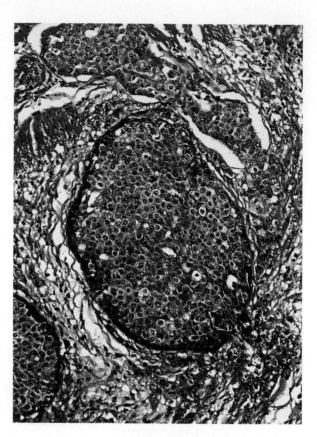

Figure 6-82
UNDIFFERENTIATED CARCINOMA
Higher magnification of one of the nodules in figure 6-81 shows uniformity of the neoplastic cells and similarity to lobular carcinoma of the breast.

membrane antigen and focally positive for cytokeratin, whereas the multinucleated giant cells are positive for histiocytic markers such as CD68. This suggests that the osteoclast-like multinucleated giant cells are probably reactive rather than neoplastic. Undifferentiated carcinomas with numerous osteoclast-like giant cells have also been described in the extrahepatic bile ducts and the ampulla of Vater, where they can produce bone (70). A small proportion of undifferentiated carcinomas, spindle and giant cell type, contain a moderate number of osteoclast-like giant cells.

MOLECULAR PATHOLOGY

The immunohistochemical demonstration of a high incidence of p53 immunoreactivity in gallbladder carcinoma suggested that molecular abnormalities of this tumor suppressor gene are important in the pathogenesis of gallbladder cancer (86,88,90). Subsequent studies showed loss of heterozygosity and mutations of the p53 gene in most invasive carcinomas (89a,91). Moreover, loss of heterozygosity of the p53 gene was the only molecular abnormality detected in 6 of 22 (27 percent) carcinomas. Likewise, loss of heterozygosity at 8p (44 percent) and 9p (50 percent) loci and the 18q gene (31 percent) was also detected in gallbladder carcinomas (91). These mutations were considered frequent and early events while *ras* mutations and loss of heterozygosity at 3p, rb, and 5q occurred less frequently and were considered late events, probably related to tumor progression. The c-*erb*β-2 gene, a glycoprotein structurally similar to the epidermal growth factor receptor and related to cell growth, has recently been investigated in gallbladder carcinoma (85). Amplification of the

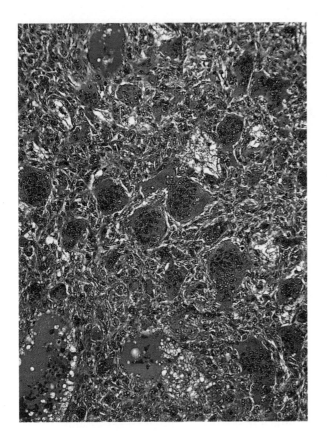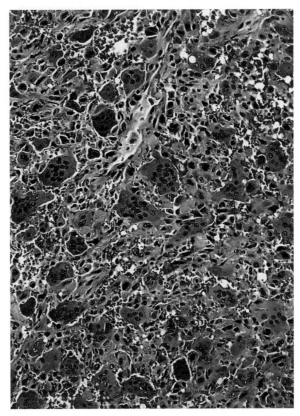

Figure 6-83
UNDIFFERENTIATED CARCINOMA WITH OSTEOCLAST-LIKE GIANT CELLS
Left: The histologic features of this tumor resemble those of giant cell tumor of bone.
Right: The mononuclear cells of this tumor show considerable nuclear atypia.

c-*erb*β-2 gene was detected in 30 of 43 (69.8 percent) invasive carcinomas (85). However, no correlation between c-*erb*β-2 gene amplification and prognosis was found.

Although the frequency of K-*ras* mutations in gallbladder carcinomas has differed widely in different studies, from 0 to 34 percent (82), most investigators have found these mutations to be significantly higher in extrahepatic bile duct tumors than in gallbladder carcinomas (83,84,87). However, the incidence of K-*ras* mutations is greater in gallbladder carcinomas associated with an anomalous junction of the pancreaticobiliary duct than in carcinomas not so associated (82). These molecular pathology findings support the concept that gallbladder carcinogenesis requires a number of genetic alterations involving activation of oncogenes or inactivation of tumor suppressor genes (89).

SPREAD

Malignant tumors of the gallbladder are insidious in their spread, often metastasizing early, before a diagnosis is made. Because of the location of the gallbladder, these tumors can spread by direct extension, through lymphatic and vascular channels, transcoelomically, along small nerves, and possibly by intraluminal implantation (92).

By contiguous growth, tumors can extend directly into the liver; invade the stomach, duodenum, or colon; or implant on peritoneal surfaces. Invasion of an adjacent viscus frequently leads to a biliary-enteric fistula, the clinical manifestations of which may be the first indication of cancer. Viable fragments may break away from the main tumor mass after it has penetrated the wall of the gallbladder and implant in the pelvic area or on other peritoneal surfaces, leading

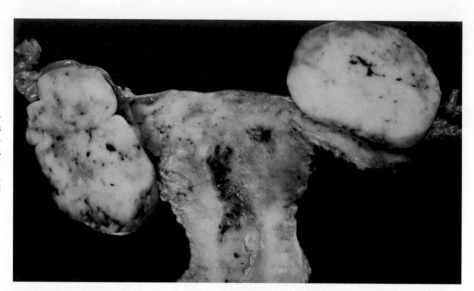

Figure 6-84
METASTATIC TUMOR
The ovaries are enlarged, although their overall shape is preserved. Both have been replaced by gray white tumor that originated in the gallbladder. (Figures 6-84 and 6-85 are from the same patient.) (Fig. 102 from Fascicle 22, 2nd Series.)

eventually to intra-abdominal carcinomatosis. In the late nonresectable stages of the disease, there may be widespread intra-abdominal metastases and ascites.

Metastasis to the regional lymph nodes occurs early and is one reason for the bad prognosis (95). Identified through dye injection studies, lymph nodes draining the gallbladder include the cystic node, pericholedochal nodes, lymph nodes superior and posterior to the head and neck of the pancreas, and retroportal, celiac, superior mesenteric, and interaortocaval nodes adjacent to the left renal vein (103). Tumors usually spread, at least initially, to the cystic or pericholedochal lymph nodes and later to the parapancreatic and preaortic nodes. The frequency of lymph node involvement correlates with the depth of invasion of the primary tumor (106). Later, distant metastases appear in the mediastinal, tracheobronchial, or supraclavicular nodes. Nodal metastases are found in approximately 50 percent of patients at the time of diagnosis, although this figure varies from 25 to 90 percent in different studies.

Carcinomas of the gallbladder can metastasize to the ovary (figs. 6-84, 6-85). In our series, 6 percent of patients had ovarian metastasis, most of whom also had peritoneal involvement. Occasionally, the ovarian metastasis is the first manifestation of gallbladder cancer (108). Clinically and pathologically, the metastasis may simulate a malignant ovarian tumor. Intestinal types of gallbladder cancer can resemble ovarian mucinous cystadenocarcinomas when meta-

static to the ovary. Moreover, conventional types of gallbladder carcinoma can mimic endometrioid or Sertoli-Leydig cell tumors of the ovary (108). Such resemblance can complicate the histologic interpretation of ovarian tumors. Metastatic carcinoma of the gallbladder can also mimic a primary carcinoma of the endometrium and of the uterine cervix (101).

Carcinomas of the gallbladder frequently invade small nerves. Usually demonstrated histologically, it is uncertain how important this mode of spread is clinically. It is also suspected that carcinomas spread by intraductal implantation. Although an uncommon event, it is thought that tumor cells that exfoliate from inside the gallbladder implant on the mucosal surface of the extrahepatic bile ducts leading eventually to multifocal tumors (92,96,97,106). Most multifocal tumors, however, are likely to be the result of a field change within the biliary epithelium. Multiple tumors do occur. Carcinomas of the gallbladder have been found in 6 percent of patients with extrahepatic bile duct cancer (100).

A complication associated with high mortality and morbidity is perforation of the gallbladder with secondary peritonitis, pericholecystic abscess, or fistula (98). There are many reports of patients who died from peritonitis and who were found at autopsy to have a perforated carcinomatous gallbladder. Most patients with perforated gallbladders, however, follow a chronic course, with abscess formation or fistula to the colon or duodenum.

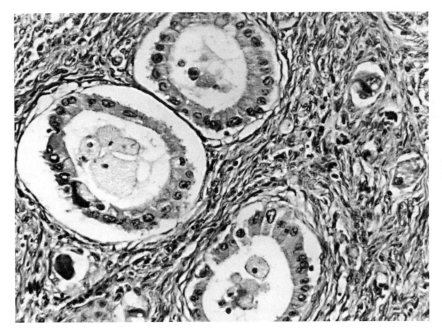

Figure 6-85
METASTATIC TUMOR
Sections from the tumor shown in figure 6-84. In addition to the well-formed neoplastic glands, the stroma appears hyperplastic and contains scattered tumor cells. (Fig. 103 from Fascicle 22, 2nd Series.)

Hematogenous dissemination occurs, but except for the liver and lung, it is unimportant compared to the other routes of metastatic spread.

Meningeal carcinomatosis, an exceedingly rare form of hematogenous dissemination, can occur in carcinoma of the gallbladder. It has been reported as the first manifestation of the tumor in a few patients (104a).

By the time of postmortem examination, more than 90 percent of patients have liver involvement (direct extension and/or metastasis) and 80 percent have regional lymph node metastasis (95). The lungs, colon, duodenum, pleura, diaphragm, and peritoneum are other common sites of metastatic spread (104).

Early Spread. The apparent ease by which gallbladder cancer spreads can be explained by the anatomy. The gallbladder has a thin wall with a narrow lamina propria and a single muscle layer through which the tumor must pass. Extension into the perimuscular connective tissue gives the tumor access to major lymphatic and vascular channels that facilitate spread.

This proclivity for early spread before the appearance of signs and symptoms applies to all types of malignant tumors known to occur in the gallbladder, with the possible exception of papillary carcinoma.

Liver Involvement. Found in 24 to 70 percent of patients at the time of surgical evaluation,

involvement of the liver usually precludes complete resection of the tumor (fig. 6-86). Not only does proximity to the liver favor direct and early extension, but tumor can also invade through vascular and lymphatic channels. Of these three routes, direct extension is the most common followed by lymphatic spread (95,102). A localized mass in the liver in the region of the gallbladder fossa is considered evidence for direct invasion. Owing to obstruction of the biliary tract by tumor, other intrahepatic lesions such as cholestasis and cholangitic abscess can occur (fig. 6-87).

Cancer Discovered After Laparoscopic Cholecystectomy. Occasionally, invasive carcinoma is found in gallbladders removed by laparoscopic surgery. Not recognized clinically or by imaging techniques, tumor is discovered during pathologic evaluation of the resected specimen. In these cases, the surgeon usually does not request an intraoperative consultation. An alarming consequence is tumor spillage with seeding along the endoscopic tract or intra-abdominal dissemination (96). Tumor has also implanted in the umbilicus (93,94,99). Even carcinoma in situ can be implanted if the organ is torn during dissection (107). Because of these complications it has been proposed that patients with radiographic gallbladder changes suggestive of carcinoma or with suspicious lesions of malignancy

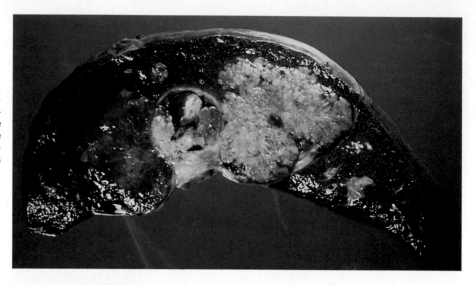

Figure 6-86
INVASION OF THE LIVER
Direct extension of gallbladder carcinoma into the liver is the most common type of spread. Small satellite nodules that represent metastases are also present.

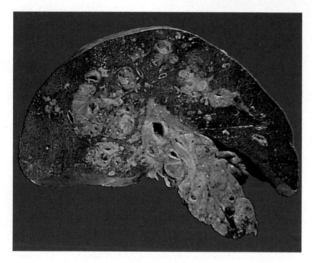

Figure 6-87
CHOLANGITIC ABSCESSES
An adenocarcinoma of the gallbladder had been previously excised from the patient. The tumor recurred and invaded the extrahepatic bile ducts, leading to obstruction and ascending cholangitis. (Pl. IIIB, Fascicle 22, 2nd Series.)

noted during laparoscopic cholecystectomy should undergo an open cholecystectomy (107).

Since few patients with carcinoma confined to the gallbladder are correctly diagnosed preoperatively and as laparoscopic cholecystectomy becomes more widely used, pathologists can expect more cases of early gallbladder cancer resected by this surgical procedure. The utility of surgical reexploration following a diagnosis of invasive

carcinoma in a laparoscopic cholecystectomy specimen has recently been addressed (96a). The survival rate of 16 patients with T2 and T3 tumors subjected to subsequent segmental liver resection and portal lymphadenectomy was better than that of patients in whom this surgical procedure was not possible because of tumor dissemination. However, larger series and longer follow-up are needed to determine whether the second surgical procedure is curative in these patients.

PROGNOSTIC FACTORS

Several prognostic factors have been identified for carcinomas of the gallbladder. These factors have little or no predictive advantage in cases of regional or metastatic disease.

Histologic Type. Papillary carcinomas, although infrequent, have the best prognosis and should be specifically identified (113–115). The 5-year relative survival rate is 36 percent, which is significantly greater than that for other histologic types (fig. 6-88). The favorable survival rate persists; at 10 years survival is 30 percent. This favorable survival probably reflects the fact that many of these tumors are noninvasive. Patients with undifferentiated or small cell carcinomas invariably survive less than a year.

Histologic Grade. Figure 6-89 shows a correlation between survival and grade. Patients with tumors assigned grade 1 (well differentiated) maintain a survival advantage for 10 years. Most patients whose tumors are assigned

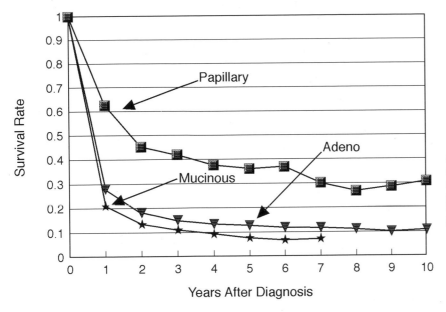

There were 2414 cases of adenocarcinoma (adeno), 137 cases of papillary carcinoma, and 165 cases of mucinous carcinoma. All stages and grades are combined. Data from the Surveillance, Epidemiology, and End Results Program, National Cancer Institute.

Figure 6-89
TEN-YEAR SURVIVAL
FOR CANCERS OF THE
GALLBLADDER ACCORDING
TO HISTOLOGIC GRADE

All stages and histologic types are combined. The number of cases for grade 1 was 327; for grade 2, 626; for grade 3, 731; and for grade 4, 85. Data taken from the Surveillance, Epidemiology, and End Results Program, National Cancer Institute, for the years 1981–1990.

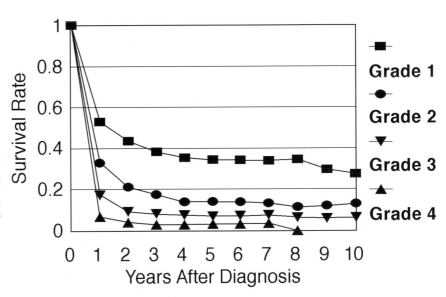

grade 3 (poorly differentiated) or grade 4 (undifferentiated) die within the first year after diagnosis. Histologic grade 3 is the one most commonly recorded. The criteria for grading are presented on page 68.

Vascular Invasion. Vascular invasion, either within blood vessels or lymphatic channels, has an adverse affect on outcome (113). Overall, vascular invasion as seen histologically has the effect of reducing outcome to the next stage of disease (fig. 6-90). For this reason, pathologists should specifically include the presence or absence of vascular

invasion in their reports, especially for tumors that have not ostensibly spread to the liver.

Stage of Disease. The single most important factor having the greatest effect on survival is the extent of disease, or stage, at the time of diagnosis (113). For staging, we recommend the TNM (Tumor, Lymph Node, Metastatic) system which has been published by the American Joint Committee on Cancer and the International Union Against Cancer (112,116). Because gallbladder cancer is relatively uncommon and usually diagnosed late, physicians have tended to ignore

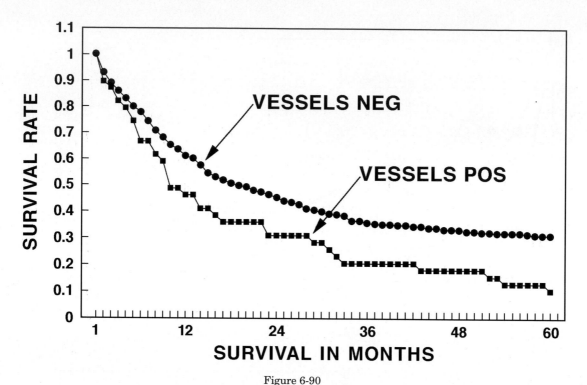

Figure 6-90
SURVIVAL RATES BASED ON PRESENCE OR ABSENCE OF BLOOD VESSEL INVASION
Rates are for localized disease only. Invaded vessels were recorded in 37 patients. (Fig. 2 from Henson DE, Albores-Saavedra J, Corle D. Carcinoma of the gallbladder: histologic types, stage of disease, grade, survival rates. Cancer 1992;70:1493–7. Data taken from Surveillance, Epidemiology, and End Results Program, National Cancer Institute.)

pathologic staging, even though its importance for survival, management, and prognosis has been repeatedly stressed (110,111,115).

Molecular Markers. Amplification of the c-*erbB*-2 oncogene or overexpression of the c-erbB-2 protein have not proven to be useful prognostic factors (117). Likewise p53 protein immunoreactivity does not correlate with histologic type or with the depth of invasion. Furthermore, DNA ploidy status has not provided useful prognostic information (109). Because survival is so short, most prognostic factors have minimal clinical value.

Survival. Unfortunately, overall survival for patients with advanced disease is no better now than it was in 1894 (118). For those patients with known lymph node and liver metastases at the time of surgery, the median survival period is 5.2 months (120). Because of this, most surgeons hold a pessimistic view for the surgical treatment of gallbladder carcinoma. However, in recent years radical surgery has improved the prognosis of patients with this tumor. Figure 6-91 shows a relation between the relative 5-year

survival rate and the stage of disease. The 10-year survival rate for patients with tumors confined to the gallbladder is 36 percent. For patients with regional disease or distant metastases, the 10-year survival rate is less than 10 percent. In one small series, the 5-year rate for patients with gallbladder carcinoma that has not spread beyond the muscle layer treated with cholecystectomy alone was 100 percent (121). For patients with regional node metastasis, the 5-year survival rate was 49 percent with cholecystectomy and regional node dissection. Others have advocated cholecystectomy, en bloc dissection of the regional nodes, wedge resection of the gallbladder bed, and resection of the suprahepatic segment of the extrahepatic bile duct for patients with lymph node metastases (119,122). The 5-year survival rate in this group of patients has varied from 45 to 63 percent.

Adjuvant chemotherapy and radiotherapy have been advocated to improve patient survival (119a,122a), but have not proven to be efficacious in controlled studies.

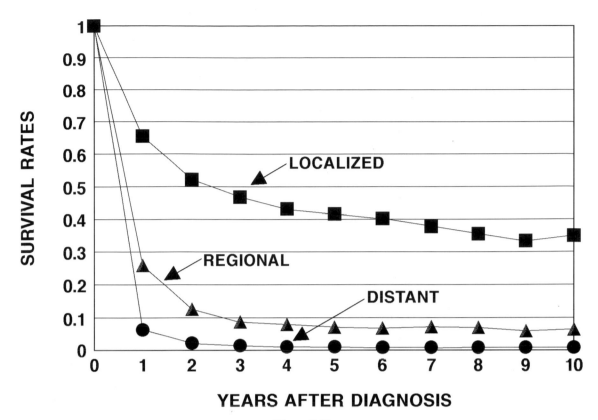

Figure 6-91
TEN-YEAR RELATIVE SURVIVAL RATES ACCORDING TO
STAGE OF DISEASE FOR CANCERS OF THE GALLBLADDER

There were 768 cases with localized, 987 with regional, and 1154 with distant disease. The 5-year relative survival rates were 42 percent for localized, 7 percent for regional, and 1 percent for distant disease. Data include all histologic types. Data taken from the Surveillance, Epidemiology, and End Results Program, National Cancer Institute.

REFERENCES

Invasive Carcinoma

1. Cowley LL, Wood V. Carcinoma developing in a remnant of the gallbladder. Ann Surg 1964;159:465–8.
2. Henson DE, Albores-Saavedra J, Corle D. Carcinoma of the gallbladder. Histologic types, stage of disease and survival rates. Cancer 1992;70:1493–7.
3. Tanga MR, Bouchard A, Ewing JB. Carcinoma developing in gallbladder remnants. J Indian Med Assoc 1973;61:132–3.

Well- to Moderately Differentiated Adenocarcinoma and Unusual Histologic Types

4. Abu-Farsakh H, Fraire AE. Adenocarcinoma and (extragonadal) choriocarcinoma of the gallbladder in a young woman. Hum Pathol 1991;22:614–6.
5. Adachi H, Aki T, Yoshida H, Yumoto T, Wakahara H. Combined choriocarcinoma and adenocarcinoma of the lung. Acta Pathol Jpn 1989;39:147–52.
6. Albores-Saavedra J, Henson DE, Angeles-Angeles A. Enteroendocrine cell differentiation in carcinoma of the gallbladder and mucinous cystadenocarcinoma of the pancreas. Pathol Res Pract 1989;183:169–75.
7. Albores-Saavedra J, Henson DE, Sobin LH. Histological typing of tumors of the gallbladder and extrahepatic bile ducts. World Health Organization. Springer-Verlag, Berlin, 1991.
8. Albores-Saavedra J, Molberg K, Henson DE. Unusual malignant epithelial tumors of the gallbladder. Sem Diag Pathol 1996;13:326–38.
9. Albores-Saavedra J, Nadji M, Henson DE. Intestinal type adenocarcinoma of the gallbladder. A clinicopathologic and immunohistochemical study of seven cases. Am J Surg Pathol 1986;10:19–25.

10. Banerjee SS, Eyden BP, Wells S, McWilliam LJ, Harris M. Pseudoangiosarcomatous carcinoma: a clinicopathological study of seven cases. Histopathology 1992;21:13–23.

11. Baretton G, Blasenbreu S, Vogt T, Lohrs U, Rau H, Schmidt M. DNA ploidy in carcinoma of the gallbladder. Prognostic significance and comparison of flow and image cytometry on archival tumor material. Path Res Pract 1994;190:584–92.

12. Donohue JH, Nagorney DM, Grant CS, Tsushiima K, Ilstrup DM, Adson MA. Carcinoma of the gallbladder. Does radical resection improve outcome? Arch Surg 1990;125:237–41.

13. Evett RD, Higgins JA, Brown AL Jr. The fine structure of normal mucosa in human gallbladder. Gastroenterology 1964;47:49–60.

14. Fujii K, Yasui W, Shimamoto OF, et al. Immunohistochemical analysis of nm23 gene product in human gallbladder carcinomas. Virchows Arch 1995;426:355–9.

15. Hickey WF, Seiler MW. Ultrastructural markers of colonic adenocarcinoma. Cancer 1981;47:140–5.

16. Kawamura J, Rhinsho K, Taki Y, et al. Choriocarcinoma and undifferentiated cell carcinoma of the bladder with gonadotrophin secretion. J Urol 1979;121:684–6.

17. Koga A, Momii S, Eguchi M, Makino T. Ultrastructure of well-differentiated adenocarcinoma of the gallbladder. Ultrastr Pathol 1991;15:41–8.

18. Kubosawa H, Nagao K, Kondo Y, Ishige H, Inaba N. Co-existence of adenocarcinoma and choriocarcinoma in the sigmoid colon. Cancer 1984;54:866–8.

19. Larraza-Hernandez O, Henson DE, Albores-Saavedra J. The ultrastructure of gallbladder carcinoma. Acta Morphol Hung 1984;32:279–93.

20. Lee CS, Pirdas A. Epidermal growth factor receptor immunoreactivity in gallbladder and extrahepatic biliary tract tumors. Path Res Pract 1995;191:1087–91.

21. Marcus PB, Martin JH, Green RH, Krouse MA. Glycocalyceal bodies and microvillous core rootlets. Arch Pathol Lab Med 1979;103:89–92.

22. McKechnie JC, Fechner RE. Choriocarcinoma and adenocarcinoma of the esophagus with gonadotropin secretion. Cancer 1971;27:694–702.

23. Nappi O, Swanson PE, Wick M. Pseudovascular adenoid squamous cell carcinoma of the lung: clinicopathologic study of three cases and comparison with true

pleuropulmonary angiosarcoma. Hum Pathol 1994;25:373–8.

24. Ohta T, Nagakawa T, Fonseca L, et al. Stromal distribution of CA 19-9 as a predictor of lymph node metastases in gallbladder cancer without serosal invasion. Oncology 1994;51:238–43.

25. Parker GW, Joffe N. Calcifying primary mucus-producing adenocarcinoma of the gallbladder. Br J Radiol 1972;45:468–9.

26 Pushchak MJ, Farhi DC. Primary choriocarcinoma of the lung. Arch Pathol Lab Med 1987;111:477–9.

27. Ramponi A, Angeli G, Arceci F, Puzzuoli R. Gastric choriocarcinoma: an immunohistochemical study. Path Res Pract 1986;181:390–6.

28. Rogers LF, Lastra MP, Lin KT, Bennett D. Calcifying mucinous adenocarcinoma of the gallbladder. Am J Gastroenterol 1973;59:441–5.

29. Soon Lee C, Pirdas-Zivcic A. nm23-H1 protein immunoreactivity in cancers of the gallbladder, extrahepatic bile ducts and ampulla of Vater. Pathology 1994;26:448–52.

30. Tatematsu M, Ichinose M, Miki K, et al. Gastric phenotypic expression in human gallbladder cancers revealed by pepsinogen immunohistochemistry and mucin histochemistry. Virchows Arch [A] 1988;413:25–32.

31. Teh M, Wee A, Raju GC. An immunohistochemical study of p53 protein in gallbladder and extrahepatic bile duct/ampullary carcinomas. Cancer 1994;74:1542–5.

32. Velu TJ, Beguinot L, Vass EC, et al. Epidermal-growth-factor-dependent transformation by a human EGF receptor proto-oncogene. Science 1987;238:1408–10.

33. Wee A, Teh M, Raju GC. Clinical importance of p53 protein in gallbladder carcinoma and its precursor lesions. J Clin Pathol 1994;47:453–6.

34. Wistuba I, Gazdar AF, Roa I, Albores-Saavedra J. p53 protein over-expression in gallbladder carcinoma and its precursor lesions: an immunohistochemical study. Hum Pathol 1996;27:360–5.

35. Yamaguchi K, Enjoji M. Carcinoma of the gallbladder. A clinicopathology of 103 patients and a newly proposed staging. Cancer 1988;62:1425–32.

36. Yamamoto M, Nakajo S, Tahara E. Immunohistochemical analysis of estrogen receptors in human gallbladder. Acta Pathol Jpn 1990;40:14–21.

37. Yamamoto M, Oda N, Tahara E. DNA ploidy patterns in gallbladder adenocarcinoma. Jpn J Clin Oncol 1990;20:83–6.

Clear Cell Adenocarcinoma

38. Albores-Saavedra J, Molberg K, Henson DE. Unusual malignant epithelial tumors of the gallbladder. Sem Diag Pathol 1996;13:326–38.

39. Bennington JL, Kradjian R. Renal carcinoma. Philadelphia: WB Saunders, 1967:38–42.

40. Bittinger A, Altekrüger I, Barth P. Clear cell carcinoma of the gallbladder. A histological and immunohistochemical study. Path Res Pract 1995;191:1259–65.

41. Maruiwa M, Yano H, Kataoke A, et al. Heterotransplantation of an alpha-fetoprotein producing human gallbladder carcinoma into nude mice. Acta Pathol Jpn 1988;38:501–13.

42. Satoh H, Iyama A, Hidaka K, et al. Metastatic carcinoma of the gallbladder from renal cancer presenting as intraluminal polypoid mass. Dig Dis Sci 1991;36:520–3.

43. Sugaya Y, Sugaya H, Kuronuma Y, et al. A case of gallbladder carcinoma producing both alpha-fetoprotein (AFP) and carcinoembryonic antigen (CEA). Gastroenterol Jpn 1989;24(3):325–31.

44. Vardaman C, Albores-Saavedra J. Clear cell carcinoma of the gallbladder and extrahepatic bile ducts. Am J Surg Pathol 1995;19:91–9.

45. Watanabe M, Hari Y, Najimi T, et al. Alpha-fetoprotein-producing carcinoma of the gallbladder. Dig Dis Sci 1993;38:561–4.

46. Weiss L, Harlos JP, Torhorst J, et al. Metastatic patterns of renal carcinoma: an analysis of 687 necropsies. J Cancer Res Clin Oncol 1988;114:605–12.

Adenosquamous Carcinoma

47. Albores-Saavedra J, Henson DE. Tumors of the gallbladder and extrahepatic bile ducts. Atlas of Tumor Pathology, 2nd Series, Fascicle 22. Washington, D.C.: Armed Forces Institute of Pathology, 1986:84–6.
48. Albores-Saavedra J, Nadji M, Henson DE, Angeles-Angeles A. Enteroendocrine cell differentiation in carcinoma of the gallbladder and mucinous cystadenocarcinoma of the pancreas. Pathol Res Pract 1989;183:169–75.
49. Grosso LE, Gonzalez JG. Stromal osteoclast-like giant cells in an adenosquamous carcinoma of the gallbladder. Hum Pathol 1992;23:703–6.
50. Nishihara K, Nagai E, Izumi Y, et al. Adenosquamous carcinoma of the gallbladder. A clinicopathological immunohistochemical and flow cytometric study of twenty cases. Jpn J Cancer Res 1994;85:389–99.
51. Nishihara K, Takashima M, Haraguchi M, Tsuneyoshi M. Adenosquamous carcinoma of the gallbladder with gastric foveolar-type epithelium. Pathol Internat 1995;45:250–6.
52. Steele VE, Nettesheim P. Unstable cellular differentiation in adenosquamous cell carcinoma. JNCI 1981;67:149–54.
53. Suster S, Huszar M, Herczeg E, Bubis JJ. Adenosquamous carcinoma of the gallbladder with spindle cell features. A light microscopic and immunohistochemical study of a case. Histopathology 1987;11:209–14.

Small Cell Carcinoma

54. Albores-Saavedra J, Cruz-Ortiz H, Alcantara-Vazques A, Henson DE. Unusual types of gallbladder carcinoma. A report of 16 cases. Arch Pathol Lab Med 1981;105:287–93.
54a. Albores-Saavedra J, Henson DE. Tumors of the gallbladder and extrahepatic bile ducts. Atlas of Tumor Pathology, 2nd Series, Fascicle 22. Washington, D.C.: Armed Forces Institute of Pathology, 1986:84–6.
55. Albores-Saavedra J, Molberg K, Henson DE. Unusual malignant epithelial tumors of the gallbladder. Sem Diag Pathol 1996;13:326–38.
56. Albores-Saavedra J, Soriano J, Larraza-Hernandez O, Aguirre J, Henson DE. Oat cell carcinoma of the gallbladder. Hum Pathol 1984;15:639–46.
57. Burke AB, Skekitka KM, Sobin LH. Small cell carcinomas of the large intestine. Am J Clin Pathol 1991;95:315–21.
58. Cavazzana AO, Fassina AS, Tollot M, Ninfo V. Small-cell carcinoma of the gallbladder. An immunocytochemical and ultrastructural study. Pathol Res Pract 1991;187:472–6.
59. Duan HJ, Ishigame H, Ishii Z, Itoh N, Shigematsu H. Small cell carcinoma of the gallbladder combined with adenocarcinoma. Acta Pathol Jpn 31:1991;841–6.
60. Guo KJ, Yamaguchi K, Enjoji M. Undifferentiated carcinoma of the gallbladder: a clinicopathologic, histochemical, and immunochemical study of 21 patients with a poor prognosis. Cancer 1988;1872–9.
61. Iida Y, Tsutsumi Y. Small cell (endocrine cell) carcinoma of the gallbladder with squamous and adenocarcinomatous components. Acta Pathol Jpn 1992;119–25.
61a. Kuwabara H, Uda H. Small cell carcinoma of the gallbladder with intestinal metaplastic epithelium. Pathol Int 1998;48:303–6.
62. Nishihara K, Nagai E, Tsuneyoshi M, Nagashima M. Small cell carcinoma combined with adenocarcinoma of the gallbladder. Arch Pathol Lab Med 1994;118:177–81.
63. Nishihara K, Tsuneyoshi M. Small cell carcinoma of the gallbladder. A clinicopathological, immunohistochemical and flow cytometrical study of 15 cases. Int J Oncol 1993;3:901–8.
64. Ron IG, Wigler N, Llie B, Chaitchik S. Small cell carcinoma of the gallbladder: clinical course and response to chemotherapy. Tumori 1992;78:207–10.
65. Spence RW, Burns-Cox CJ. ACTH-secreting "apudoma" of gallbladder. Gut 1975;16:473–6.
66. Zamboni G, Franzin G, Bonetti F, et al. Small-cell neuroendocrine carcinoma of the ampullary region. A clinicopathologic, immunohistochemical, and ultrastructural study of three cases. Am J Surg Pathol 1990;14:703–13.

Undifferentiated Carcinoma

67. Addis BI, Dewar A, Thurlow NP. Giant cell carcinoma of the lung. Immunohistochemical and ultrastructural evidence of dedifferentiation. J Pathol 1991;155:231–40.
68. Albores-Saavedra J, Alcantara-Vazquez A, Meza-Chavez L, et al. Carcinoma anaplastico de celulas fusiformes y gigantes del tiroides. Prensa Med Mex 1972;37:421–9.
69. Albores-Saavedra J, Cruz-Ortiz H, Alcantara-Vazques A, Henson DE. Unusual types of gallbladder carcinoma. A report of 16 cases. Arch Pathol Lab Med 1981;105:287–93.
70. Albores-Saavedra J, Molberg K, Henson DE. Unusual malignant epithelial tumors of the gallbladder. Sem Diag Pathol 1996;13:326–38.
71. Appelman HD, Coopersmith N. Pleomorphic spindle cell carcinoma of the gallbladder: relation to sarcoma of the gallbladder. Cancer 1970;25:535–41.
72. Bak M, Teglbjaerg PS. Pleomorphic (giant cell) carcinoma of the intestine. An immunohistochemical and electron microscopic study. Cancer 1989;64:2557–64.
73. Carcangiu ML, Steeper T, Zampi G, Rosai J. Anaplastic thyroid carcinoma. A study of 70 cases. Am J Clin Pathol 1985;83:135–58.
74. Caruso RA, Famulari C, Giuffré G, Mazzeo G. Pleomorphic carcinoma of the gallbladder. Tumori 1991;77:523–6.
75. Diebold-Berger S, Vaiton JC, Pache JC, Emanuele S, d'Amore G. Undifferentiated carcinoma of the gallbladder. Report of a case with immunohistochemical findings. Arch Pathol Lab Med 1995;119:279–82.
76. Fishback NF, Travis WP, Moran CA, et al. Pleomorphic (spindle giant cell) carcinoma of the lung. A clinicopathologic correlation of 78 cases. Cancer 1994;73:2936–45.
77. Guo KJ, Yamaguchi K, Enjoji M. Undifferentiated carcinoma of the gallbladder. A clinicopathologic, histochemical, and immunohistochemical study of 21 patients with a poor prognosis. Cancer 1988;61:1872–9.
78. Nishihara K, Tsuneyoshi M. Undifferentiated spindle cell carcinoma of the gallbladder: a clinicopathologic, immunohistochemical and flow cytometric study of 11 cases. Hum Pathol 1993;24:1298–305.

79. Suarez-Vilela D, Izquierdo-Garcia FM, Nieves-Diez C, Salas-Valien Y, Gonzalez-Moran MA. Tumor rabdoide maligno de vesícula biliar. Estudio inmunohisto-químico y ultraestructural de un caso. Patología (Esp) 1996;20:263–67.

80. Tschang T, Garza-Garza R, Kissane JM. Pleomorphic carcinoma of the pancreas: an analysis of 15 cases. Cancer 1977;39:2114–26.

81. Yamaguchi K, Enjoji M. Carcinoma of the gallbladder. A clinicopathology of 103 patients and a newly proposed staging. Cancer 1988;62:1425–32.

Molecular Pathology

82. Hanada K, Itoh M, Fujii K, et al. K-ras and p53 mutations in stage I gallbladder carcinoma with an anomalous junction of the pancreaticobiliary duct. Cancer 1996;77:452–8.

83. Imai M, Hoshi T, Ogawa K. K-ras codon 12 mutations in biliary tract tumors detected by polymerase chain reaction denaturing gradient gel electrophoresis. Cancer 1994;73:2727–33.

84. Malats N, Porta M, Pinol J, Corominas JM, Real FX. Ki-ras mutations as a prognostic factor in extrahepatic bile system cancer. J Clin Oncol 1995;13:1679–86.

85. Suzuki T, Takano Y, Kakita A, Okudaira M. An immunohistochemical and molecular biological study of c-erbß-2 amplification and prognostic relevance in gallbladder cancer. Path Res Pract 1993;189:283–92.

86. Teh M, Wee A, Raju GC. An immunohistochemical study of p53 protein in gallbladder and extrahepatic bile duct/ampullary carcinomas. Cancer 1994;74:1542–5.

87. Watanabe M, Asaka M, Tanaka J, Kwosawa M, Kasai M, Miyazaki T. Point mutation of K-ras gene codon 12 in biliary tract tumors. Gastroenterology 1994;107:1147–53.

88. Wee A, Teh M, Raju GC. Clinical importance of p53 protein in gallbladder carcinoma and its precursor lesions. J Clin Pathol 1994;47:453–6.

89. Weinberg RA. Oncogenes, antioncogenes and the molecular basis of multistep carcinogenesis. Cancer Res 1989;49:3713–21.

89a. Witsuba I, Albores-Saavedra J. Genetic abnormalities involved in the pathogenesis of gallbladder carcinoma. J Hepatobiliary Pancreat Surg (in press).

90. Wistuba I, Gazdar AF, Roa I, Albores-Saavedra J. p53 protein over-expression in gallbladder carcinoma and its precursor lesions. An immunohistochemical study. Hum Pathol 1996;27:360–5.

91. Wistuba I, Sugio K, Hung J, et al. Allele-specific mutations involved in the pathogenesis of endemic gallbladder carcinoma in Chile. Cancer Res 1995;55:2511–5.

Spread

92. al Qudah MS. Intraluminal implantation of gallbladder cancer into the bile ducts. Br J Surg 1994;81:590.

93. Baer HU, Metzger A, Glattli A, Klaiber C, Ruchti C, Czerniak A. Subcutaneous periumbilical metastasis of a gallbladder carcinoma after laparoscopic cholecystectomy. Surg Laparos Endos 1995;5:59–63.

94. Clair DG, Lautz DB, Brooks DC. Rapid development of umbilical metastases after laparoscopic cholecystectomy for unsuspected gallbladder carcinoma. Surgery 1993;113:355–8.

95. Fahim RB, McDonnell JR, Richards JC, Ferris DO. Carcinoma of the gallbladder: a study of its modes of spread. Ann Surg 1962;156:114–24.

96. Fong Y, Brennan MF, Turnbull AT, Colt D, Blumgart LH. Gallbladder cancer discovered during laparoscopic surgery. Potential for iatrogenic tumor dissemination. Arch Surg 1993;128:1054–6.

96a. Fong Y, Heffernan N, Blumgart LH. Gallbladder carcinoma discovered during laparoscopic cholecystectomy: aggressive resection is beneficial. Cancer 1998;83:423–7.

97. Kirshbaum JD, Kozoll DD. Carcinoma of the gallbladder and extrahepatic bile ducts. Surg Gynec Obstet 1975;55:531–6.

98. Kotorac V. Biliary peritonitis resulting from a perforated carcinomatous gallbladder. Gastroenterology 1972;63:328–30.

99. Nally C, Preshaw RM. Tumour implantation at umbilicus after laparoscopic cholecystectomy for unsuspected gallbladder carcinoma. Canad J Surg 1994;37:243–4.

100. Ohtani T, Shirai Y, Tsukuda K, Hatakeyama K, Muto T. The association between extrahepatic biliary carcinoma and the junction of the cystic duct and the biliary tree. Europ J Surg 1994;160:37–40.

101. Schust DJ, Moore DH, Baird DB, Novotny DB. Primary adenocarcinoma of the gallbladder presenting as primary gynecologic malignancy: a report of two cases. Obstet Gynecol 1994;83:83:1–4.

102. Shirai Y, Tsukada K, Ohtani T, Watanabe H, Hatakeyama K. Hepatic metastases from carcinoma of the gallbladder. Cancer 1995;75:2063–8.

103. Shirai Y, Yoshida K, Tsukada K, Ohtani T, Muto T. Identification of the regional lymphatic system of the gallbladder by vital staining. Br J Surg 1992;79:659–62.

104. Sons HU, Borchard F, Joel BS. Carcinoma of the gallbladder: autopsy findings in 287 cases and review of the literature. J Surg Oncol 1985;28:199–206.

104a. Tuas RJ, Kousdtaal J, Koeler PJ. Meningeal carcinomatosis as presenting symptom of a gallbladder carcinoma. Clin Neurol Neurosurg 1993;95:253–6.

105. Tsukada K, Kurosaki I, Uchida K, et al. Lymph node spread from carcinoma of the gallbladder. Cancer 1997;80:661–7.

106. Vazquez-Echarri J, Peydro Blasco J, Garcia-Garcia S, et al. Embolic implantation of a cancer of the gallbladder into the distal choledochus. A rare cause of obstructive jaundice. Rev Esp Enferm Dig 1985;68:61–5.

107. Wibbenmeyer LA, Wade TP, Chen RC, Meyer RC, Turgeon RP, Andrus CH. Laparoscopic cholecystectomy can disseminate in situ carcinoma of the gallbladder. J Am Coll Surg 1995;181:504–10.

108. Young RH, Scully RE. Ovarian metastases from carcinoma of the gallbladder and extrahepatic bile ducts simulating primary tumors of the ovary. A report of six cases. Int J Gynecol Pathol 1990;9:60–72.

Prognostic Factors

109. Baretton G, Blasenbreu S, Vogt T, Löhrs U, Schmidt M. DNA ploidy in carcinoma of the gallbladder. Prognostic significance and comparison of flow and image cytometry on archival tumor material. Pathol Res Pract 1994;190:584–92.

110. Bergdahl L. Gallbladder carcinoma first diagnosed at microscopic examination of gallbladders removed for presumed benign disease. Ann Surg 1980;191:19–22.

111. Bivins BA, Meeker WR Jr, Griffen WO Jr. Importance of histologic classification of carcinoma of the gallbladder. Am Surg 1975;41:121–4.

112. Fleming DI, Cooper JS, Henson DE, et al. AJCG Cancer staging manual, 5th ed., Philadelphia: Lippincott-Raven, 1997.

113. Henson DE, Albores-Saavedra J, Corle D. Carcinoma of the gallbladder. Histologic types, stage of disease, and survival rates. Cancer 1992;70:1498–501.

114. Hisatomi K, Haratake J, Horie A, Ohsato K, Relation of histopathological features to prognosis of gallbladder cancer. Am J Gastroenterol 1990;85:567–72.

115. Nevin JE, Moran TJ, Kay S, King R. Carcinoma of the gallbladder: staging, treatment, and prognosis. Cancer 1976;37:141–8.

116. Sobin LH, Wittekind CH. TNM classification of malignant tumours. 5th ed, New York: Wiley-Liss, 1997.

117. Suzuki T, Takano Y, Kakita A, Okudaira M. An immunohistochemical and molecular biological study of c-erbB-2 amplification and prognostic relevance in gallbladder cancer. Pathol Res Pract 1993;189:283–92.

Survival

118. Ames D. Primary carcinoma of the gallbladder. Johns Hopkins Hosp Bull 1984;5:74–80.

119. Onoyama H, Yamamoto M, Tseng A, Ajiki T, Saitoh Y. Extended cholecystectomy for carcinoma of the gallbladder. World J Surg 1995;19:758–63.

119a. Morrow CE, Sutherland DE, Florack G, Eisenberg MM, Grage TB. Primary gallbladder carcinoma: significance of subserosal lesions and results of aggressive surgical treatment and adjuvant chemotherapy. Surgery 1983;94:709–14.

120. Perpetuo MM, Valdivieso M, Heilbrun LK, et al. Natural history study of gallbladder cancer: a review of 36 years experience at M.D. Anderson Hospital and Tumor Institute. Cancer 1978;42:330–5.

121. Shimada H, Endo I, Togo S, Nakano A, Izumi T. The role of lymph node dissection in the treatment of gallbladder carcinoma. Cancer 1997;79:892–9.

122. Shirai Y, Yoshida K, Tsukada K, Muto T, Watanabe H. Radical surgery for gallbladder carcinoma. Long-term results. Ann Surg 1992;216:565–8.

122a. Todoroki T. Radiation therapy for primary gallbladder cancer. Hepatogastroenterology 1997;44:1229–39.

✧✧✧

7

ENDOCRINE TUMORS AND TUMORS OF PARAGANGLIA

ENDOCRINE TUMORS

Carcinoid Tumors

Carcinoid tumors of the gallbladder are neoplasms of the diffuse endocrine cell system that usually exhibit trabecular, insular, or nesting growth patterns, with occasional tubule formation (2). However, as in other segments of the gastrointestinal tract, carcinoids of the gallbladder show a broad morphologic spectrum. The cell population includes different neuroendocrine cell types. Moreover, the metastatic potential is probably related to the size of the tumor rather than to its histologic structure. Immunohistochemistry has increased the accuracy of diagnosing carcinoid tumors because it allows identification of their secretory products. However, most carcinoid tumors of the gallbladder synthesize more than one substance, including serotonin and one or more peptide hormones. Some of these tumors are reactive only for the general neuroendocrine markers, such as chromogranin and synaptophysin. Functional classification, therefore, is of little practical value, except in those rare cases in which only a single peptide hormone is detected (somatostatinoma, gastrinoma). Rarely, carcinoid tumors of the gallbladder are associated with the Zollinger-Ellison syndrome or with multiple endocrine neoplasia type 1 (MEN 1).

Although rare, the incidence of carcinoid tumors of the gallbladder is difficult to determine because the terminology of endocrine tumors of the biliary tract is controversial and the criteria for diagnosis and classification differ among pathologists. Among 3,557 carcinoid tumors of the gastrointestinal tract collected by the Surveillance, Epidemiology, and End Results (SEER) Program of the National Cancer Institute from 1973 to 1991, there were 18 (0.5 percent) carcinoids of the gallbladder (15). A variety of malignant epithelial tumors with endocrine differentiation have been erroneously designated as carcinoid tumors. For example, adenocarcinomas of the gallbladder containing numerous endocrine cells (3) have been interpreted as carcinoid tumors (28). This interpretation is further complicated by the focal solid and nesting growth patterns exhibited by some of these adenocarcinomas which can simulate endocrine or carcinoid features. Small cell carcinomas with prominent trabecular or ribbon patterns have also been designated as malignant carcinoid tumors (6,12); signet ring cell carcinomas containing endocrine cells have even been interpreted as signet ring cell carcinoids (21). The tubular variant of carcinoid tumor has been confused with well-differentiated adenocarcinoma (1,2). Moreover, carcinoid tumors have been reported as APUDomas and the term "neuroendocrine carcinoma" has been used indiscriminately as a synonym for carcinoid tumor or for small cell carcinoma (9,13).

At least 25 well-documented examples of carcinoid tumors of the gallbladder have been reported (22), and, as mentioned, 18 cases have been collected by the SEER Program during a 19-year period (15).

Clinical Features. Small carcinoid tumors are usually incidental findings in gallbladders removed for cholelithiasis. Most, however, are symptomatic; they give rise to cholecystitis-like symptoms and can be visualized by ultrasonography, computed tomography, and angiography (10,11). Three patients with liver metastases developed the carcinoid syndrome (5,24,25). The Zollinger-Ellison syndrome was caused by a gastrin-secreting carcinoid tumor (4,17). In contrast to somatostatinomas of the pancreas, somatostatin-producing carcinoids of the biliary tree are not clinically functioning tumors. To our knowledge, there has been only one patient reported with carcinoid tumors of the gallbladder and stomach associated with the Zollinger-Ellison syndrome and MEN 1 (4). High serum levels of somatostatin, secretin, calcitonin, and 5-hydroxyindoleacetic acid have occasionally been found (18).

Second primary tumors are not unusual in patients with carcinoid tumors of the gallbladder. In addition to the carcinoid tumor, one patient had an intracranial meningioma (8). Another patient had two malignant tumors, a hepatocellular carcinoma and a colonic adenocarcinoma (14). Another had carcinoma of the uterine cervix and a

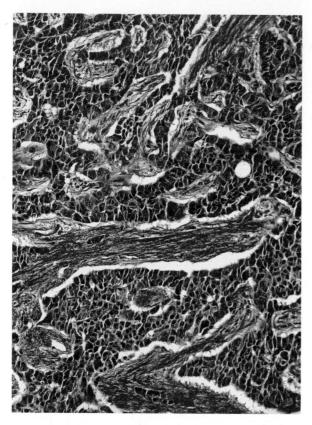

Figure 7-1
CARCINOID TUMOR
This carcinoid tumor of the gallbladder displays a trabecular growth pattern. The trabeculae are separated by fibrous bands.

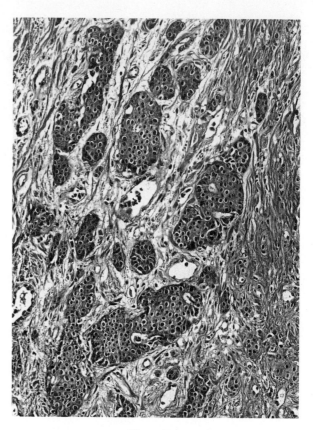

Figure 7-2
CARCINOID TUMOR
The characteristic insular pattern is shown.

breast carcinoma (22). One carcinoid tumor coexisted with and was in close proximity to a multifocal carcinoma in situ of the gallbladder (23). Two patients had multicentric carcinoid tumors in the gallbladder and the small intestine (1,25).

Gross Findings. Carcinoid tumors measuring 3 to 5 mm appear as small nodular or polypoid elevations of the mucosa. Because of their small size these lesions can easily be overlooked on gross examination of cholecystectomy specimens (22). Larger neoplasms are nodular or polypoid submucosal masses that infiltrate the full thickness of the wall and may even extend into the liver or adjacent hollow viscera. Most carcinoid tumors are gray-white or yellow and measure less than 2 cm. They can arise in any part of the gallbladder.

Microscopic Findings. Most carcinoid tumors of the gallbladder exhibit the characteristic organoid pattern described for such tumors in

other anatomic locations. The tumor cells are often arranged in small nests, cords, or trabeculae separated by delicate fibrous bands (figs. 7-1–7-3). Occasionally, microtubular structures that contain extracellular mucin are present. The neoplastic cells are small and uniform, and contain round or oval nuclei with finely granular chromatin and inconspicuous nucleoli (fig. 7-4). The cytoplasm is eosinophilic and granular or clear. We have seen a carcinoid tumor composed predominantly of cells with oncocytic features. Likewise, the tubular variant of carcinoid tumor, similar to that found in the appendix, has been described in the gallbladder (fig. 7-5) (1,2). Since this tumor consists predominantly of tubular structures lined by cuboidal or columnar cells, it can be confused with a well-differentiated adenocarcinoma (1,2). The Grimelius stain reveals cytoplasmic argyrophil granules in most carcinoid tumors of the gallbladder while argentaffin granules are present in a small number of tumors.

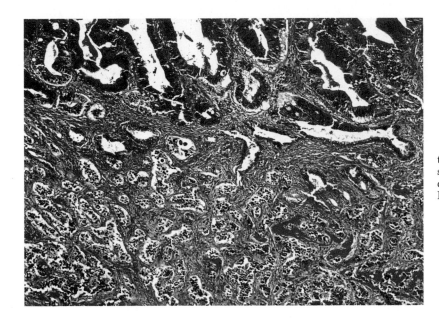

Figure 7-3
CARCINOID TUMOR
This carcinoid is composed of cords and trabeculae separated by dense fibrous tissue and is growing beneath an in situ carcinoma of the gallbladder. (Courtesy of Dr. M.B. Resnick, Boston, MA.)

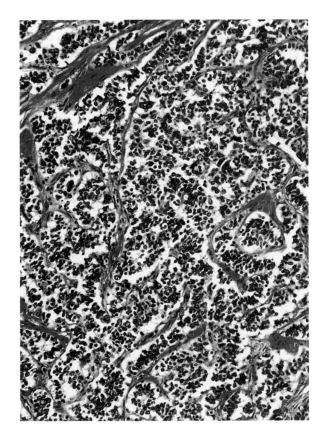

Figure 7-4
CARCINOID TUMOR
This carcinoid tumor is composed of small round cells and therefore can be confused with small cell carcinoma.

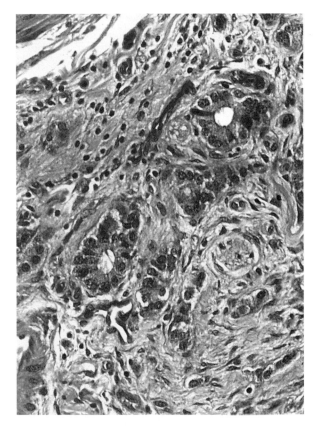

Figure 7-5
TUBULAR CARCINOID
Small tubular structures lined by cuboidal cells and thin cords lie in a fibrous stroma.

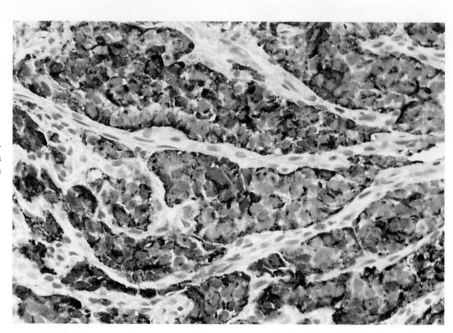

Figure 7-6
CARCINOID TUMOR
Diffuse and strong immunoreactivity for chromogranin is seen
in the carcinoid tumor shown in
figure 7-4.

Immunohistochemical and Electron Microscopic Findings. The few carcinoid tumors that have been studied with immunohistochemical techniques, including five of our own, have shown diffuse reactivity for the general neuroendocrine markers including chromogranin, synaptophysin, and neuron-specific enolase (fig. 7-6) (23). Some tumors have also expressed reactivity for serotonin (23), somatostatin (9,14), pancreatic polypeptide (9,26), or gastrin (17). More than one substance has been detected in most tumors. Numerous round neurosecretory granules of variable density and measuring between 150 and 300 nm have been found in the cytoplasm of tumor cells by electron microscopy.

Prognosis. The biologic behavior of carcinoid tumors of the gallbladder is not well known because most cases are reported soon after diagnosis and follow-up is short. None of the patients with tumors less than 1 cm had metastases at the time of publication. However, lymph node and liver metastases have been reported with larger tumors. The 5-year survival rate of the 18 patients with symptomatic carcinoid tumors of the gallbladder from the SEER program was 41.3 percent (15). Of these 18 patients, 38.9 percent had carcinoid tumors confined to the gallbladder wall.

We have previously reported a unique neoplasm of the gallbladder with features of an atypical carcinoid tumor as described in the lung (1). In addition to the characteristic organoid pattern and cytologic features of a carcinoid tumor, it had atypical areas with increased mitotic activity and foci of necrosis. The tumor behaved aggressively; the patient died with multiple metastases 14 months after diagnosis. Whether this atypical carcinoid tumor requires separation from the classic carcinoid tumor remains to be determined.

Composite or combined adenocarcinoma-carcinoid tumors have been reported in the gallbladder (7,16,18–20,27). However, a critical analysis of these cases has led us to conclude that the majority were adenocarcinomas with numerous endocrine cells (3) or small cell carcinomas with foci of adenocarcinoma. In composite tumors, the adenocarcinomatous and carcinoid components are easily recognized with conventional stains. In adenocarcinomas with endocrine cells, the latter elements are not detected in hematoxylin and eosin–stained sections (3). Identification of the endocrine cells requires immunohistochemistry or electron microscopy. Occasionally, adenocarcinomas may even show a solid growth pattern with endocrine cells, resembling a carcinoid tumor. The cytologic features of the solid areas, however, are similar to those of the glandular component.

TUMORS OF PARAGANGLIA

Paraganglioma

This exceedingly rare benign tumor of the gall-bladder is composed of chief and sustentacular cells arranged in a nesting pattern. The only two reported examples and two of our own were incidentally found in cholecystectomy specimens (31,33). Most likely, the tumor arises from the small paraganglia located within the perimuscular connective tissue (29,30,32). Grossly, it appears as a small nodule that measures less than 1 cm and protrudes from the external surface. Microscopically, paragangliomas are well or poorly demarcated and composed predominantly of chief cells arranged in a nesting or "zellballen" pattern (figs. 7-7, 7-8). The chief cells have abundant eosinophilic or clear cytoplasm and round

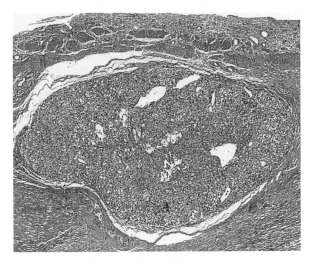

Figure 7-7
PARAGANGLIOMA
This paraganglioma appears as a well-demarcated nodule in the perimuscular connective tissue of the gallbladder.

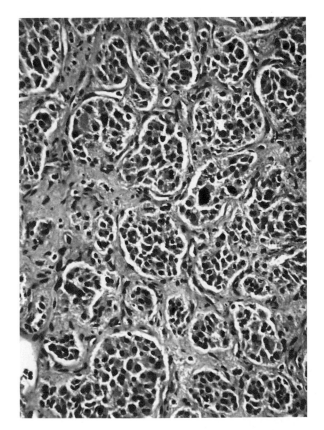 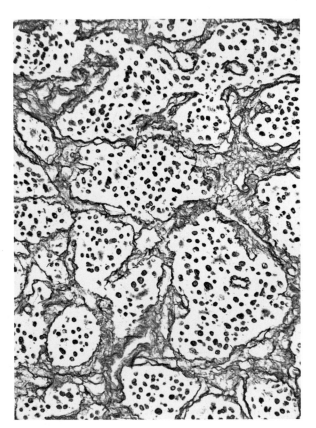

Figure 7-8
PARAGANGLIOMA
Left: This tumor contains nests of polygonal cells, some with large hyperchromatic nuclei. The nests are separated by thin fibrous septa containing capillaries.
Right: Reticulin stain shows a zellballen pattern and intervening vascular septa. (Courtesy of Dr. H.D. Appelman, Ann Arbor, MI.)

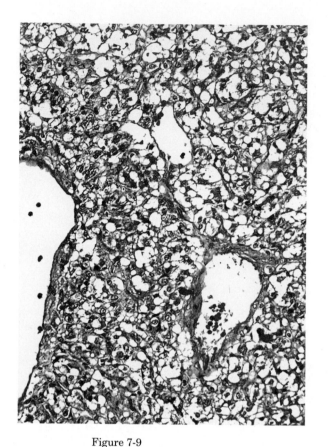

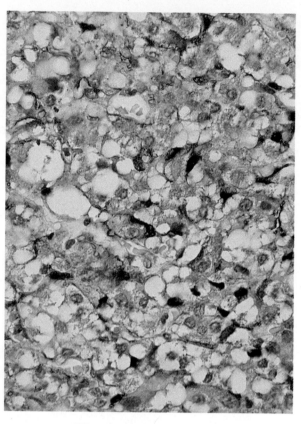

Figure 7-9
PARAGANGLIOMA
This paraganglioma is composed predominantly of clear cells.

Figure 7-10
PARAGANGLIOMA
S-100 protein immunostain highlights the sustentacular cells of this paraganglioma of the gallbladder.

hyperchromatic nuclei (fig. 7-9). Small nests of chief cells are surrounded by sustentacular cells which can be highlighted with the S-100 protein stain (fig. 7-10). The chief cells are immunoreactive for neuron-specific enolase and chromogranin. We were not able to detect peptide hormones by immunohistochemistry in two paragangliomas of the gallbladder.

REFERENCES

Carcinoid Tumors

1. Albores-Saavedra J, Henson DE. Tumors of the gallbladder and extrahepatic bile ducts. Atlas of Tumor Pathology, 2nd Series, Fascicle 22. Washington, D.C.: Armed Forces Institute of Pathology, 1986.
2. Albores-Saavedra J, Henson DE, Sobin LH. In: WHO histological typing of tumours of the gallbladder and extrahepatic bile ducts. Berlin: Springer-Verlag, 1991.
3. Albores-Saavedra J, Nadji M, Henson DE, Angeles-Angeles A. Entero-endocrine cell differentiation in carcinomas of the gallbladder and mucinous cystadenocarcinomas of the pancreas. Path Res Pract 1988;183: 169–75.
4. Barone GW, Schaefer RF, Counce JS, Eidt JF. Gallbladder and gastric argyrophil carcinoid associated with a case of Zollinger-Ellison syndrome. Am J Gastroenterol 1992;87:392–4.
5. Bergdahl L. Carcinoid tumor of the biliary tract. Aust NZ J Surg 1976;46:136–8.
6. Bosl GJ, Yagoda A, Camara-Lopez LH. Malignant carcinoid of the gallbladder. Third reported case and review of the literature. J Surg Oncol 1980;13:215–22.
7. Fish DE, Al-Izzi M, George PP, Whitaker B. Combined endocrine cell carcinoma and adenocarcinoma of the gallbladder. Histopathology 1990;17:471–2.

8. Gaffney PR, Coyle LJ. Carcinoid tumor of the gallbladder associated with a meningioma. Ir J Med Sci 1978;147:318–21.

9. Heymann MF, Fiche M, Dubois-Gordeeff A, et al. Endocrine cell carcinoma (carcinoid tumour) of the gallbladder producing pancreatic polypeptide and somatostatin. Histopathology 1997;30:606–7.

10. Jutte DL, Bell RH, Penn I, et al. Carcinoid tumors of the biliary system. Dig Dis Sci 1986;32:763–9.

11. Kitagawa K, Takashima T, Matsui O, Kadoya M, Karatake KJ, Tsuji M. Angiographic findings in two carcinoid tumors of the gallbladder. Gastrointest Radiol 1986;11:51–5.

12. Kumar S, Agarwal S, Bhargava SK, Minocha VR. Malignant carcinoid tumor of the gallbladder: a case report and review of literature. Tropical Gastroenterol 1992;13:78–84.

13. McLean CA, Pedersen JS. Endocrine cell carcinoma of the gallbladder. Histopathology 1991;19:173–6.

14. Mochizuki M. Minute carcinoid tumor of the gallbladder. Acta Pathol Jpn 1991;41:383–5.

15. Modlin IM, Sandor A. An analysis of 8305 cases of carcinoid tumors. Cancer 1997;79:813–29.

16. Muto Y, Okamoto K, Uchimura M. Composite tumor (ordinary adenocarcinoma, typical carcinoid and goblet cell adcnocarcinoid) of the gallbladder: a variety of composite tumor. Am J Gastroenterol 1984;79:645–9.

17. Nakamura S, Tajima S, Sato K. An autopsied case of malignant Zollinger-Ellison syndrome due to gastrinoma of the gallbladder accompanied by giant intrahepatic metastases. Gan no Rinsho 1978;24:152–61.

18. Noda M, Miwa A, Kitagawa M. Carcinoid tumors of the gallbladder with adenocarcinomatous differentiation: a morphologic and immunohistochemical study. Am J Gastroenterol 1989;84:953–7.

19. Ohmori T, Furuya K, Okada K, Tabei R, Tao S. Adenoendocrine cell carcinoma of the gallbladder: a histochemical and immunohistochemical study. Acta Pathol Jpn 1993;43:268–74.

20. Olinici CD, Vasiu R. Composite endocrine cell, typical adenocarcinoma and signet ring carcinoma of the gallbladder. Rom J Morphol Embryol 1991;37:171–3.

21. Papotti M, Galliano D, Monga G. Signet-ring cell carcinoid of the gallbladder. Histopathology 1990;17:255–9.

22. Porter JM, Kalloo AN, Abernathy EC, Yeo AJ. Carcinoid tumor of the gallbladder: laparoscopic resection and review of the literature. Surgery 1992;112:100–5.

23. Resnick MB, Jacobs DO, Brodsky GL. Multifocal adenocarcinoma in situ with underlying carcinoid tumor of the gallbladder. Arch Pathol Lab Med 1994;118:933–4.

24. Salimi Z, Sharafuddin M. Ultrasound appearance of primary carcinoid tumor of the gallbladder associated with carcinoid syndrome. J Clin Ultrasound 1995;23:435–7.

25. Slany J, Wonger R, Kuhlmayer R. Multiple primary carcinoid of the gallbladder, pancreas and ileum with cardiac metastases. Z Gastroenterol 1969;7:213–9.

26. Tanaka K, Lida Y, Tsutsumi Y. Pancreatic polypeptide-immunoreactive gallbladder carcinoid tumor. Acta Pathol Jpn 1992;115–8.

27. Wada A, Ishiguro S, Tateishi R, et al. Carcinoid tumor of the gallbladder associated with adenocarcinoma. Cancer 1983;51:1911–7.

28. Yamamoto M, Nakajo S, Miyoshi N, Nakais S, Tahara E. Endocrine cell carcinoma (carcinoid) of the gallbladder. Am J Surg Pathol 1989;13:292–302.

Paraganglioma

29. Fine G, Raju UB. Paraganglia in the human gallbladder. Arch Pathol Lab Med 1980;104:265–8.

30. Kuo T, Anderson CB, Rosai J. Normal paraganglia in the human gallbladder. Arch Pathol 1974;97:46–7.

31. Miller TA, Weber TR, Appelman HD. Paraganglioma of the gallbladder. Arch Surg 1972;105:637–9.

32. Raju UB, Fine G. Ultrastructure of the gallbladder paraganglia. Arch Pathol Lab Med 1980;104:379–83.

33. Wolff M. Paraganglia of the gallbladder [Letter]. Arch Surg 1973;107:493.

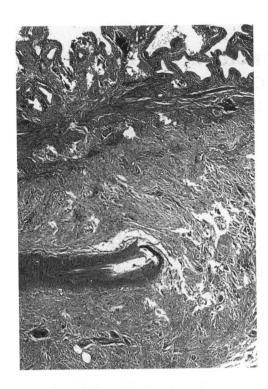

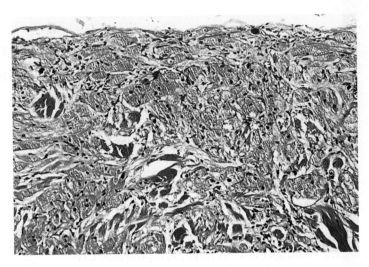

Figure 8-2
GRANULAR CELL TUMOR
Left: Low-power view of a granular cell tumor that involved predominantly the muscular layer and the subserosal connective tissue of the gallbladder.
Above: Higher magnification showing sheets of granular cells, some of which have large hyperchromatic nuclei.

described (14,15). Grossly, they appear as intramural nodules or as polypoid lesions measuring less than 1 cm in diameter; microscopically, they do not differ from neurofibromas seen in other anatomic sites. We have observed a plexiform neurofibroma in the wall of the gallbladder from a 62-year-old woman.

Neurofibromatosis

Involvement of the gallbladder by neurofibromatosis is distinctly uncommon. Only a few cases, usually associated with neurofibromatosis type I, have been mentioned in review papers (16). However, no pathologic description has been reported. We have had the opportunity to study two patients: a 28-year-old female with type II neurofibromatosis, and a 53-year-old male with type I neurofibromatosis. In both patients the involved segment of gallbladder wall was polypoid and covered with an intact smooth mucosa (fig. 8-3). Microscopically, polypoid nodules of spindle cells with wavy nuclei, identified as Schwann cells, expanded the lamina propria and were covered by a normal mucosa (figs. 8-4, 8-5). The spindle cells had a fascicular growth pattern and were S-100 protein positive (fig. 8-6). A few ganglion cells were recognized in the first case.

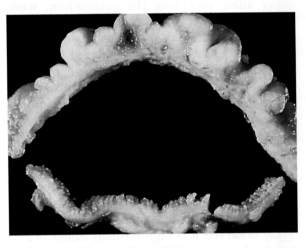

Figure 8-3
NEUROFIBROMATOSIS
Polypoid nodules are covered by intact gallbladder mucosa.

Ganglioneuromatosis

Ganglioneuromatosis of the gallbladder is found in some patients with type 2b multiple endocrine neoplasia syndrome (18,19). The basic histologic changes, which are similar to those found in the small and large intestine, include Schwann cell and ganglion cell proliferation, primarily in the lamina propria, as well as enlarged and distorted

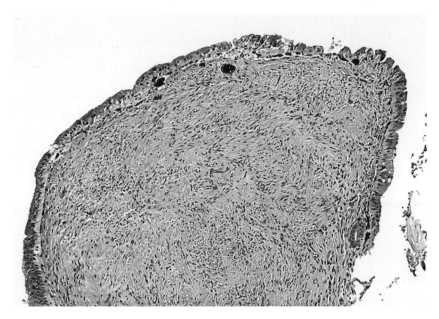

Figure 8-4
NEUROFIBROMATOSIS
A polypoid nodule covered by normal gallbladder epithelium is composed of spindle-shaped cells separated by abundant fibrous stroma.

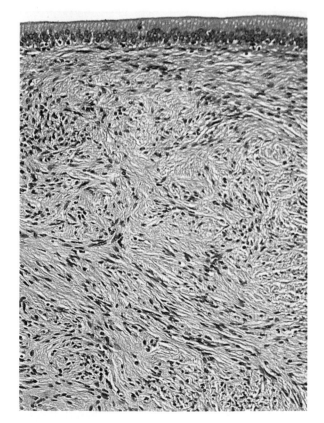

Figure 8-5
NEUROFIBROMATOSIS
Higher magnification of neurofibromatosis of the gallbladder. Fascicles of spindle-shaped cells expand the lamina propria.

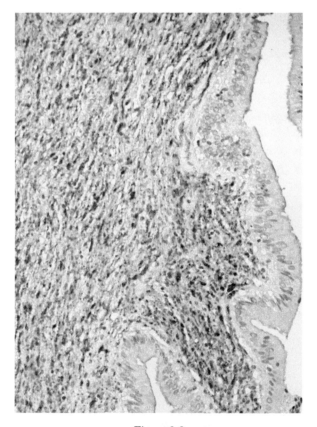

Figure 8-6
NEUROFIBROMATOSIS
Nearly all spindle-shaped cells are immunoreactive for S-100 protein.

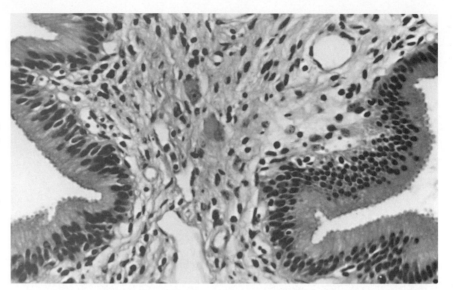

Figure 8-7
GANGLIONEUROMATOSIS
A small group of ganglion cells is visible in the lamina propria. (Fig. 25 from Fascicle 22, 2nd Series.)

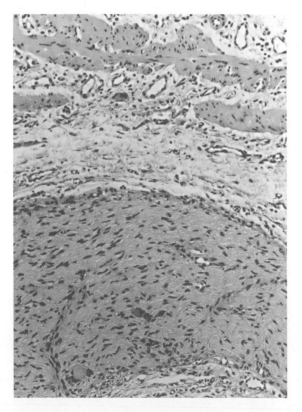

Figure 8-8
GANGLIONEUROMATOSIS
An enlarged nerve trunk is present in the perimuscular connective tissue. A few ganglion cells are also visible. (Fig. 26 from Fascicle 22, 2nd Series.)

nerves with a plexiform appearance in the muscle layer and perimuscular connective tissue (figs. 8-7, 8-8). Lesions have been observed in children and adults, and may cause biliary tract symptoms. In adults, ganglioneuromatosis coexisting with cholelithiasis has been documented (17). The ganglioneuromatosis might have led to poor contraction, resulting in bile stasis and formation of gallstones.

Involvement of the gallbladder should be considered in patients who are known to have the syndrome and who develop symptoms related to the biliary tract.

MALIGNANT MESENCHYMAL TUMORS

Malignant mesenchymal tumors of the gallbladder are so rare as to constitute pathologic curiosities. Many of these tumors reported in the older literature, especially those in which no specific cell type was recognized or which were considered spindle, pleomorphic, or round cell sarcomas, were probably undifferentiated spindle and giant cell carcinomas or the spindle cell variant of squamous carcinoma. As emphasized by others, undifferentiated spindle and giant cell carcinomas can be mistaken for sarcomas (21–23).

We have personally studied a rhabdomyosarcoma, a malignant fibrous histiocytoma, and an angiosarcoma of the gallbladder. The rhabdomyosarcoma occurred in a 2-year-old girl, was of

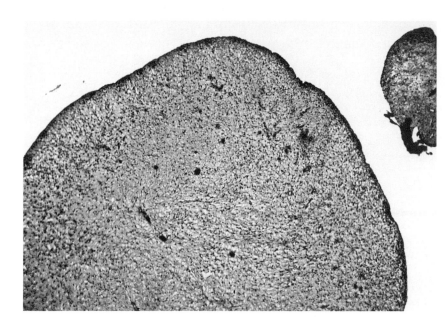

Figure 8-9
EMBRYONAL
RHABDOMYOSARCOMA
(SARCOMA BOTRYOIDES)
The polypoid structure is composed of loose myxoid stroma and contains many dilated blood vessels. This structure is characteristic of sarcoma botryoides and should not be mistaken for a benign polyp.

embryonal type, had typical botryoid features, and invaded the liver by direct extension, but not the extrahepatic bile ducts (figs. 8-9–8-11). Immunohistologic stains revealed that many neoplastic round cells, especially those with an abundant eosinophilic cytoplasm, contained desmin and myoglobin, which have also been found in cells from embryonal rhabdomyosarcomas in other sites (fig. 8-12). An example of rhabdomyosarcoma considered to be primary in the gallbladder also involved the common bile duct (26). In cases like this, it is impossible to ascertain whether the gallbladder tumor represents an extension of the rhabdomyosarcoma of the common bile duct or vice versa. Embryonal rhabdomyosarcoma is less common in the gallbladder than in the extrahepatic bile ducts. Less than five well-documented cases have been reported in the gallbladder.

The malignant fibrous histiocytoma was a gray-white necrotic mass that coexisted with lithiasis. It replaced most of the gallbladder from a 60-year-old woman. The tumor extended to the liver, did not metastasize, but caused the death of the patient. It was a densely cellular neoplasm composed of histiocytes and fibroblasts arranged in bundles and showing the characteristic storiform pattern (fig. 8-13). Numerous collagen fibers were seen between the neoplastic cells which were negative for cytokeratin and epithelial membrane antigen.

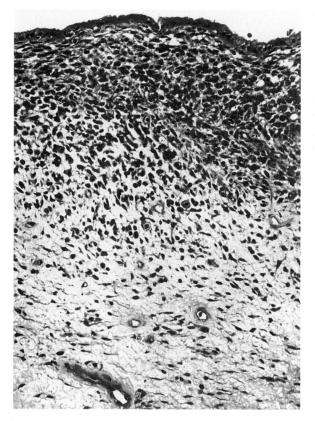

Figure 8-10
EMBRYONAL RHABDOMYOSARCOMA
(SARCOMA BOTRYOIDES)
Immediately beneath the biliary epithelium is a concentration of primitive mesenchymal cells that forms the cambium layer. Myxoid areas are present in the deeper part of the tumor.

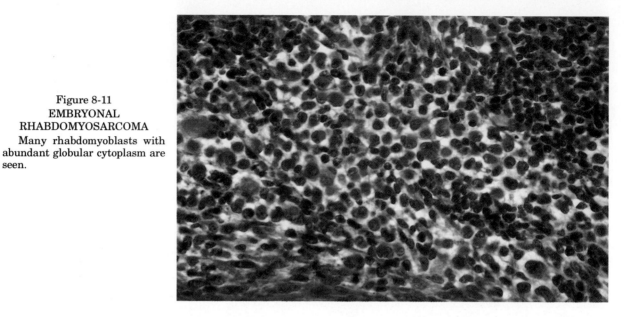

Figure 8-11
EMBRYONAL
RHABDOMYOSARCOMA
Many rhabdomyoblasts with abundant globular cytoplasm are seen.

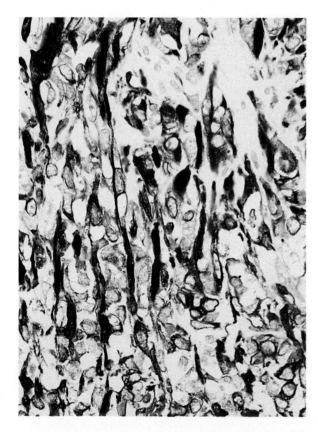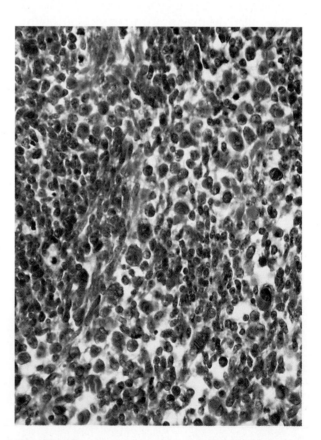

Figure 8-12
EMBRYONAL RHABDOMYOSARCOMA
Left: The strap rhabdomyoblasts are desmin positive. Cross-striations are visible in some of the cells.
Right: Myoglobin-positive rhabdomyoblasts are seen in this embryonal rhabdomyosarcoma.

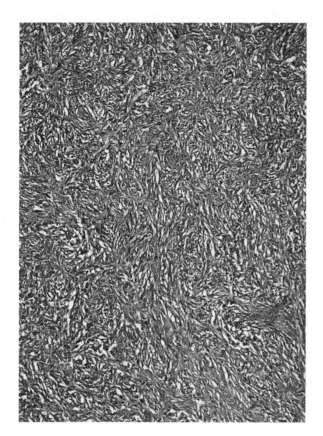 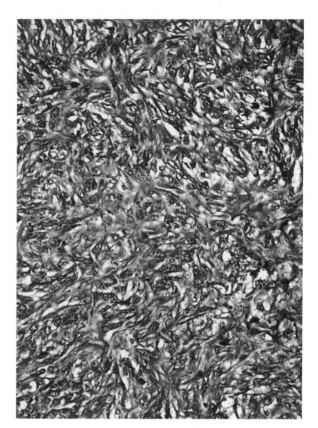

Figure 8-13
MALIGNANT FIBROUS HISTIOCYTOMA
Left: Spindle cells mixed with histiocytes are arranged in bundles with areas showing a storiform pattern.
Right: Detail of spindle cells with vesicular nuclei. Abundant collagen fibers and well-defined storiform pattern are also seen.

A few primary leiomyosarcomas, which probably originated in the muscle layer, have been reported (24,27,29,30). Their histologic structure and antigenic profile are similar to those of leiomyosarcomas in other sites, and they can cause the same problems in diagnosis (figs. 8-14, 8-15). We had the opportunity to review an epithelioid leiomyosarcoma from the Armed Forces Institute of Pathology (AFIP) files that was muscle-specific actin and desmin positive.

The first reported example of angiosarcoma appeared as a small hemorrhagic nodule in the body of a gallbladder that was removed from a 62-year-old woman because of symptoms of chronic cholecystitis (20). Metastatic lesions appeared in the liver and omentum several months after diagnosis. The histologic features of the tumor did not differ from those of angiosarcomas in other locations. Two additional angiosarcomas of the gallbladder have been documented (25,28):

one occurred in a 56-year-old man and the other in an 81-year-old woman. Although the latter tumor showed epithelioid features, the neoplastic cells were positive for factor VIII–related antigen and CD31, but negative for cytokeratin, epithelial membrane antigen, and carcinoembryonic antigen. This immunohistochemical profile excluded a moderately differentiated adenocarcinoma with angiosarcoma-like areas.

Kaposi's Sarcoma

Because of the AIDS (acquired immunodeficiency syndrome) epidemic, Kaposi's sarcoma is now the most common sarcoma of the gallbladder in adults. We have seen six cases, two of which also involved the liver and the extrahepatic bile ducts. These tumors were incidental autopsy findings. Two AIDS patients with symptomatic Kaposi's sarcoma of the gallbladder in the absence of

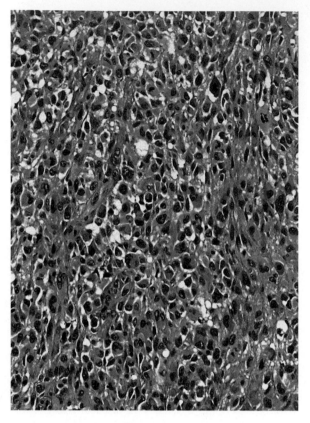

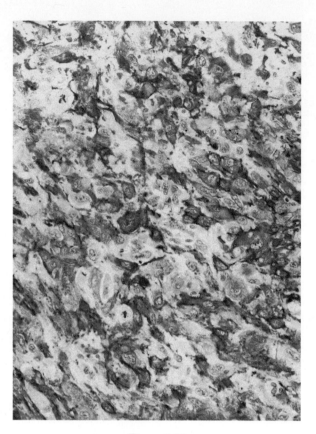

Figure 8-14
EPITHELIOID LEIOMYOSARCOMA
This leiomyosarcoma was composed predominantly of epithelial smooth muscle cells that were cytokeratin negative, but stained with the smooth muscle markers.

Figure 8-15
LEIOMYOSARCOMA
Most neoplastic cells of the leiomyosarcoma shown on figure 8-14 are smooth muscle actin positive.

cutaneous or gastrointestinal involvement have been reported (31,32). The hemorrhagic lesions are usually located in the subserosa or muscular wall of the gallbladder, and show the characteristic spindle cells and vascular slits.

MISCELLANEOUS MALIGNANT TUMORS

Carcinosarcoma

Carcinosarcomas are composed of variable proportions of both carcinomatous and sarcomatous elements (33–35,37–41). Characteristically, the sarcomatous component contains heterologous elements and lacks epithelial markers by immunocytochemistry or electron microscopy. Found in the same age groups as carcinomas and usually associated with stones, these tumors represent less than 1 percent of all malignant neoplasms of the gallbladder.

Gross Findings. Carcinosarcomas are polypoid tumors that measure from 3 to 15 cm, and can fill most of the gallbladder lumen (fig. 8-16). They are either pedunculated or sessile and often arise in the fundus. The cut surface shows gray-white or yellow tissue, usually with extensive areas of necrosis and hemorrhage. Cartilage can be recognized as small, blue-white, glistening nodules.

Microscopic Findings. The epithelial elements are both glandular and squamous. The glandular component is a constant feature, while foci of keratinizing malignant squamous cells are found in only one third of the tumors. The neoplastic glands are lined by cuboidal or columnar cells and separated by abundant malignant stroma containing heterologous elements (figs. 8-17, 8-18). These cuboidal or columnar epithelial cells may also display cord or trabecular

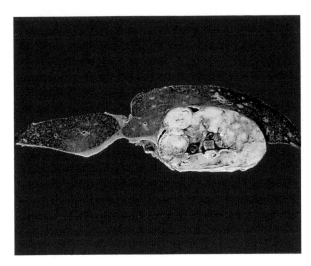

Figure 8-16
CARCINOSARCOMA
This large and partially necrotic carcinosarcoma filled and distended the gallbladder but did not invade the liver.

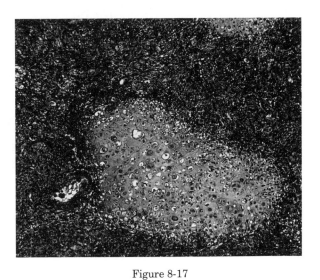

Figure 8-17
CARCINOSARCOMA
A focus of malignant cartilage and neoplastic glands is surrounded by a spindle cell sarcoma. (Courtesy of Dr. J.C. Mandard, Cain, France.)

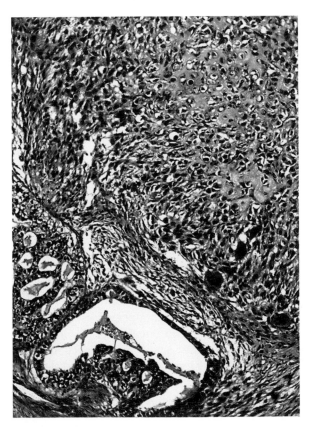

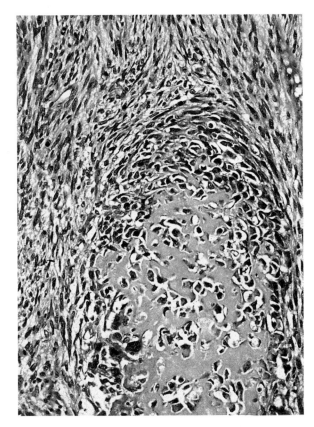

Figure 8-18
CARCINOSARCOMA
Left: Neoplastic glands, osteoid material surrounded by spindle cells, and osteoclast giant cells are seen.
Right: A well-defined focus of osteoid is surrounded by a spindle cell sarcoma.

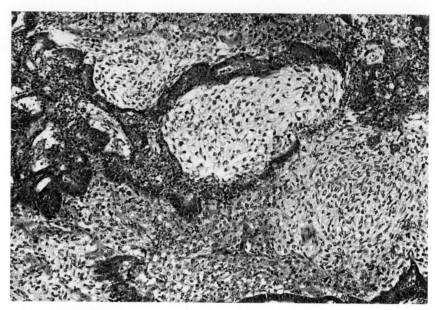

Figure 8-19
CARCINOSARCOMA
Anastomosing cords and glands are surrounded and compressed by a myxoid sarcoma. This tumor showed areas of hepatoid differentiation adjacent to clear cells.

growth patterns. In one of our cases, neoplastic glands and anastomosing cords of epithelial cells were focally compressed and surrounded by a malignant myxoid stroma, which also showed small nests and cords of glycogen-rich clear cells with hepatoid differentiation (fig. 8-19). These hepatoid areas expressed alpha-fetoprotein by immunohistochemistry. A component of small cell carcinoma with endocrine differentiation was present in one of nine carcinosarcomas we have examined. The malignant stroma comprises undifferentiated spindle cells arranged in broad interlacing bundles or displaying a storiform pattern. Occasionally, multinucleated giant cells with hyperchromatic nuclei are mixed with the spindle cells. The mesenchymal component also includes areas of malignant cartilage and bone. Rarely, foci of rhabdomyosarcoma have been identified by conventional stains and confirmed by electron microscopy and immunohistochemistry (38). Between these cellular elements there are many collagen and reticulin fibers. Blood vessel invasion and numerous mitotic figures, some abnormal, are readily identified.

The presence of heterologous elements distinguishes carcinosarcoma from undifferentiated spindle and giant cell carcinomas. Likewise, epithelial markers such as cytokeratin and epithelial membrane antigen are not present in the mesenchymal component of carcinosarcomas, but

are present in at least some of the spindle and giant cells of most undifferentiated carcinomas.

The origin of the stroma is uncertain and controversial, but the fact that cytokeratin and carcinoembryonic antigen are present only in the glandular and squamous components suggests that the spindle cells and heterologous elements might truly be of mesenchymal origin (fig. 8-20). However, we should note that poorly differentiated carcinomas arising in other organs such as breast, pancreas, and thyroid are known to produce cartilage and bone, which has been explained on the basis of a metaplastic process. Some pathologists believe that carcinosarcomas and undifferentiated carcinomas, spindle and giant cell type, regardless of their site of origin, are closely related and probably originate from the same cell. For this reason the unifying term "sarcomatoid carcinoma" has been proposed for these two tumors (42). However, since current histologic classifications are not based on histogenesis but on cell phenotype we prefer to retain the term "carcinosarcoma."

Analysis of the few reported cases and those we have examined personally indicates that carcinosarcomas are highly aggressive neoplasms that behave like carcinomas. Seven of nine patients from our series died with metastases, one is living with recurrence, and only one is disease free. Of 11 patients collected by the SEER program, 9 died as a result of the tumor (36). Direct extension

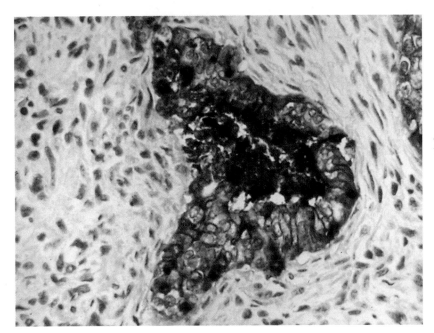

Figure 8-20
CARCINOSARCOMA
The neoplastic gland is carcinoembryonic antigen positive while the sarcomatous stroma is negative.

into the liver is common. Lymph node and pulmonary metastases occur in some patients. Both the carcinomatous and sarcomatous components have been recognized in metastatic deposits (37).

Malignant Melanoma

Most malignant melanomas of the gallbladder are metastatic and often incidental findings at autopsy (45,46,50). Only 17 patients with primary melanoma of the gallbladder have been reported (44,44a,47,51–53). Five had symptoms of cholecystitis and one had a perforated gallbladder. These patients fulfilled the following criteria: 1) despite a meticulous search, no other primary tumor was found; 2) they survived many years after cholecystectomy or died from metastatic melanoma months or years after the diagnosis; and 3) the gallbladder melanoma was a solitary polypoid mass that showed junctional activity and contained melanin pigment.

Primary malignant melanomas of gallbladder are usually solitary, polypoid masses that are heavily pigmented. Histologically, they are similar to the more common cutaneous melanomas. The junctional activity, which is characteristic for a primary melanoma, is seen along the epithelium overlying the tumor (figs. 8-21, 8-22). However, pagetoid spread, mimicking junctional activity, has been documented in metastatic ma-

lignant melanoma (48). Large expanding tumors that ulcerate the gallbladder mucosa do not show the junctional changes, consequently, a primary site in the gallbladder cannot be confirmed.

The immunohistochemical profile of melanoma of the gallbladder is similar to that of melanoma from other sites. They are S-100 protein and HMB-45 positive. Electron microscopy in one case revealed melanosomes in tumor cells as well as in adjacent normal gallbladder epithelium (49). Melanocytes, which are the origin of melanomas, have been observed in the normal human gallbladder (43).

Ideally, cases of primary malignant melanoma of the gallbladder should be confirmed by autopsy or long-term follow-up. Because of the unpredictable biologic behavior of melanoma and the presence of pagetoid spread in the epithelium adjacent to metastatic deposits, some have questioned the existence of this tumor in the gallbladder (48).

We have seen examples of undifferentiated carcinoma, spindle and giant cell type, that had been confused with primary malignant melanoma of the gallbladder. However, undifferentiated carcinomas lack junctional activity and do not contain melanin. Moreover, these epithelial tumors are cytokeratin positive and S-100 protein and HMB-45 negative.

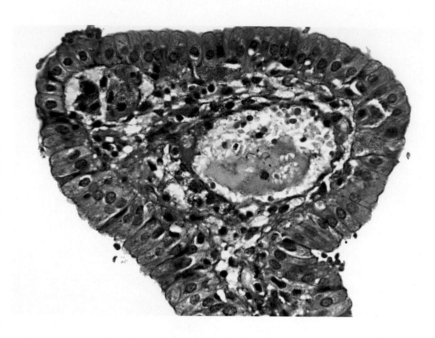

Figure 8-21
PRIMARY
MALIGNANT MELANOMA
Normal gallbladder mucosa shows foci of junctional activity. Note the presence of pigmented melanocytes wedged between the columnar mucosal cells. (Fig. 7 from Peison B, Rabin L. Malignant melanoma of the gallbladder. Cancer 1976;37:2448-54).

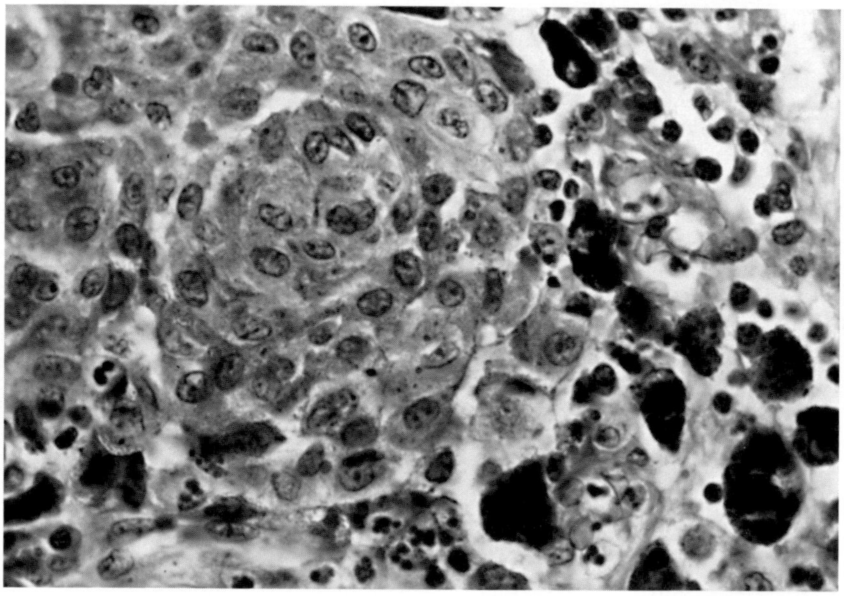

Figure 8-22
PRIMARY
MALIGNANT MELANOMA
This malignant melanoma shows nuclear hyperchromasia and cytoplasmic melanin granules. (Fig. 9 from Peison B, Rabin L. Malignant melanoma of the gallbladder. Cancer 1976;37:2448-54).

Malignant Lymphoma

Malignant lymphomas of any type may infiltrate the gallbladder, usually as part of a systemic process (57,61). Often, the tumor is an incidental finding in gallbladders removed for cholelithiasis. Rarely, patients with secondary lymphomas present with symptoms of acute or chronic cholecystitis (61). Primary malignant lymphomas of the gallbladder are exceedingly rare (54–56,60,62).

We reported five cases that involved the gallbladder, and in only one case was the lymphoma considered primary (54). This was a small lymphocytic diffuse B-cell malignant lymphoma that infiltrated the full thickness of the wall, but did not spread to regional lymph nodes or to adjacent organs (fig. 8-23). The patient has remained disease free 7 years after cholecystectomy. In the remaining four cases, the lymphomas were secondary and of B-cell phenotype. They were classified as large cell, small lymphocytic, immunoblastic, and follicular lymphoma (figs. 8-24, 8-25). Although very few examples of primary lymphomas of the gallbladder have been recorded, most can be classified as low-grade malignant lymphoma of mucosa-associated lymphoid tissue (MALToma) which appears to be the most common type of primary lymphoma of the gallbladder (54,55,60,62). Some of these tumors arise in a background of chronic cholecystitis with lymphoid hyperplasia (59).

A single example of angiotropic intravascular lymphoma in a 68-year-old woman has been reported (58). The malignant lymphoid cells were found predominantly within the small blood vessels of the gallbladder wall. Immunoreactivity for leukocyte common antigen and the pan B-cell markers confirmed the lymphoid nature of the neoplastic cells. Another example of an intravascular lymphoma recently reviewed by us occurred in a 64-year-old man with cholelithiasis. The tumor had histologic and immunohistochemical features of a large B-cell lymphoma (figs. 8-26, 8-27).

Grossly, malignant lymphomas are infiltrative gray-white lesions that produce thickening of the wall and may lead to ulceration of the mucosa. Despite the massive neoplastic lymphoid infiltration of the wall, the villous structure of the gallbladder is often preserved. As with lymphomas in other hollow viscera, regional

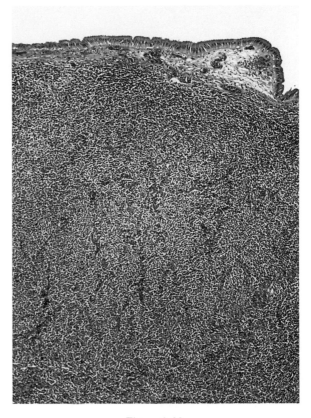

Figure 8-23
MALIGNANT LYMPHOMA,
SMALL CELL LYMPHOCYTIC TYPE
This malignant lymphoma, small lymphocytic type, infiltrated the full thickness of the gallbladder wall.

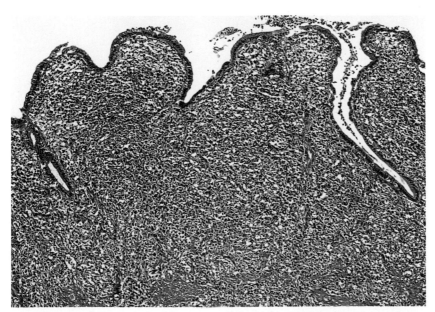

Figure 8-24
MALIGNANT LYMPHOMA,
LARGE CELL TYPE
Malignant lymphoma, large cell type, diffusely infiltrated the gallbladder. The surface epithelium is normal.

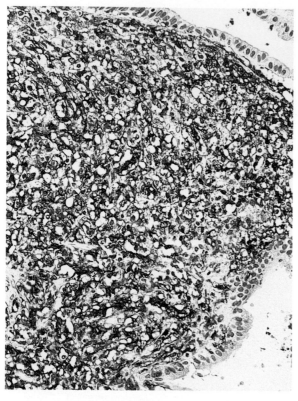

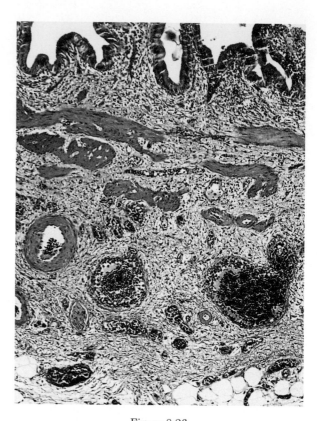

Figure 8-25
LARGE B-CELL MALIGNANT LYMPHOMA

The neoplastic cells are leukocyte common antigen positive and expand the lamina propria. The overlying biliary epithelium is normal.

Figure 8-26
INTRAVASCULAR LYMPHOMA

Low-power view shows many vessels of the gallbladder wall filled with tumor cells.

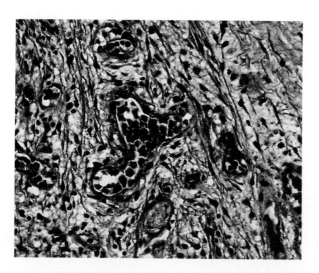

Figure 8-27
INTRAVASCULAR LYMPHOMA

Left: High magnification of small vessels in the lamina propria of the gallbladder filled with neoplastic lymphoid cells that had a B-cell phenotype.

Right: Large vessel in the perimuscular connective tissue of the gallbladder is partially filled with neoplastic lymphoid cells.

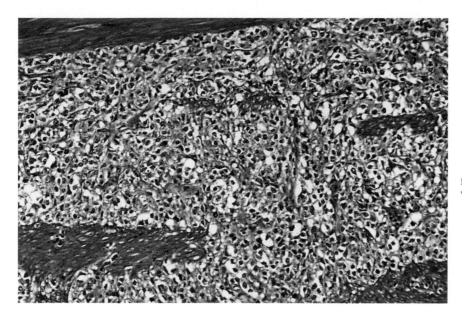

Figure 8-28
DIFFUSE INFILTRATION OF
THE MUSCULAR WALL OF
THE GALLBLADDER BY A
LARGE B-CELL LYMPHOMA
This type of lymphomatous in-
filtration should not be confused
with undifferentiated carcinoma.

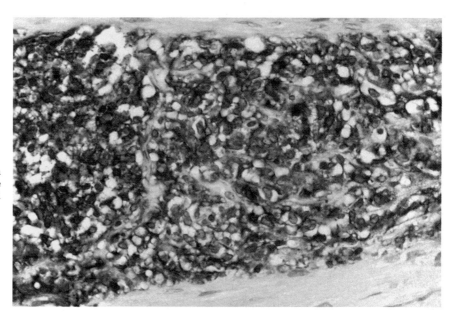

Figure 8-29
DIFFUSE INFILTRATION OF
THE MUSCULAR WALL OF
THE GALLBLADDER BY A
LARGE B-CELL LYMPHOMA
The cells of the lymphoma
shown in figure 8-28 are positive
for leukocyte common antigen and
negative for epithelial markers.

lymph nodes may be involved. Large cell lymphomas that show a trabecular or linear growth
pattern can be confused with undifferentiated
carcinomas, especially in small biopsy specimens (fig. 8-28). However, immunohistochemistry usually clarifies the diagnosis (figs. 8-25,
8-29). Immunostains for leukocyte common antigen and B- or T-cell markers are positive in
lymphomas, whereas cytokeratin and, less fre-

quently, carcinoembryonic antigen stains are
positive in carcinomas.

Currently, we know of no way to histologically
differentiate primary lymphoma from secondary
lymphoma in the gallbladder. All lymphomas
discovered in cholecystectomy specimens should
be presumed secondary and a diagnosis of primary lymphoma made only after careful exclusion (57).

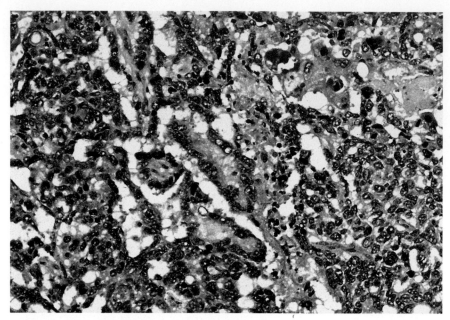

Figure 8-30
YOLK SAC TUMOR
Yolk sac tumor showing papillary structures covered by poorly differentiated cuboidal and columnar cells.

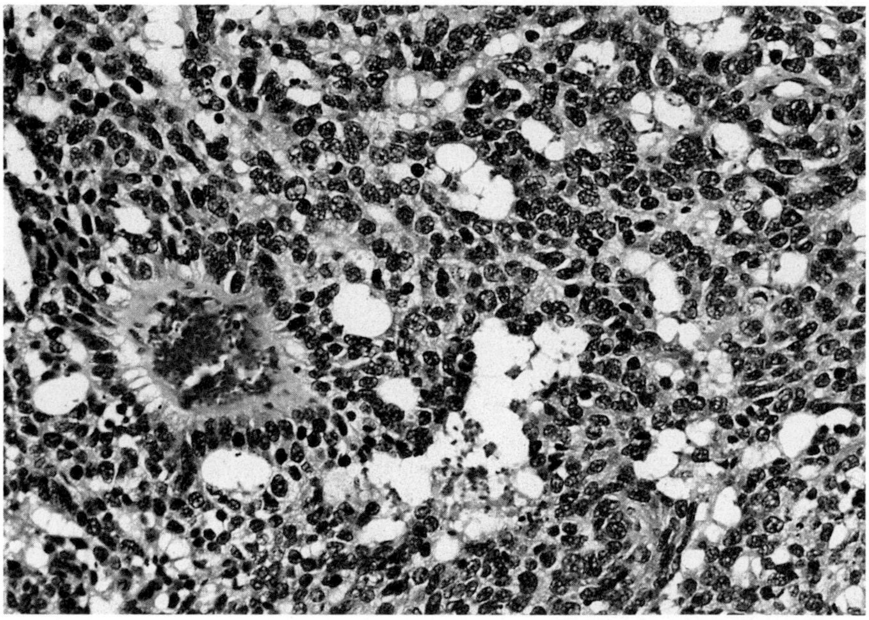

Figure 8-31
YOLK SAC TUMOR
Anastomosing cords and a perivascular arrangement of tumor cells are shown here.

Yolk Sac Tumor

Yolk sac tumors are uncommon but distinctive germ cell neoplasms that usually arise in the ovary or testis. Rarely, they occur in extragonadal sites as a result of abnormal migration of germ cell elements (64). A few examples of yolk sac tumor have been reported in the liver (63,65). We reviewed one case from the AFIP files that arose in a gallbladder with multiple calculi from a 36-year-old woman. Its histologic structure and immunohistochemical profile were similar to those of gonadal yolk sac tumors (figs. 8-30, 8-31).

DEFINITION OF TNM

T: Primary Tumor

TX   Primary tumor cannot be assessed

T0   No evidence of primary tumor

Tis   Carcinoma in situ

T1   Tumor invades lamina propria or muscle layer

     T1a   Tumor invades lamina propria

     T1b   Tumor invades muscle layer

T2   Tumor invades the perimuscular connective tissue, no extension beyond serosa or into liver

T3   Tumor perforates the serosa (visceral peritoneum) or directly invades one adjacent organ, or both (extension 2 cm or less into liver)

T4   Tumor extends more than 2 cm into liver, and/or into two or more adjacent organs (stomach, duodenum, colon, pancreas, omentum, extrahepatic bile ducts, any involvement of liver)

N: Regional Lymph Nodes

NX   Regional lymph nodes cannot be assessed

N0   No regional lymph node metastasis

N1   Metastasis in cystic duct, pericholedochal, and/or hilar lymph nodes (i.e., in the hepatoduodenal ligament)

N2   Metastasis in peripancreatic (head only), periduodenal, periportal, celiac, and/or superior mesenteric lymph nodes

M: Distant Metastasis

MX   Presence of distant metastasis cannot be assessed

M0   No distant metastasis

M1   Distant metastasis

STAGE GROUPING

Stage 0	Tis	N0	M0
Stage I	T1	N0	M0
Stage II	T2	N0	M0
Stage III	T1	N1	M0
	T2	N1	M0
	T3	N0, N1	M0
	T3	N1	M0
Stage IVA	T4	N0, N1	M0
Stage IVB	Any T	N2	M0
	Any T	Any N	M1

THE SURGICAL PATHOLOGY REPORT

The information included in the surgical pathology report of a cholecystectomy specimen should contain the required data to stage the tumor according to the TNM staging system for gallbladder cancer. This information not only has diagnostic, prognostic, and therapeutic implications, but can also be used for research purposes. The following features should be described:

1. Whether the gallbladder is received fresh or formalin fixed, has been previously opened or not.

2. Characteristics of the external surface including dimensions, color, presence of congestion, hemorrhage, focal or diffuse calcifications of the wall (porcelain gallbladder), adhesions or masses.

3. Measurements of the thickness of the wall and amount of bile, mucinous, or serous fluid found in the gallbladder. When present, number, size, and color of stones; these should be classified into pigmented or cholesterol stones.

4. Location of the tumor (fundus, body, or neck), size, color, consistency, necrosis. Polypoid, nodular, diffusely infiltrating, or combined gross features should be reported.

5. Appearance of adjacent non-neoplastic mucosa: smooth, granular, polypoid, hemorrhagic or ulcerated; cholesterolosis.

6. Histologic type, grading, and pathologic staging of tumor. Extension into lamina propria, muscular wall, perimuscular connective tissue, or serosa should be stated. Dysplasia or carcinoma in situ should be mentioned. The presence of perineural lymphatic and blood vessel invasion should be recorded because they correlate with prognosis. When present, squamous, pyloric gland or intestinal metaplasia should be recorded.

7. Cystic node status: presence or absence of metastases.

8. Cystic duct margin: free or involved by tumor.

9. Status of liver if small fragment is attached to the serosa or if portion of liver is separately submitted.

10. Status of other lymph nodes (porta hepatis, retroduodenal, peripancreatic), if separately submitted.

11. The results of immunoperoxidase stains, flow cytometry, and electron microscopic examination should be included.

REFERENCES

Benign Nonepithelial Tumors

1. Arbab AA, Brasfield R. Benign tumors of the gallbladder. Surgery 1967;61:535–40.
2. Boman F, Gultekin H, Dickman PS. Latent Epstein-Barr virus infection demonstrated in low-grade leiomyosarcomas of adults with acquired immunodeficiency syndrome, but not adjacent Kaposi's lesion or smooth muscle tumors in immunocompetent patients. Arch Pathol Lab Med 1997;121:834–38.
3. Chen KT. Osteomas of the gallbladder. Arch Pathol Lab Med 1994;118:755-6.
4. Furukawa H, Kanai Y, Mukai K. Arteriovenous hemangioma of the gallbladder. CT and pathologic findings [Letter]. AJR Am J Roentgenol 1997;168:1383.
5. Huff DS, Lischner HW, Go HC, deLeon GA. Unusual tumors in two boys with Wiskott-Aldrich-like syndrome. Lab Invest 1979;40:305.
6. Lee ES, Locker J, Nalesnik M, et al. The association of Epstein-Barr virus with smooth muscle tumors occurring after organ transplantation. N Engl J Med 1995;332:19–25.

7. Mayorga F, Hernando M, Val-Bernal F. Diffuse expansive cavernous hemangioma of the gallbladder. Gen Diagn Pathol 1996;142:211–5.

7a. Ortiz-Hidalgo C, DeLeon Bojorge B, Albores-Saavedra J. Stromal tumor of the gallbladder with pheotype of interstitial cells of Cajal. A previously unrecognized neoplasm. Am J Surg Pathol 2000 (in press).

8. Toma P, Loy A, Pastorino C, Derchi LE. Leiomyomas of the gallbladder and splenic calcifications in an HIV-infected child. Pediatr Radiol 1997;27:92–4.

Granular Cell Tumors

9. Aisner SC, Khaneja S, Ramirez O. Multiple granular cell tumors of the gallbladder and biliary tree. Arch Pathol Lab Med 1982;106:470–1.

10. Lindberg G, Saboorian H, Housini I, Ashfaq R, Albores-Saavedra J. The clinicopathologic spectrum of granular cell tumors [Abstract]. Lab Invest 1996;74:9A.

11. Sanchez JA, Nauta RJ. Resection of a granular cell tumor at the hepatic confluence. A precarious location of a benign tumor. Am Surg 1991;57:446–50.

12. Yamaguchi K, Kuroki S, Daimaru Y, Hashimoto H, Enjoji M. Granular cell tumor of the gallbladder. Report of a case. Acta Pathol Jpn 1985;35:687–91.

13. Yamashina M, Stemmerman GN. Granular cell tumor: unusual cause for mucocele of gallbladder. Am J Gastroenterol 1984;79:701–3.

Neurofibroma

14. Eggleston JF, Goldman RL. Neurofibroma and elastosis of the gallbladder. Report of an unusual case. Am J Gastroenterol 1982;77:335–7.

15. Morizumu H, Sano T, Hirose T, Hizawa K. Neurofibroma of the gallbladder seen as a papillary polyp. Acta Pathol Jpn 1988;38:259–68.

Neurofibromatosis

16. Rutgeerts P, Hendricks H, Geboes K, Ponette E, Broeckaert L, Vantrappen G. Involvement of the upper digestive tract by systemic neurofibromatosis. Gastrointest Endosc 1981;1:22–5.

Ganglioneuromatosis

17. Carney JA, Sizemore GW, Hayles AM. Multiple endocrine neoplasia, type 2b. Pathobiol Annu 1978;8:105–53.

18. Chetty R, Clark SP. Cholecystitis, cholelithiasis, and ganglioneuromatosis of the gallbladder: an unusual presentation of MEN type 2b. J Clin Pathol 1993;46:1061-3.

19. Floquet J, Rauber G, Prenat T. L'adenomatose polyendocrinienne ou multiple endocrine neoplasia de type 2b. Nouv Presse Med 1979;8:2758–9.

Malignant Mesenchymal Tumors

20. Albores-Saavedra J, Henson DE. Tumors of the gallbladder and extrahepatic bile ducts. Atlas of Tumor Pathology, 2nd Series, Fascicle 22. Washington D.C.: Armed Forces Institute of Pathology, 1986.

21. Appelman HD, Coopersmith, N. Pleomorphic spindle-cell carcinoma of the gallbladder. Cancer 1970;25:535–41.

22. Carpentier Y, Lambilliotte JP. Primary sarcoma of the gallbladder. Cancer 1973;32:493-7.

23. Edmondson HA. Tumors of the gallbladder and extrahepatic bile ducts. Atlas of Tumor Pathology, 1st Series, Fascicle 26. Washington, D.C.: Armed Forces Institute of Pathology, 1967.

24. Kumar S, Gupta A, Shrivastava UK, Bhargava SK. Leiomyosarcoma of gallbladder: a case report. Indian J Pathol Microbiol 1993;36:78–80.

25. Kumar A, Lal BK, Singh MK, Kapur BM. Angiosarcoma of the gallbladder. Am J Gastroenterol 1989;84:1431–3.

26. Mihara S, Matsumoto H, Tokunaga F, Yano H, Ota M, Yamashita S. Botryoid rhabdomyosarcoma of the gallbladder in a child. Cancer 1982;49:812–8.

27. Newmark H, Kliewer K, Curtis A, DenBensten L, Enestein W. Primary leiomyosarcoma of gallbladder seen on computed tomography and ultrasound. Am J Gastroenterol 1986;8:202–4.

28. White K, Chan YF. Epithelioid angiosarcoma of the gallbladder. Histopathology 1994;24:269–71.

29. Willen R, Willen H. Primary sarcoma of the gallbladder. A light and electron microscopical study. Virchows Arch [A] 1982;396:91–102.

30. Yasuma T, Yanaka M. Primary sarcoma of the gallbladder—report of three cases. Acta Pathol Jpn 1971;21:285–304.

Kaposi's Sarcoma

31. Enad JG, Lapa JC, Jaklic B, Nellestein ME, Ghosh BC. Kaposi's sarcoma of the gallbladder. Milit Med 1992;157:559–61.

32. Lesman AL, Golub R, Giron JA, Ilardi CF. Primary Kaposi's sarcoma of the gallbladder in AIDS. J Clin Gastroenterol 1993;17:352–3.

141

Carcinosarcoma

33. Albores-Saavedra J, Henson DE, Sobin LH. Histological typing of tumors of the gallbladder and extrahepatic bile ducts. World Health Organization. Springer-Verlag, Berlin, 1991.
34. Born MW, Ramey WG, Ryan SF, Gordon PE. Carcinosarcoma and carcinoma of the gallbladder. Cancer 1984;53:2171–7.
35. Fagot H, Fabre JM, Ramos J, et al. Carcinosarcoma of the gallbladder. A case report and review of the literature. J Clin Gastroenterol 1994;18:314–6.
36. Henson DE, Albores-Saavedra J, Corle D. Carcinoma of the gallbladder. Histologic types, stage of disease and survival rates. Cancer 1992;70:1493–7.
37. Inoshita, S, Iwashita A, Enjoji M. Carcinosarcoma of the gallbladder. Report of a case and review of the literature. Acta Pathol Jpn 1986;36:913–20.
38. Ishihara T, Kawano H, Takahashi M, et al. Carcinosarcoma of the gallbladder. A case report with immunohistochemical and ultrastructural studies. Cancer 1990;66:992–7.
39. Mansori KS, Cho SY. Malignant mixed tumor of the gallbladder. Am J Clin Pathol 1980;73:709–11.
40. Mehrotra TN, Gupta SC, Naithani YP. Carcinosarcoma of the gallbladder. J Pathol 1971;104:145–8.
41. von Kuster LC, Cohen C. Malignant mixed tumors of the gallbladder: report of two cases and review of the literature. Cancer 1982;50:1166–70.
42. Wick MR, Swanson PE. Carcinosarcomas: current perspectives and an historical review of nosological concepts. Semin Diag Pathol 1993;10:118–27.

Malignant Melanoma

43. Breathnach AS. Normal and abnormal melanin pigmentation of the skin. In: Wolman M, ed. Pigments in pathology. New York: Academic Press, 1969:353–94.
44. Carle G, Lessells AM, Best PV. Malignant melanoma of the gallbladder. Cancer 1981;48:2318–22.
44a. Dong XD, DeMatos P, Prieto VG, Siegler HF. Melanoma of the gallbladder. A review of cases seen at Duke University Medical Center. Cancer 1999;85:32–9.
45. Goldin EG. Malignant melanoma metastatic to the gallbladder. Case report and review of the literature. Am Surg 1990;56:369–73.
46. Hatae Y, Kikuchi M, Segawa M, Yonemitsu K. Malignant melanoma of the gallbladder. Pathol Res Pract 1978;163:281–7.
47. Heath DI, Womack C. Primary malignant melanoma of the gallbladder. J Clin Pathol 1988;41:1073–7.
48. Higgins CM, Strutton CM. Malignant melanoma of the gallbladder—does primary melanoma exist? Pathology 1995;27:312–4.
49. Laitio M. Melanogenic metaplasia of the gallbladder epithelium. Acta Chir Scand 1975;141:57–60.
50. McFadden PM, Krementz ET, McKinnon WM, Pararo LL, Ryan RF. Metastatic melanoma of the gallbladder. Cancer 1979;44:1802–8.
51. Peison B, Rabin L. Malignant melanoma of the gallbladder: report of three cases and review of the literature. Cancer 1976;37:2448–54.
52. Seul B, Luchtrath H. Malignes melanomes der gallenblase. Chirug 1984;55:179–81.
53. Verbanck JJ, Rutgeerts LJ, Van Aelst, et al. Primary malignant melanoma of the gallbladder, metastatic to the common bile duct. Gastroenterology 1986;91:214–8.

Malignant Lymphoma

54. Albores-Saavedra J, Gould E, Manivel-Rodriguez C, Angeles-Angeles A, Henson DE. Chronic cholecystitis with lymphoid hyperplasia. Rev Invest Clin (Mex) 1989;41:159–64.
55. Botha JB, Kahn LB. Primary lymphoma of the gallbladder. S Afr Med J 1974;48:1345–8.
56. Friedman EP, Lazda E, Davis J. Primary lymphoma of the gallbladder. Postgrad Med J 1993;69:585–7.
57. Gillespie JJ, Ayala AG, MacKay B, Silliman YE. Diagnosis of lymphoma from a cholecystectomy specimen: case report and review of the literature. South Med J 1977;70:353–4.
58. Laurino L, Melato M. Malignant angioendotheliomatosis (angiotropic lymphoma) of the gallbladder. Virchows Arch [A] 1990;417:243–6.
59. McCluggage WG, Mackel E, McCusker G. Primary low grade malignant lymphoma of mucosa-associated lymphoid tissue of gallbladder. Histopathology 1996;29:285–7.
60. Mosnier JF, Brousse N, Sevestre C, et al. Primary low-grade B-cell lymphoma of the mucosa-associated lymphoid tissue arising in the gallbladder. Histopathology 1992;20:273–5.
61. Tishler M, Rahmani R, Shilo R, et al. Large cell lymphoma presenting as acute cholecystitis. Acta Haematol 1987;77:51–2.
62. VanSlyck EJ, Schuman BM. Lymphocytic lymphosarcoma of the gallbladder. Cancer 1972;30:810–6.

Yolk Sac Tumor

63. Craig JR, Petus RL, Edmondson HA. Tumors of the liver and intrahepatic bile ducts. Atlas of Tumor Pathology. Second Series. Fascicle 26. Washington, D.C.; Armed Forces Institute of Pathology, 1989.
64. Huntington RW Jr, Bullock WK. Yolk sac tumors of extragonadal origin. Cancer 1970;25:1368–76.
65. Weinberg AG, Finegold MJ. Primary hepatic tumors of childhood. Hum Pathol 1983;14:512–37.

9
SECONDARY TUMORS OF GALLBLADDER

Metastatic tumors of the gallbladder are uncommon, usually asymptomatic, and either discovered at autopsy or incidentally during laparotomy (2). The majority result from transcelomic spread and are usually associated with metastatic lesions elsewhere in the abdomen. Grossly, they appear as small, single or multiple nodules attached to the serosal surface. The most common primary sites for metastatic carcinomas in the gallbladder are the stomach, pancreas, ovary, bile ducts, colon, and breast.

Bloodborne metastases to the gallbladder are even less common than those of transcelomic spread. They have been reported with malignant melanoma and with carcinomas of the kidney, lung, breast, esophagus, and nasopharynx. These metastatic lesions are single or multiple, commonly invade the mucosa, and may appear several years following removal of the primary tumor. They often begin as submucosal nodules that eventually become pedunculated.

The most commonly encountered metastatic tumor in both autopsy and surgical material is malignant melanoma (4,4a,8). Secondary deposits of melanoma comprise 50 to 66 percent of all gallbladder metastases (1). In a study of 125 patients with malignant melanoma, 19 (15 percent) had gallbladder metastasis (4) and in another study of 78 patients, 11 (14 percent) had metastatic lesions in the gallbladder (12).

Patients with resected metastatic melanoma have also been reported (8). Most of these patients have biliary symptoms and a history of melanoma that had been excised from the skin or the eye (7). The polypoid masses are usually detected by ultrasound examination or computed tomography (3,10). The time from diagnosis of the primary tumor to the presentation of gallbladder metastasis has varied from 6 months to 13 years, with a mean of 3 to 4 years (7).

Two neoplasms, malignant melanoma and renal cell carcinoma, commonly give rise to symptomatic, solitary, polypoid metastases that closely mimic primary malignant gallbladder tumors. A single intraluminal polypoid metastasis is usually confused with a primary gallbladder carcinoma by ultrasound or computed tomography (fig. 9-1). This is especially true when the gallbladder metastasis is the first manifestation of the primary tumor.

Grossly, a solitary metastasis of melanoma usually involves the mucosa and muscle coat (12). Mucosal lesions are polypoid and protrude into the lumen of the gallbladder (fig. 9-2). Microscopically, the tumor is not difficult to recognize since it is often heavily pigmented. In contrast to primary malignant melanoma of the gallbladder, metastatic deposits lack junctional activity (fig. 9-3). However, pagetoid spread mimicking junctional activity has been reported. Involvement of the gallbladder is usually associated with involvement of the liver and sometimes with metastatic lesions in the extrahepatic bile ducts.

We have seen a single example of a solitary polypoid metastasis in the gallbladder as the first manifestation of a renal cell carcinoma in a kidney transplant recipient (figs. 9-4, 9-5). A solitary synchronous metastasis of renal cell carcinoma was detected during a radical nephrectomy and excised several months later (11). Several cases of gallbladder metastases of renal cell

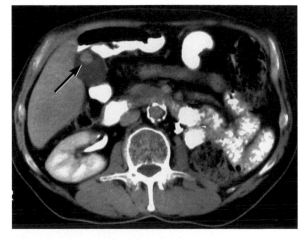

Figure 9-1
METASTATIC RENAL CELL CARCINOMA
Computed tomography depicting a single polypoid mass arising from the wall of the gallbladder which proved to be a metastatic renal cell carcinoma (arrow).

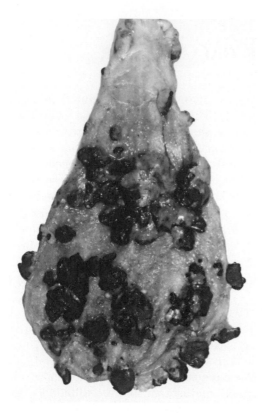

Figure 9-2
METASTATIC MELANOMA

The gallbladder lumen is exposed. Numerous polypoid melanomatous deposits are shown. (Fig. 3 from Shimkin PM, Soloway MS, Jaffe E. Metastatic melanoma of the gallbladder. Am J Roentgenol Rad Ther Nucl Med 1972;116:393-5).

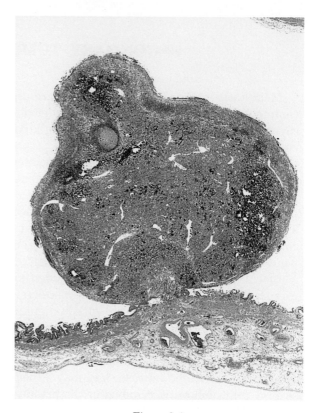

Figure 9-4
METASTATIC RENAL
CELL CARCINOMA

A solitary polypoid metastatic renal cell carcinoma from a kidney recipient. The gallbladder metastasis was the first manifestation of the tumor.

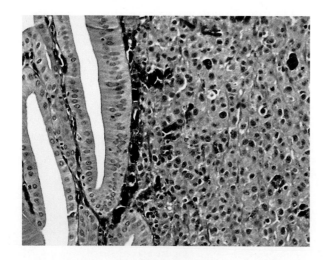

Figure 9-3
METASTATIC MALIGNANT MELANOMA

The tumor contains melanin pigment and lacks junctional activity.

carcinoma years after resection of the primary tumor have been reported (5,6,9,13).

Carcinomas from adjacent organs such as the colon or stomach may occasionally extend into the wall of the gallbladder. Primary carcinomas of the liver rarely may spread to the gallbladder by direct extension, appearing as a polypoid mass (13). We have seen a solitary hepatic metastasis of a colonic adenocarcinoma that invaded the gallbladder by direct extension and mimicked a primary gallbladder carcinoma (fig. 9-6).

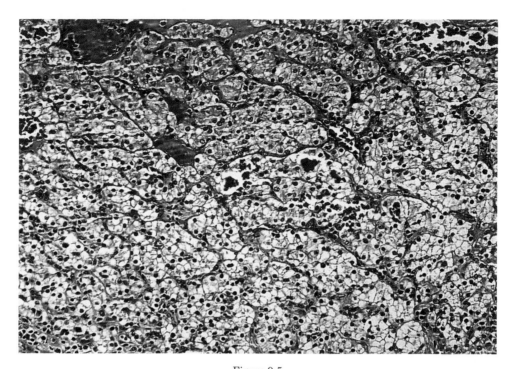

Figure 9-5
METASTATIC RENAL CELL CARCINOMA
Higher magnification of the tumor shown on figure 9-4. Nests of neoplastic cells with clear cytoplasm are shown.

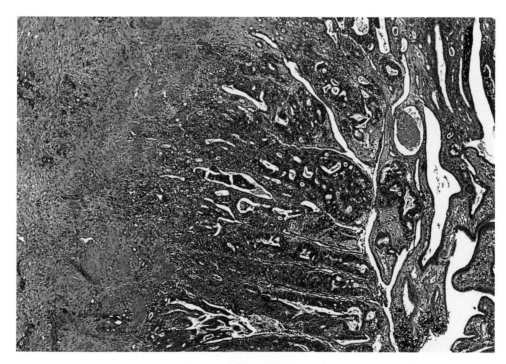

Figure 9-6
METASTATIC COLONIC ADENOCARCINOMA
The tumor represents a direct extension from a hepatic metastasis of a colonic adenocarcinoma.

REFERENCES

1. Backman H. Metastases of malignant melanoma in the gastrointestinal tract. Geriatrics 1969;24:112–20.
2. Botting AJ, Harrison EG, Black BM. Metastatic hypernephroma masquerading as a polypoid tumor of the gallbladder and review of metastatic tumors of the gallbladder. Proc Mayo Clin 1963;38:225–32.
3. Bundy AL, Ritchie WW. Ultrasonic diagnosis of metastatic melanoma of the gallbladder presenting as acute cholecystitis. J Clin Ultrasound 1982;10:285–7.
4. DasGupta T, Brasfield R. Metastatic melanoma. Cancer 1964;17:1323–39.
4a. Dong XD, DeMatos P, Prieto VG, Siegler HF. Melanoma of the gallbladder. A review of cases seen at Duke University Medical Center. Cancer 1999;85:32–9.
5. Fullarton GM, Burgoyne M. Gallbladder and pancreatic metastases from bilateral renal carcinoma presenting with hematobilia and anemia. Urology 1991:38:184–6.
6. Golbey S, Gerard PS, Frank RG. Metastatic hypernephroma masquerading as acute cholecystitis. Clin Imaging 1991;15:293–5.
7. Lang RG, Bailey EM, Sober AJ. Acute cholecystitis from metastatic melanoma to the gallbladder in a patient with a low risk melanoma. Br J Dermatol 1997;136:279–82.
8. McFadden PM, Krementz ET, McKinnon WM, Pararo LL, Ryan RF. Metastatic melanoma of the gallbladder. Cancer 1979;44:1802–8.
9. Nagler J, McSherry CK, Miskovitz P. Asymptomatic metachronous metastatic renal cell adenocarcinoma to the gallbladder. Report of a case and guidelines for evaluation of intraluminal polypoid gallbladder masses. Dig Dis Sci 1994;39:2476–9.
10. Phillips G, Pochaczevsky R, Goodman J, Kumari S. Ultrasound patterns of metastatic tumors in the gallbladder. J Clin Ultrasound 1982;10:379–83.
11. Satoh H, Iyama A, Hidaka K, Nakashiro H, Harada S, Hisatsugu ST. Metastatic carcinoma of the gallbladder from renal cancer presenting as intraluminal polypoid mass. Dig Dis Sci 1991;36:520–3.
12. Shimkin PM, Soloway MS, Jaffe E. Metastatic melanoma of the gallbladder. Am J Roentgenol Rad Ther Nucl Med 1972;116:393–5.
13. Terasaki S, Nakanuma Y, Terada T, Unoura M. Metastasis of hepatocellular carcinoma to gallbladder presenting massive intraluminal growth: report of an autopsy case. J Clin Gastroenterol 1990;12:714–5.

10
TUMOR-LIKE LESIONS OF GALLBLADDER

A number of tumor-like lesions occur in the gallbladder and extrahepatic bile ducts. Some of these lesions are inflammatory in nature and may be mistaken for neoplasms because of their gross features or appearance on cholecystograms, computed tomography, or ultrasonography. Others, such as adenomyomatous hyperplasia or mucocele, may be confused with cancer histologically. With some exceptions, these lesions are asymptomatic and usually discovered in specimens removed for cholecystitis. Some are important because they may be precursors of cancer.

CHANGES IN CHOLECYSTITIS

The epithelial changes in chronic cholecystitis are not constant, but vary greatly in structure, severity, and topographic distribution. Moreover, their incidence is often a reflection of sampling, the number of sections examined, and the technique of study. We believe that pathologists should become familiar with these changes, otherwise an inexperienced observer may confuse them with carcinoma. It has been suggested that some of these lesions, especially intestinal metaplasia and squamous metaplasia, play an important role as precursors of carcinoma of the gallbladder (4,11,12).

Chronic cholecystitis, with or without ulceration, may be accompanied by proliferation of hypertrophic nerve bundles in the muscular and perimuscular connective tissue. Sometimes this change is so pronounced as to simulate a traumatic neuroma or a plexiform neurofibroma.

REACTIVE EPITHELIAL ATYPIA

Accelerated cell proliferation in the mucosa of the human gallbladder during cholelithiasis has been shown by autoradiography (16). Twenty-three times more tritiated thymidine is incorporated into the epithelium of lithiferous gallbladders than normal ones. From a morphologic point of view, however, the most constant epithelial abnormality seen in cholecystitis is an increase in the number of mucin-producing cells. In other words, there is tendency for the epithelium to assume a greater secretory, rather than an absorptive, function (7,8). Ulceration of the mucosa often occurs and is usually followed by epithelial regeneration. These regenerating cells can appear atypical, showing vesicular or hyperchromatic nuclei, prominent nucleoli, basophilic or eosinophilic cytoplasm, and even mitotic figures (figs. 10-1–10-3). In contrast to dysplastic cells, reactive atypical epithelial cells are p53 negative by immunohistochemistry. In addition, focal atrophy is often noted; the epithelium becomes cuboidal or flattened and loses microvilli. Other changes include pseudostratification and multilayering. Hyperplasia of the penciloid cells can also occur (fig. 10-4). All these changes probably represent a reaction of the surface epithelium to injury (7) and should not be mistaken for dysplasia or carcinoma in situ (3).

INTESTINAL METAPLASIA

Approximately one third of gallbladders excised for cholelithiasis show intestinal metaplasia, which is more common in females, and appears to increase with age, and perhaps more importantly, with duration of the gallstones (1a,3,5,9–11). The initial lesion begins with the appearance of a few goblet cells at the tip of the mucosal folds. When fully developed, it consists of variable proportions of goblet cells, columnar cells with a brush border, Paneth cells, and endocrine cells. Goblet cells usually predominate (1a). As the lesion progresses, the metaplastic cells extend downward along the lateral surfaces replacing several or multiple mucosal folds. Gland-like structures lined by intestinal metaplastic epithelium eventually fill and expand the lamina propria, forming nodular elevations of the mucosa (fig. 10-5). Intestinal metaplasia often coexists with foci of foveolar gastric type epithelium and metaplastic pyloric type glands (fig. 10-6).

Since cholelithiasis induces active proliferation of epithelial cells we speculate that this favors the appearance of stem cells that have the ability to differentiate into cells with mature intestinal and gastric phenotypes. This would explain the transition from normal columnar

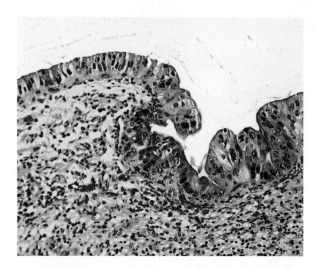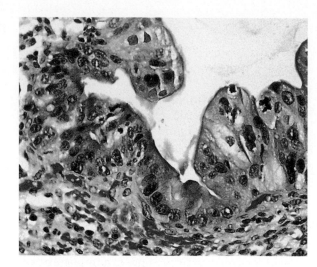

Figure 10-1
REACTIVE EPITHELIAL ATYPIA
Left: The surface gallbladder epithelium shows columnar cells with clear or basophilic cytoplasm, penciloid cells, and intraepithelial polymorphonuclear leukocytes.
Right: Higher magnification shows epithelial pseudostratification and abnormal mitotic figures.

cells to cells with slender microvilli similar to those of the intestine (13), the presence of cells with both cytoplasmic mucin and Paneth granules, as well as the common coexistence of intestinal metaplasia with foci of foveolar gastric type epithelium and hyperplasia of pyloric type glands (1a)

Metaplastic epithelium contains several substances found in normal and abnormal intestinal epithelium. For example, metaplastic cells contain intestinal-associated antigens (5,6), which also occur in well- to moderately differentiated adenocarcinomas. They contain carcinoembryonic antigen (2) and a neutral or acidic non-sulfated mucin (15), which also occur in carcinomas of the gallbladder and intestine. In contrast to dysplasia and carcinoma in situ, metaplastic epithelium does not show p53 overexpression by immunohistochemistry (17). However, genetic analysis of metaplastic lesions has shown the same molecular abnormalities described in gallbladder carcinomas suggesting that metaplastic epithelium is a cancer precursor (18).

Several types of endocrine cells, including enterochromaffin cells (EC) and enterochromaffin-like cells (ECL), have been described in metaplastic epithelium (1a,14). Intermixed with columnar and goblet cells, these endocrine cells rest on the basal lamina and are located near capillaries. They can be identified by the Fon-

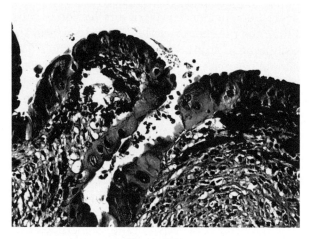

Figure 10-2
REACTIVE EPITHELIAL ATYPIA
The surface epithelium, which shows nuclear atypia, is low cuboidal, penciloid, and columnar. This heterogeneity of the epithelial cell population is characteristic of reactive atypia.

tana-Masson and Grimelius stains, immunohistochemistry, or by electron microscopy (figs. 10-7, 10-8). With immunohistochemical methods, we have found serotonin and a variety of peptide hormones in the endocrine cells. Serotonin-containing cells are the most common endocrine cells (1a). Less frequently, endocrine cells show

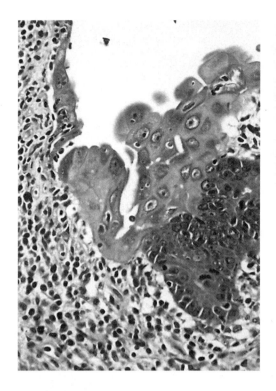

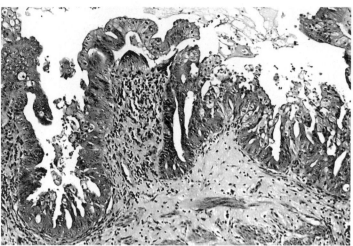

Figure 10-3
REACTIVE EPITHELIAL ATYPIA

Left: The surface gallbladder epithelium is atypical and contains both basophilic and eosinophilic cells with vesicular nuclei and prominent nucleoli. Atrophic epithelium is also present.

Above: Hyperplastic epithelial changes are seen in reactive atypia. Many of the cells have vesicular nuclei, prominent nucleoli, and abundant basophilic or clear cytoplasm.

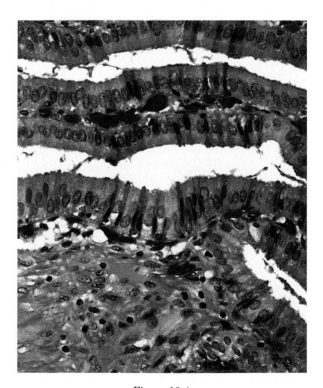

Figure 10-4
PENCILOID CELLS

An increased number of penciloid cells in a case of chronic cholecystitis.

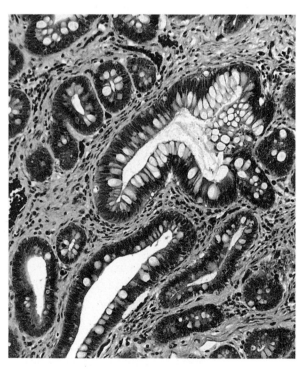

Figure 10-5
INTESTINAL METAPLASIA

The epithelium at the top has been replaced by mature goblet cells. Both the surface epithelium and the gland-like structures in the lamina propria are lined by mature goblet cells.

149

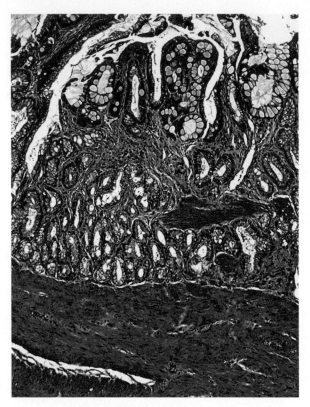

Figure 10-6
INTESTINAL AND PYLORIC GLAND METAPLASIA
Both intestinal and pyloric gland metaplasia coexist in this gallbladder.

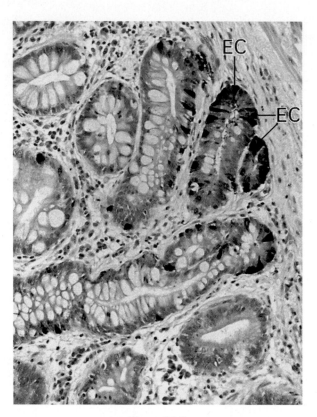

Figure 10-7
ENDOCRINE CELLS IN AREAS
OF INTESTINAL METAPLASIA
Many serotonin-containing (EC) cells are admixed with the goblet cells.

immunoreactivity for somatostatin, pancreatic polypeptide, gastrin, and motilin (1a).

Rarely, dysplastic changes occur in the metaplastic cells with intestinal phenotype and dysplastic intestinal metaplasia can be seen adjacent to adenocarcinomas. For this reason, *dysplastic intestinal metaplasia* has been regarded by some as a premalignant lesion.

Intestinal metaplasia of the gallbladder should be distinguished from ectopic gastric mucosa, a developmental abnormality which is less common and contains chief and parietal cells not present in intestinal metaplasia.

PYLORIC GLAND METAPLASIA

This is the most common metaplastic lesion associated with cholelithiasis. It has been estimated that 50 percent of gallbladders with chronic inflammation or lithiasis exhibit hyperplasia of the pyloric type glands which may be found in the neck, lateral walls, or fundus. The initial change consists in the branching of a crypt close to the base. Secondary budding occurs, forming additional glands which may be arranged as poorly defined lobules or grow in a diffuse manner (11).

These glands are usually confined to the lamina propria, but occasionally may extend through the muscle layer to the serosal surface and even invade nerve trunks (fig. 10-9A,B) (1). They are lined by columnar cells with basal nuclei and a vacuolated cytoplasm which contains non-sulfated acid mucin. In some cases, endocrine and Paneth cells are also found between these mucin-containing cells. Some of the endocrine cells are argentaffin, while others are argyrophilic and are immunoreactive for serotonin and peptide hormones (fig. 10-9C) (1a).

Rarely, desquamated mucin-containing cells from metaplastic pyloric glands may acquire a signet ring cell morphology, mimicking signet

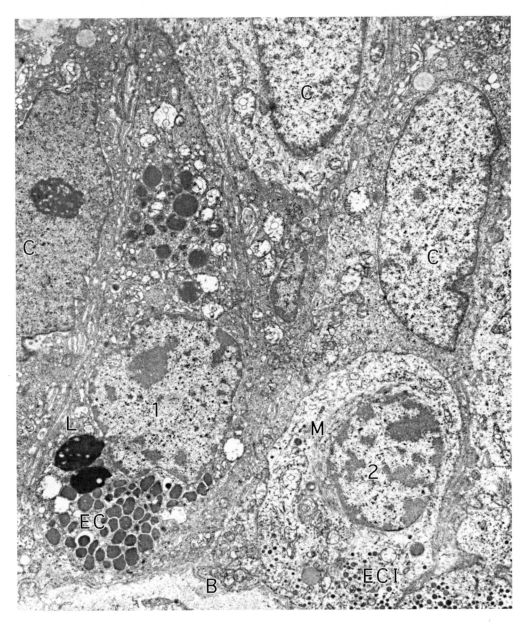

Figure 10-8
ULTRASTRUCTURE OF ENDOCRINE CELLS

Metaplastic gallbladder epithelial cells show two types (types 1 and 2) of enterochromaffin cells. Both cells rest on the basal lamina (B). The secretory granules in the cell type 1 (EC) are large and slightly irregular in outline, whereas the secretory granules in the cell type 2 (ECL) are small and perfectly round. There are bundles of microfilaments (M) around the nucleus in the cell type 2 and large lysosomal dense bodies (L) in the cell type 1. Both types of enterochromaffin cells are closely associated with the columnar epithelial cells (C) of the gallbladder mucosa. (Fig. 136 from Fascicle 22, 2nd Series.)

ring cell carcinoma in situ. Although these desquamated cells contain mucin and are cytokeratin positive they lack nuclear atypia and are carcinoembryonic antigen negative (fig. 10-9D).

Pyloric type glands which result from metaplasia are morphologically and histochemically distinct from the glands that normally occur in the gallbladder neck. Hyperplasia of pyloric type glands may coexist with fully developed intestinal metaplasia, tubular adenoma, or carcinoma. Dysplastic changes are occasionally seen in pyloric type glands adjacent to adenocarcinomas,

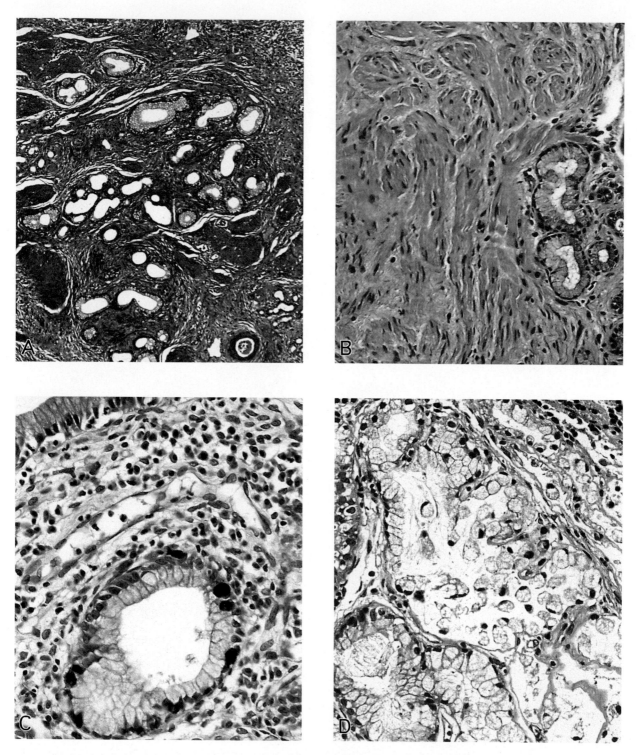

Figure 10-9
HYPERPLASIA OR METAPLASTIC PYLORIC TYPE GLANDS

A: Lobules of metaplastic pyloric type glands extend into the muscle layer of the gallbladder, simulating adenocarcinoma.

B: Perineural and intraneural "invasion" by metaplastic pyloric glands which are lined by benign-appearing mucin-producing columnar cells.

C: Serotonin-containing cells in a metaplastic pyloric gland located in the lamina propria of the gallbladder.

D: Desquamated mucin-containing cells from metaplastic pyloric glands mimic signet ring cell carcinoma in situ.

suggesting that some of these tumors arise from these glands. The absence of fundic gastric mucosa with parietal and chief cells allows separation of metaplastic pyloric type glands from ectopic gastric mucosa.

PAPILLARY HYPERPLASIA

We divide papillary hyperplasia into two types: primary and secondary. The former is exceedingly rare and occurs in patients without cholelithiasis, cholecystitis, primary sclerosing cholangitis, or inflammatory bowel disease. Clinically, the patients develop symptoms similar to those of chronic cholecystitis. The papillary lesions may be focal, segmental, or diffuse. When diffuse, they may involve the entire mucosa of the gallbladder and extrahepatic bile ducts. Grossly, there is focal or diffuse thickening of the mucosa, which appears granular. Histologically, the crowded and tall columnar mucosal folds and papillary structures are lined by columnar cells similar to those of normal gallbladder and bile duct epithelium (fig. 10-10) (19,22). Some of the columnar cells may contain subnuclear vacuoles (19). Cells with intestinal phenotypes and dysplastic changes have not been described in this form of papillary hyperplasia, although the number of reported cases is small.

The most common form of papillary hyperplasia is secondary to gallstone disease or specific infectious cholecystitis. Usually a focal lesion, it has been reported in 0.4 to 5.0 percent of all gallbladders removed for lithiasis. Microscopically, papillary hyperplasia is characterized by numerous crowded mucosal folds and well-developed papillary structures. The mucosal folds are longer than normal and tend to branch (fig. 10-11). They are lined by tall columnar cells with regular basal nuclei. Occasionally, a few goblet and Paneth cells are seen admixed with the columnar cells.

Papillary hyperplasia secondary to ulcerative colitis and primary sclerosing cholangitis appears to have distinctive features. It is usually segmental or diffuse. The papillary structures are lined by mucus-secreting columnar cells that may show nuclear atypia. Admixed with the columnar cells are collections of Paneth cells and endocrine cells. Until 1993, only three cases had been recorded (19a,20). A case of papillary hyper-

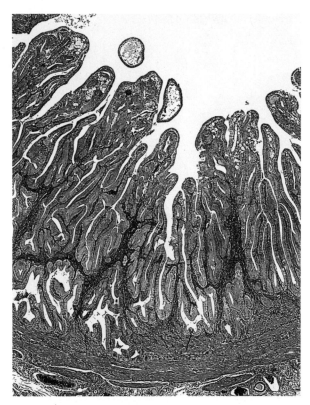

Figure 10-10
PRIMARY PAPILLARY HYPERPLASIA
Crowded and tall mucosal folds and papillary structures are seen.

plasia coexisting with tuberculosis of the gallbladder showed similar histologic features (21).

SQUAMOUS METAPLASIA

Replacement of the surface columnar epithelium by stratified squamous epithelium results in an exceedingly rare lesion. We have seen four cases, all of which were associated with lithiasis (23). In one patient, the gallbladder showed only chronic inflammation. The other three patients had, in addition, a malignant tumor: two cases of squamous cell carcinoma and one of malignant fibrous histiocytoma. Histologically, the squamous epithelium appeared to be mature, with a normal granular and keratin layer (fig. 10-12). Focal progression to dysplasia and carcinoma in situ was observed in the two cases associated with the squamous cell carcinoma. All gallbladders showing squamous metaplasia should be carefully studied for incipient carcinoma.

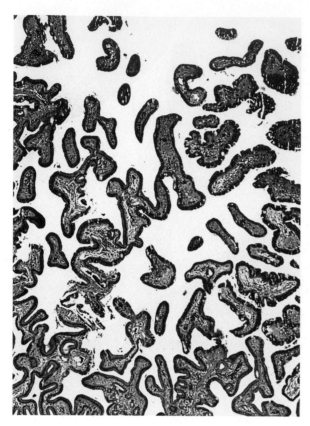
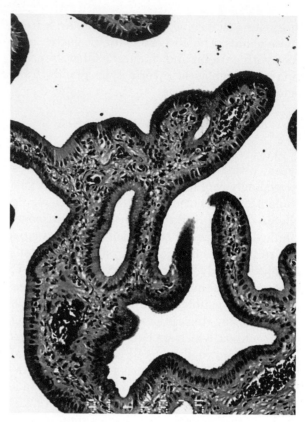

Figure 10-11
PAPILLARY HYPERPLASIA SECONDARY TO CHOLELITHIASIS
Left: Tall branching mucosal folds project into the lumen of the gallbladder.
Right: Higher magnification of papillary structures lined by normal biliary epithelium.

Figure 10-12
SQUAMOUS METAPLASIA
The gallbladder epithelium has been replaced by mature, keratinized, squamous epithelium. Normal epithelium is seen at the top. (Courtesy of Dr. J. Aguirre, Mexico City, Mexico.)

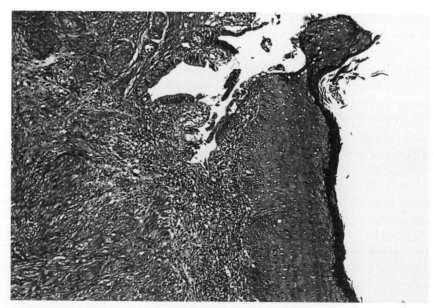

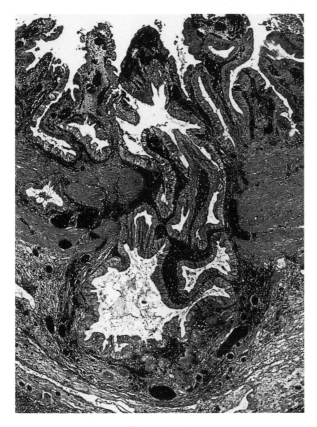

Figure 10-13
ROKITANSKY-ASCHOFF SINUS
The gallbladder mucosa has herniated through the muscle layer into the perimuscular connective tissue.

ROKITANSKY-ASCHOFF SINUSES

Rokitansky-Aschoff sinuses, or crypts, are epithelial invaginations that may penetrate the muscle layer and reach the perimuscular connective tissue. They are analogous to the diverticula that develop in other hollow viscera, such as the colon or urinary bladder (fig. 10-13) (24,25,31,32). In contrast to adenomyomatous hyperplasia, the muscle layer is not hyperplastic (27,29,34).

Occasionally visualized on cholecystograms, they are often seen in cases of chronic cholecystitis and less frequently in normal gallbladders. Their etiology and pathogenesis are still controversial (26). Increased intraluminal pressure and a weak muscle layer are thought to be important pathogenetic factors.

Histologically, the sinuses are long and tortuous, tend to branch, and are lined by a single layer of columnar cells. It is unlikely they will ever be confused with a well-differentiated adenocarcinoma. Occasionally, however, and especially in the neck of the gallbladder, the marked proliferation and branching of the epithelium may simulate glands and lead to an erroneous diagnosis of carcinoma. Important features in the differential diagnosis include the lack of nuclear pleomorphism and mitotic activity, lobular orientation of the gland-like structures, absence of invasion, and demonstration of a continuity between surface epithelium and crypts.

Inflammation and fibrosis of the gallbladder wall may obliterate segments of the sinuses, which become dilated or cystic because of retained secretions. Bile, cholesterol crystals, or even stones can also accumulate in the crypts.

Rarely, carcinoma in situ arises from Rokitansky-Aschoff sinuses (28,30). More frequently, carcinoma in situ originates from the surface epithelium and extends into the sinuses. Regardless of the origin of the in situ lesion, distinction from stromal invasion becomes clinically important. In a series of 24 cases of carcinoma in situ of the gallbladder, 11 (45 percent) extended into Rokitansky-Aschoff sinuses (33). In these cases, identification of the residual benign columnar epithelium is helpful in distinguishing in situ carcinoma from stromal infiltration.

ADENOMYOMATOUS HYPERPLASIA

Adenomyomatous hyperplasia (*diverticular disease*) is a common lesion of the gallbladder and characterized by invaginations or saccular outpouchings of the mucosa (Rokitansky-Aschoff sinuses) accompanied by smooth muscle hyperplasia (36b–d,35,38). Although the prevalence of this condition varies in different series, during the last decade it has risen considerably, probably because of the use of new and more sensitive imaging techniques (37,39). In a recent series of 3,197 consecutive cholecystectomies, adenomyomatous hyperplasia was found in 279 (8.7 percent) (42); older series have reported a lower incidence that has varied from 0.8 to 2.8 percent (38,41).

Clinically it may be either asymptomatic or produce symptoms indistinguishable from those of chronic cholecystitis. Even though more than 90 percent of the cases are associated with stones, in some series the disease was reported

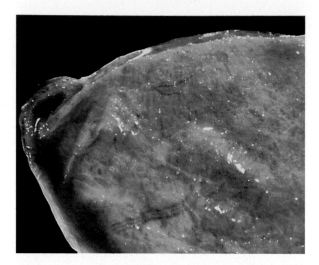

Figure 10-14
LOCALIZED FORM OF
ADENOMYOMATOUS HYPERPLASIA
The fundus of the gallbladder contains a nodular lesion
with a central dimple and cystically dilated structures.

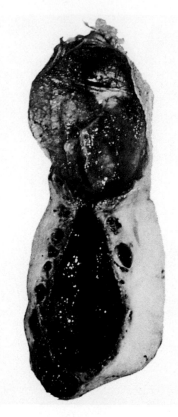

Figure 10-15
SEGMENTAL ADENOMYOMATOUS HYPERPLASIA
A sharply circumscribed adenomyomatous hyperplasia
is separated from the normal part of the gallbladder by a
stricture. The thick wall of the distal locules contains cystic
spaces in which there are many pigmented calculi. (Fig. 141
from Fascicle 22, 2nd Series.)

to be slightly more common in adult men (36b, 42). In our experience as in most reported series, however, it has been more common in adult females (43). Although adenomyomatous hyperplasia can be visualized by cholecystography, computed tomography, and ultrasonography, correct diagnosis is rarely made preoperatively (37,41).

According to the extent of involvement, adenomyomatous hyperplasia is divided into three forms: localized, segmental, and diffuse. The *localized form*, also known as *adenomyoma*, is the most common and is usually found at the tip of the fundus. Grossly, it appears as a well-circumscribed, umbilicated nodule bulging into the lumen or projecting toward the serosal surface. The cut surface is composed of gray or yellow-white rubbery tissue, with numerous small cystic spaces causing a honeycomb appearance (fig. 10-14). In the *segmental and diffuse forms*, there is a thickening of part or all of the gallbladder wall and small cystic spaces (fig. 10-15). Close inspection of the mucosa may reveal slit-like spaces or small orifices that communicate with the cystic spaces of the wall (fig. 10-16).

The basic histologic changes consist of branching duct or gland-like structures in the wall of the gallbladder and hyperplasia of smooth muscle cells (fig. 10-17). The epithelial structures, which may contain inspissated bile,

mucus, or stones, represent mucosal invaginations or outpouchings. Therefore, they are lined by a single layer of tall columnar cells similar to those of the surface epithelium. Foveolar and intestinal metaplasia rarely occur. Perineural invasion by benign ductal structures has recently been reported in adenomyomatous hyperplasia and should not be confused with adenocarcinoma (figs. 10-18, 10-19) (36). Continuity between the ductal or gland-like structures and the surface epithelium is often seen. Inflammation and fibrosis, which often accompany this lesion, can obstruct and even obliterate the epithelial-lined spaces. Obstruction enhances dilatation of the distal portion of the gland-like structures, which may then become cystic. Secondary gland formation sometimes occurs in the form of small pyloric type glands. When these glands

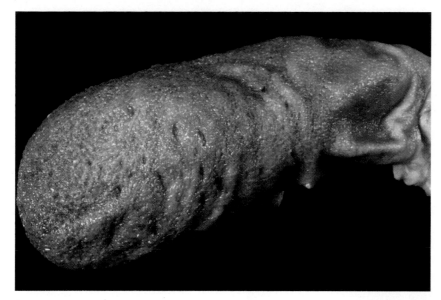

Figure 10-16
DIFFUSE FORM OF
ADENOMYOMATOUS
HYPERPLASIA
Numerous small openings of the
diverticula are visible in the mucosa
of the gallbladder.

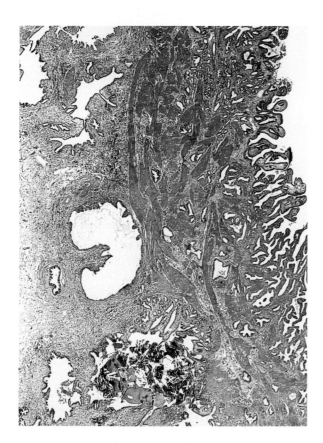

Figure 10-17
ADENOMYOMATOUS HYPERPLASIA
The cystically dilated ductal structures are most prominent in the perimuscular connective tissue. The hyperplastic
muscle layer also contains many ducts but they are not
markedly dilated.

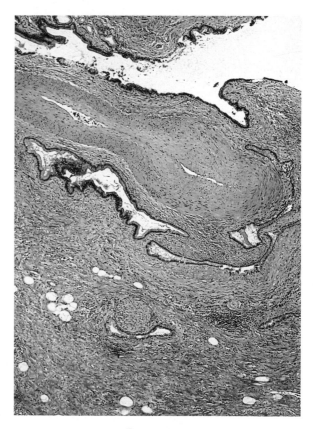

Figure 10-18
ADENOMYOMATOUS HYPERPLASIA
WITH PERINEURAL INVASION
Long and dilated ductal structures are lined by normal-ap-
pearing columnar epithelium. Perineural invasion by a small
ductal structure is seen in the subserosal connective tissue.

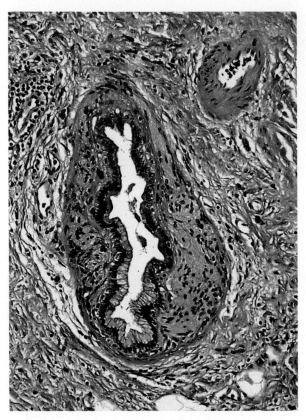

Figure 10-19
ADENOMYOMATOUS HYPERPLASIA
WITH PERINEURAL INVASION
A small ductal structure lined by benign-appearing co-
lumnar epithelium is seen within a nerve trunk. (Fig. 4 from
Albores-Saavedra J, Henson DE. Adenomyomatous hyper-
plasia of the gallbladder with perineural invasion. Arch
Pathol Lab Med 1995;119:1173–6.)

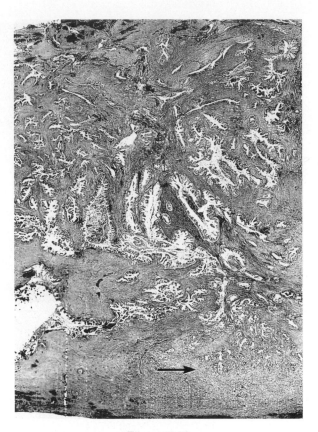

Figure 10-20
ADENOCARCINOMA ARISING IN
ADENOMYOMATOUS HYPERPLASIA
Adenocarcinoma arises in the deepest portion of a local-
ized adenomyomatous hyperplasia (arrow).

proliferate, they tend to form poorly defined lobules. The hyperplastic muscle bundles usually
surround the gland-like structures, a feature
that allows separation from Rokitansky-Aschoff
sinuses. Proliferation of distorted and hypertrophic nerve trunks occurs in some cases.

The epithelial invaginations of adenomyomatous hyperplasia may undergo neoplastic
transformation (40). Dysplastic changes and in
situ and invasive carcinomas have been reported.
The incidence of carcinoma in adenomyomatous
hyperplasia has varied from 2.0 to 6.4 percent
(42). In our own series of 48 patients, 2 (4.1
percent) had invasive adenocarcinoma. Adenocarcinomas are usually well differentiated and
are more commonly associated with the segmen-

tal or diffuse than with the localized form of
adenomyomatous hyperplasia (figs. 10-20, 10-
21). We do not consider adenomyomatous hyperplasia a premalignant lesion. In over 600 carcinomas of the gallbladder one of us (JA-S) has
examined, only 6 (1 percent) arose in adenomyomatous hyperplasia. The development of
carcinoma may be related to the presence of
stones rather than to the hyperplasia itself.

Adenocarcinomas that arise from the surface
epithelium may extend along the epithelial invaginations, mimicking invasion of the wall.
Likewise, adenomas of pyloric gland type that
originate in the lamina propria may grow along
the Rokitansky-Aschoff sinuses and simulate
malignancy. We have seen only two cases of
tubular adenoma that arose in an epithelial invagination of adenomyomatous hyperplasia.

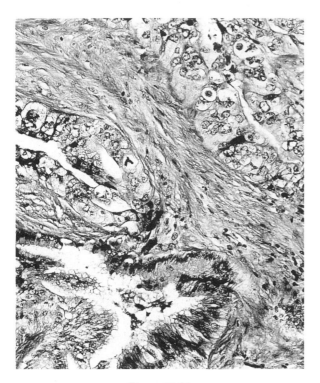

Figure 10-21
ADENOCARCINOMA ARISING
IN ADENOMYOMATOUS HYPERPLASIA
Benign-appearing columnar epithelium lines a ductal structure in close proximity to neoplastic glands. An abnormal mitosis is seen in one of the glands.

LUSCHKA'S DUCTS

Luschka's ducts represent a common developmental anomaly found in gallbladders with or without inflammation and lithiasis. They are located primarily in the perimuscular connective tissue adjacent to the liver or, less frequently, along the serosal surface. They are usually multiple and communicate with the intrahepatic bile ducts or with the abdominal cavity when located along the serosal surface. It has been claimed that these ducts also communicate with the gallbladder lumen, particularly in the region of the neck (36a). Histologically, Luschka's ducts are lined by either a cuboidal or columnar biliary type epithelium and are surrounded by concentric rings of connective tissue, which differentiates them from deep Rokitansky-Aschoff sinuses (fig. 10-22). Luschka's ducts are medium-sized or small ectopic bile ducts that are laid down during embryologic development (36c). When numerous, the small bile ducts that show reactive atypia may be mistaken for carcinoma.

MUCOCELE

Mucocele results from obstruction of the neck of the gallbladder by stones followed by excessive mucin production and distention of the lumen. Patients with cystic fibrosis may also develop

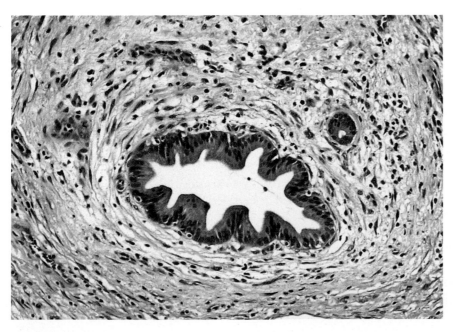

Figure 10-22
LUSCHKA'S DUCT
A dilated Luschka's duct is lined by columnar biliary type epithelium and surrounded by concentric rings of collagen fibers. Smaller bile ducts and some chronic inflammatory cells are also present in the surrounding fibrous tissue. Luschka's ducts are most common in the perimuscular connective tissue adjacent to the liver.

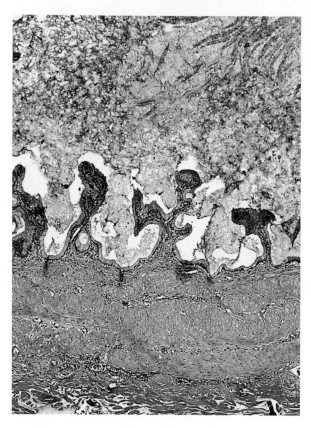

Figure 10-23
MUCOCELE OF THE GALLBLADDER
The lumen is filled with extracellular mucin. The surface epithelium appears normal.

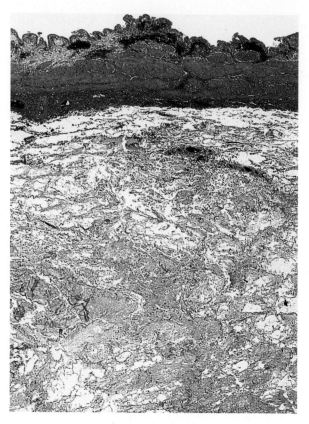

Figure 10-24
MUCOCELE OF THE GALLBLADDER
Abundant extracellular mucin is seen in the subserosal connective tissue while the lumen appears empty.

mucocele. We have seen nine cases, eight associated with cholelithiasis and one with cystic fibrosis. Microscopically, abundant mucin accumulates in the lumen and into the Rokitansky-Aschoff sinuses but the epithelium remains normal (fig. 10-23). However, the mucin may show focal calcifications and crystalloid structures. Eventually, mucosal ulceration occurs and the mucin extends into the wall and sometimes even outside the wall, a finding which often leads to confusion with mucinous adenocarcinoma. In some cases, the mucin outside the wall of the gallbladder is more abundant than that within the lumen (fig. 10-24). However, no tumor cells are seen in the extracellular mucin. Rarely, mucin-containing macrophages (muciphages) are seen floating in the extracellular mucin, mimicking signet ring cell carcinoma. However, neoplastic signet ring cells are cytokeratin and carcinoembryonic antigen-positive while the muciphages are negative for

these markers. The gallbladder wall shows varying degrees of fibrosis and chronic inflammation.

HETEROTOPIA

Ectopic tissues are occasionally found in the gallbladder or bile ducts. Except for cases of gastric or pancreatic heterotopia, they are usually not associated with clinical symptoms.

Gastric Heterotopia

By 1992, 40 examples of ectopic gastric mucosa had been described in the biliary tree, most within the gallbladder (44,47,49,50,52–59,61,64,66,67). We have examined four additional cases. In most cases, the ectopic mucosa was located in the neck, although all parts of the gallbladder have been involved (44,47,49). Although the ectopic gastric mucosa may be visualized by cholecystography, ultrasound, or computed tomography, a diagnosis

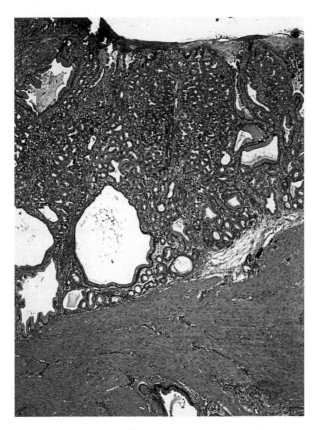

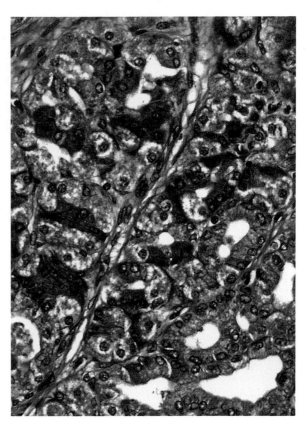

Figure 10-25
GASTRIC HETEROTOPIA
The gallbladder wall is replaced by fundic type gastric mucosa containing dilated glands and a thick muscle layer that closely resembles gastric wall.

Figure 10-26
GASTRIC HETEROTOPIA
Higher magnification of figure 10-25 shows small glands containing parietal and chief cells.

of ectopic gastric mucosa has not been made preoperatively.

According to clinical and pathologic features, patients can be separated into two groups. The first group, having no history of chronic cholecystitis or cholelithiasis, is composed of young adults, adolescents, and children complaining of epigastric distress, right upper quadrant pain, nausea, and vomiting. Three patients developed peptic ulceration and one presented with a perforation and hemorrhage (40,47,56). A few patients have had biliary obstruction and jaundice because of compression of the cystic or common bile ducts. The second group of patients is older and the heterotopic gastric mucosa is usually an incidental finding in gallbladders excised for cholecystitis. Although ectopic gastric mucosa is considered to be a congenital anomaly, children are rarely diagnosed with the anomaly (57).

Grossly, ectopic gastric tissue appears as an intramural or submucosal, polypoid, gray-white nodule, usually no greater than 2 cm in diameter and covered by an intact, often rugated mucosa. Occasionally, the nodule involves the full thickness of the gallbladder wall. An established peptic ulcer was recorded in the ectopic mucosa in three young patients (52,58). Histologically, there may be pyloric, antral, or fundic type epithelium with parietal and chief cells (figs. 10-25, 10-26). By immunohistochemistry, we have shown endocrine cells that are reactive for serotonin, somatostatin, and gastrin in two cases. A transverse and circular smooth muscle layer under the gastric epithelium has been described (58,66). In patients in whom gastric glands and muscle are present, the normal gallbladder wall appears partially replaced by stomach. A unique case of dual heterotopia in which gastric mucosa

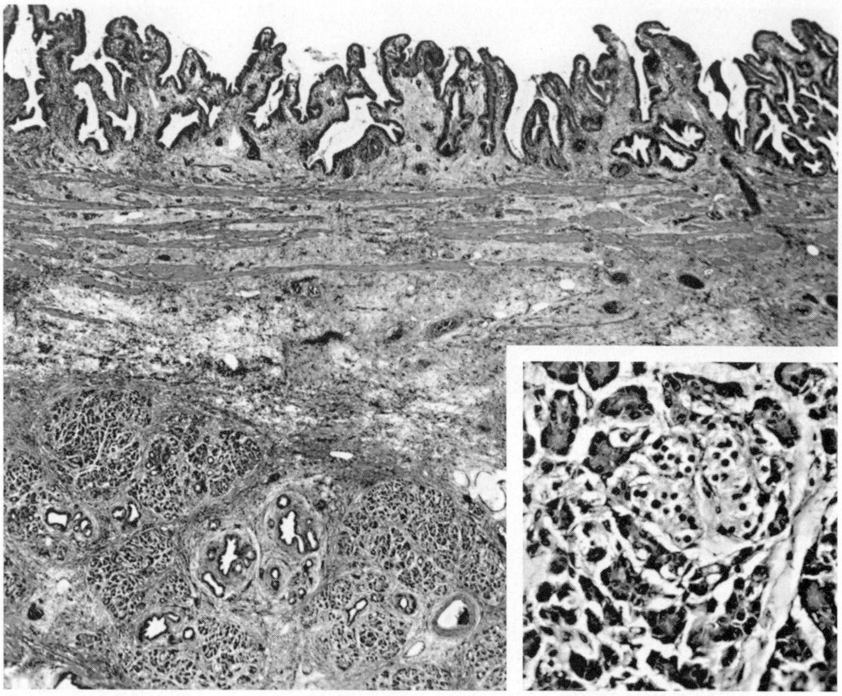

Figure 10-27
PANCREATIC HETEROTOPIA
A small focus of pancreatic tissue is present in the perimuscular connective tissue of the gallbladder. Inset: An islet surrounded by pancreatic acini is seen. (Fig. 151 from Fascicle 22, 2nd Series.)

and thyroid tissue coexisted in the wall of the gallbladder has also been documented (50).

Pancreatic Heterotopia

Pancreatic heterotopia, which occurs more often in the stomach, duodenum, or jejunum, is usually an incidental finding in the gallbladder (51). Most patients are female, and only a few have symptoms. Gallstones are present in about one third of patients. Grossly, the wall of the gallbladder may show only a focal thickening or contain a small yellow-white nodule. Histologically, all the normal pancreatic structures are present: acini, small ducts, and islets of Langerhans (fig. 10-27). The small excretory ducts usually open into the lumen of the gallbladder.

Two patients with a clinical picture of acute pancreatitis have been reported (60,65). Histologically, there was acute inflammation in the ectopic pancreas and fat necrosis in the wall of the gallbladder.

Hepatic Heterotopia

Ectopic liver is occasionally found on the serosal surface of the gallbladder (45–47,62,63). It is completely separated from the eutopic liver.

Only 19 examples have been reported to date (47). Often discovered at laparotomy or autopsy, the ectopic hepatic tissue consists of a solitary, encapsulated nodule measuring less than 1.5 cm and supported by a mesentery from the gallbladder. The ectopic liver tissue is usually normal or may show pathologic changes similar to those seen in the eutopic liver. The small fragments of normal liver torn away from the gallbladder bed during cholecystectomy should not be mistaken for ectopic liver.

Adrenal Cortical Heterotopia

Nodular rests of ectopic adrenal cortex can occur in the subserosal fat of the gallbladder wall (48). Although accessory adrenal tissue is found in many sites, location in the gallbladder is unusual.

POLYPS

Polyps that can be mistaken for benign or malignant tumors on cholecystograms, computed tomography, or ultrasonography occur in the gallbladder. As with polyps elsewhere, they are classified according to their stromal elements. They have no malignant potential. Some pathologists may prefer to call these lesions *pseudopolyps*.

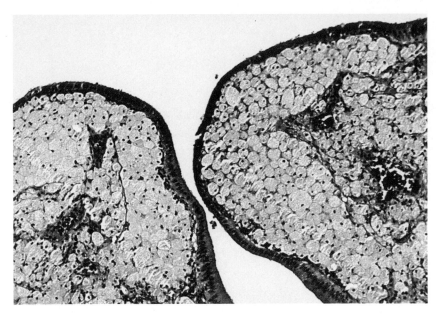

Figure 10-28
CHOLESTEROL POLYP
Two polypoid structures lined by normal gallbladder epithelium contain foam cells in the stroma.

Cholesterol Polyp

Cholesterol polyps, which may be found in any area of the gallbladder, are small tumor-like projections attached to the mucosa by a pedicle. They are usually yellow, soft textured, multilobulated nodules that rarely exceed 1 cm. The larger ones are often seen on cholecystograms or detected by sonography as mulberry-like, punctate, high echoes (68a–70). These lesions can be associated with nonspecific symptoms, such as indigestion and right upper quadrant pain, but in only a small number of cases are they associated with lithiasis or cholesterolosis. Microscopically, they are composed of foamy histiocytes which are positive with oil red O and contain cholesterol. They are covered by a single layer of columnar cells similar to those lining adjacent mucosa (fig. 10-28). Most likely, these polyps are enlarged and distended villi which become pedunculated because of the accumulation of histiocytes.

Inflammatory Polyp

These small polypoid lesions protrude into the lumen and are attached to the gallbladder wall by a broad base. They can be single or multiple, are always associated with acute and chronic cholecystitis, and are invariably denuded of the surface gallbladder epithelium (68). Because of their small size, 3 to 5 mm, and associated inflammatory changes, they are seldom visualized by cholecystography or ultrasonography. The edematous connective tissue stroma contains inflammatory cells, small dilated blood vessels, and hyperplastic epithelial invaginations. These polyps appear to be the result of enlargement and fusion of villi due to chronic inflammation.

Fibrous Polyp

This polypoid structure is larger than the granulation tissue polyp and is often detected by computed tomography or ultrasonography. Fibrous polyps usually coexist with gallstone disease and chronic cholecystitis, and consequently occur most often in females over 50 years of age. Microscopically, they show a leaf-like configuration and abundant connective tissue stroma containing scattered glands or duct-like structures which most likely result from invaginations of the surface epithelium. The stroma also contains inflammatory cells.

XANTHOGRANULOMATOUS CHOLECYSTITIS

Xanthogranulomatous inflammation is seen in 2 percent of gallbladders removed for lithiasis (78). This type of inflammatory response is most commonly seen in adult women with symptoms of acute or chronic cholecystitis (74–77). A rare complication of xanthogranulomatous cholecystitis is the formation of fistulous tracts from the

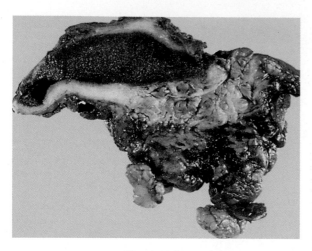

Figure 10-29
XANTHOGRANULOMATOUS CHOLECYSTITIS
A large and poorly demarcated, multinodular yellow mass involves the thickened wall of the gallbladder and extends into the adjacent soft tissues and liver.

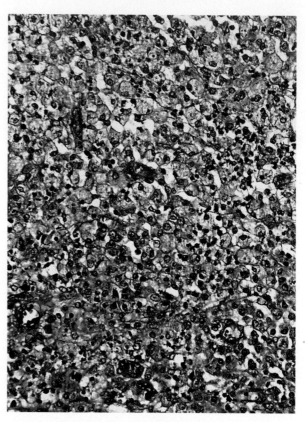

Figure 10-30
XANTHOGRANULOMATOUS CHOLECYSTITIS
Xanthogranulomatous cholecystitis showing foamy histiocytes mixed with polymorphonuclear leukocytes and plasma cells.

gallbladder to the duodenum or skin. Likewise, the inflammatory process may extend to the liver or the colon (79). Not infrequently, the findings on ultrasound examination or computed tomograms are suggestive of carcinoma (74). *Klebsiella, Escherichia coli,* and *Proteus mirabilis* have been cultured from the bile. Grossly, the lesion simulates a malignant tumor, since it appears as a poorly defined, yellow, nodular mass which often extends through the thickened wall of the gallbladder and may infiltrate adjacent organs, such as the duodenum, colon, or liver (fig. 10-29).

Histologically, the predominant cells are foamy histiocytes (which give a positive reaction to oil red O stain), lymphocytes, and plasma cells (figs. 10-30, 10-31). In addition, varying proportions of polymorphonuclear leukocytes, foreign body type giant cells, fibroblasts, bands of collagen, and cholesterol clefts are present (fig. 10-32). A storiform arrangement of the fibroblasts, reminiscent of fibrous histiocytoma, is prominent in some cases and may lead to confusion with malignancy, especially on frozen sections. However, the spindle cells lack nuclear atypia and mitotic figures are not found. The histiocytes may contain bile or ceroid pigment (71). Occasionally, they have a coarsely granular, eosinophilic cytoplasm that is strongly periodic acid–Schiff (PAS) positive. Intracellular and extracellular iron pigment, presumably the result of old hemorrhage, can be demonstrated in many cases. Xanthogranulomatous cholecystitis can coexist with carcinoma (72,75,77).

The pathogenesis of this lesion is obscure, although it has been suggested that obstruction of bile outflow by stones, mucosal ulceration, and ruptured Rokitansky-Aschoff sinuses with subsequent extravasation of bile play an important role. This pathogenetic mechanism parallels that proposed for xanthogranulomatous pyelonephritis where chronic infection, calculi, and obstruction appear to be common denominators.

Xanthogranulomatous cholecystitis can resemble malacoplakia. However, we were not able to demonstrate Michaelis-Gutmann bodies in the 58 cases we have examined. To our knowledge, only one case of malacoplakia of the gallbladder has been reported (73).

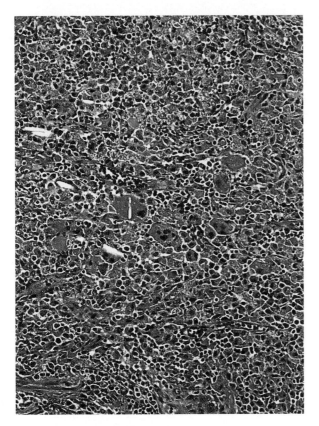

Figure 10-31
XANTHOGRANULOMATOUS CHOLECYSTITIS
Sheets of mononuclear histiocytes, with abundant eosinophilic cytoplasm, are admixed with foreign body giant cells and lymphocytes.

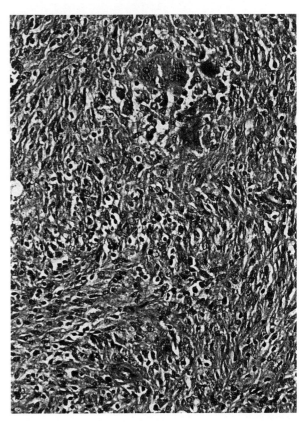

Figure 10-32
XANTHOGRANULOMATOUS CHOLECYSTITIS
Fibroblasts and histiocytes are arranged in bundles, and in some areas, they display a storiform pattern. Chronic inflammatory cells and a few multinucleated giant cells are also present. This storiform pattern may lead to confusion with a fibrous histiocytoma.

CHRONIC CHOLECYSTITIS WITH LYMPHOID HYPERPLASIA (PSEUDOLYMPHOMA)

The presence of an occasional lymphoid follicle within the inflammatory infiltrate of chronic cholecystitis is not uncommon (80,81). However, chronic cholecystitis associated with lymphoid hyperplasia extensive enough to justify the designation of "lymphoid hyperplasia" is exceedingly rare (83). Most patients with this type of cholecystitis are females with gallstones. *Klebsiella pneumoniae* and *Escherichia coli* have been isolated from the bile obtained during cholecystectomy (84a). Grossly, the mucosa of the gallbladder appears granular, nodular, or polypoid. The small nodules and polyps measure from 2 to 9 mm, are gray-white or tan, and are covered by an intact smooth mucosa. The wall of the gallbladder is thickened and fibrotic.

The polyclonal lymphoid infiltrate usually involves the lamina propria, but often extends to the muscular layer and even the serosa. It consists predominantly of normal-appearing noncleaved lymphocytes and plasma cells. Numerous varying sized lymphoid follicles with germinal centers are present throughout the inflammatory infiltrate, but are more prominent in the lamina propria (fig. 10-33). In some cases, the lymphoid tissue forms sessile or pedunculated polypoid structures, similar to those described in the rectum (fig. 10-34) (80,82,84). This lymphoid tissue is readily distinguished from malignant lymphoma on the basis of the polymorphic cell population, the presence of varying sized lymphoid follicles with germinal centers, the lack of cytologic atypia, and polyclonality. The role, if any, of this hyperplastic

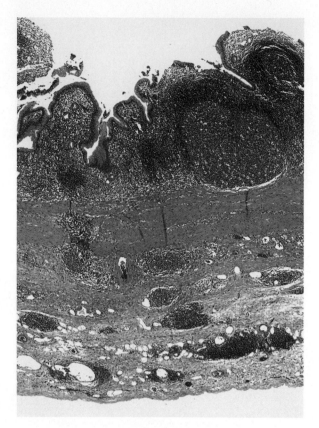

Figure 10-33
CHRONIC CHOLECYSTITIS WITH
LYMPHOID HYPERPLASIA
The lymphoid follicles, which contain germinal centers,
are more prominent in the lamina propria.

lymphoid tissue in the development of the rare primary malignant lymphoma of the gallbladder is unknown.

MYOFIBROBLASTIC PROLIFERATIONS

A heterogenous group of myofibroblastic proliferations has been described in many organs including the gallbladder, with a variety of appellations, the most common being *inflammatory pseudotumor* (85). A single example of this myofibroblastic lesion has been reported in the gallbladder and common hepatic duct of a 43-year-old man (87). The majority of these myofibroblastic proliferations mimic sarcomas. Those involving the lymph nodes and spleen appear as chronic inflammatory reactions with numerous lymphocytes and plasma cells, and a small number of myofibroblasts. The morphologic heterogeneity of these lesions probably reflects different etiologic factors. Some appear following surgical trauma, others are Epstein-Barr virus related (86), and still others are accompanied by autoimmune disorders (87). Those involving the urinary bladder have an unknown etiology.

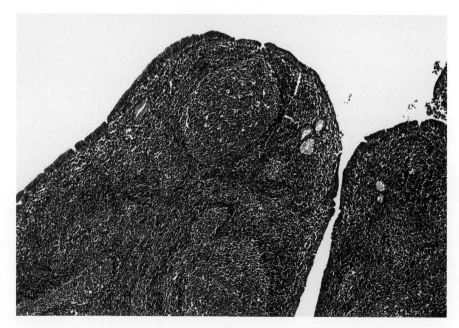

Figure 10-34
LYMPHOID HYPERPLASIA
A lymphoid polyp containing various-sized follicles with germinal centers is covered by normal gallbladder epithelium.

REFERENCES

Tumor-Like Lesions

1. Albores-Saavedra J, Henson DE. Pyloric gland metaplasia with perineural invasion of the gallbladder. A lesion that can be confused with adenocarcinoma. Cancer 1999;86:2627–31.

1a. Albores-Saavedra J, Nadji M, Henson DE, Ziegels-Weissman J, Mones JM. Intestinal metaplasia of the gallbladder: A morphologic and immunocytochemical study. Hum Pathol 1986;17:614–20.

2. Albores-Saavedra J, Nadji M, Morales AR, Henson DE. Carcinoembryonic antigen in normal, preneoplastic and neoplastic gallbladder epithelium. Cancer 1983; 52:1069–72.

3. Albores-Saavedra J, Vardaman C, Vuitch F. Non-neoplastic polypoid lesions and adenomas of the gallbladder. Pathol Ann Part I, 1993;28:145–77.

4. Azadeh B, Parai SK. Argentaffin cells, intestinal metaplasia and antral metaplasia in carcinoma of the gallbladder. Histopathology 1980;4:653–9.

5. DeBoer WG, Ma J, Rees JW, Nayman J. Inappropriate mucin production in gallbladder metaplasia and neoplasia—an immunohistological study. Histopathology 1981;5:295–303.

6. DeBoer WG, Nairn RC. Intestinal metaplasia in gallbladder: an immunohistochemical study. Pathology 1972;4:129–32.

7. Fox H. Ultrastructure of the human gallbladder epithelium in cholelithiasis and chronic cholecystitis. J Pathol 1972;108:157–64.

8. Hopwood D, Kouromalis E, Milne G, Bouchier IA. Cholecystitis: a fine structural analysis. J Pathol 1980;130:1–13.

9. Jarvi O, Lauren P. Intestinal metaplasia in the mucosa of the gallbladder and common bile duct with additional observations of pancreas heterotopy. Ann Med Exp Fenn 1967;45:213–23.

10. Kozuka S, Hachisuka K. Incidence by age and sex of intestinal metaplasia in the gallbladder. Hum Pathol 1984;15:779–84.

11. Laitio M. Goblet cells, enterochromaffin cells, superficial gastric-type epithelium and antral-type glands in the gallbladder. Beitr Pathol Bd 1975;156:343–58.

12. Laitio M. Morphology and histochemistry of non-tumorous gallbladder epithelium. Pathol Res Pract 1980;167:335–45.

13. Laitio M, Nevalainen TJ. An electron microscopic study of intestinal metaplasia in human gallbladder. Beitr Pathol Bd 1975;155:297–308.

14. Laitio M, Nevalainen TJ. Ultrastructure of endocrine cells in metaplastic epithelium of human gallbladder. J Anat 1975;120:219–25.

15. Laitio M, Terho T. Polysaccharides of metaplastic mucosa and carcinoma of the gallbladder. Lab Invest 1975;32:183–9.

16. Putz P, Willems G. Proliferative changes in the epithelium of the human lithiasic gallbladder. JNCI 1978;60:283–7.

17. Wistuba II, Gazdar AF, Roa I, Albores-Saavedra J. p53 protein overexpression in gallbladder carcinoma and its precursor lesions: an immunohistochemical study. Hum Pathol 1996;27:360–5.

18. Wistuba II, Sugio K, Hung J, et al. Allele specific mutations involved in the pathogenesis of endemic gallbladder carcinoma in Chile. Cancer Res 1995;55:2511–5.

Papillary Hyperplasia

19. Albores-Saavedra J, Defortuna SM, Smothermon WE. Primary papillary hyperplasia of the gallbladder and cystic and common bile ducts. Hum Pathol 1990;21:228–31.

19a. Albores-Saavedra J, Vardaman C, Vuitch F. Non-neoplastic polypoid lesions and adenomas of the gallbladder. Pathol Ann Part I, 1993;28:145–77.

20. Almagro UA. Diffuse papillomatosis of the gallbladder. Am J Gastroenterol 1985;80:274–8.

21. Nakajo S, Yamamoto M, Urashihara T, Kajitani T, Tahara E. Diffuse papillomatosis of the gallbladder complicated with tuberculosis. Acta Pathol Jpn 1988;38:1473–80.

22. Yamamoto M, Nakajo S, Ito M, et al. Primary mucosal hyperplasia of the gallbladder. Acta Pathol Jpn 1988;38:393–8.

Squamous Metaplasia

23. Albores-Saavedra J, Henson DE. Tumors of the gallbladder and extrahepatic bile ducts. Atlas of Tumor Pathology, 2nd Series, Fascicle 22. Washington, D.C.: Armed Forces Institute of Pathology, 1986.

Rokitansky-Aschoff Sinuses

24. Beilby JO. Diverticulosis of the gallbladder. Br J Exp Pathol 1967;48:455–61.

25. Christensen AH, Ishak KG. Benign tumors and pseudo-tumors of the gallbladder. Arch Pathol 1970;90:423–32.

26. Elfving G. Crypts and ducts in the gallbladder wall. Acta Pathol Microbiol Scand 1960;49(Suppl):1–45.

27. Fotopoulos JP, Crampton AR. Adenomyomatosis of the gallbladder. Med Clin North Am 1964;48:9–36.

28. Funabiki T, Matsumoto S, Tsukada N, et al. A patient with early gallbladder cancer derived from a Rokitansky-Aschoff sinus. Jpn J Surg 1993;23:350–5.

29. Jutras AJ, Levesque HP. Adenomyoma and adenomyomatosis of the gallbladder. Radiol Clin North Am 1966;4:483–500.

30. Kawarada Y, Sanda M, Mizumoto R, Yatani R. Early carcinoma of the gallbladder, non-invasive carcinoma originating in the Rokitansky-Aschoff sinus. A case report. Am J Gastroenterol 1986;81:61–6.

31. King ES. Cholecystitis glandularis and diverticula of the gallbladder. Br J Surg 1953;41:156–61.

32. LeQuesne LP, Ranger I. Cholecystitis glandularis proliferans. Br J Surg 1957;44:447–58.

33. Yamaguchi A, Hachisuka K, Masatoshi I, Tsubone M. Carcinoma in situ of the gallbladder with superficial extension into the Rokitansky-Aschoff sinuses and mucous glands. Gastroenterol Jpn 1992;27:765–72.

34. Young TE. So-called adenomyoma of the gallbladder. Am J Clin Pathol 1959;31:423–27.

Adenomyomatous Hyperplasia and Luschka's Ducts

35. Aguirre JR, Boher RO, Guraieb S. Hyperplastic cholecystoses: a new contribution to the unitarian theory. Am J Roentgenol 1969;107:1–13.

36. Albores-Saavedra J, Henson DE. Adenomyomatous hyperplasia of the gallbladder with perineural invasion. Arch Pathol Lab Med 1995;119:1173–6.

36a. Beilby JO. Diverticulosis of the gallbladder. Br J Exp Pathol 1967;48:455–61.

36b. Christensen AH, Ishak KG. Benign tumors and pseudotumors of the gallbladder. Arch Pathol 1970;90:423–32.

36c. Elfving G. Crypts and ducts in the gallbladder wall. Acta Pathol Microbiol Scand 1960;49(Suppl):1–45.

36d. Fotopoulos JP, Crampton AR. Adenomyomatosis of the gallbladder. Med Clin North Am 1964;48:9–36.

37. Gerard PS, Berman D, Zafaranloo S. CT and ultrasound of gallbladder adenomyomatosis mimicking carcinoma. J Comput Assist Tomogr 1990;14:490–1.

38. Jutras JA, Longtin M, Levesque HP. Hyperplastic cholecystoses. Am J Roentgenol 1960;83:795–827.

39. Kasahara Y, Sonobe N, Tomiyoshi H, et al. Adenomyomatosis of the gallbladder. A clinical survey of 30 surgically treated patients. Arch Jpn Chir 1992;61:190–8.

40. Katoh T, Nakai T, Hayashi S, et al. Noninvasive carcinoma of the gallbladder arising in localized type adenomyomatosis. Am J Gastroenterol 1988;83:670–4.

41. Meguid MM, Aun F, Bradford ML. Adenomyomatosis of the gallbladder. Am J Surg 1984;147:260–2.

42. Ootani T, Shirai Y, Tzukada K, Muto T. Relationship between gallbladder carcinoma and segmental type of adenomyomatosis of the gallbladder. Cancer 1992;69:2647–52.

43. Ram MD, Midha D. Adenomyomatosis of the gallbladder. Surgery 1975;78:224–9.

Heterotopia

44. Adam R, Fabiani B, Bismuth H. Hematobilia resulting from heterotopic stomach in the gallbladder neck. Surgery 1989;105:564–9.

45. Ashby EC. Accessory liver lobe attached to the gallbladder. Br J Surg 1969;56:311-2.

46. Bassis ML, Izenstark JL. Ectopic liver. Its occurrence in the gallbladder. Arch. Surg 1956;73:204–6.

47. Boyle L, Gallivan MV, Chun B, Lack EE. Heterotopia of gastric mucosa and liver involving the gallbladder. Report of two cases with literature review. Arch Pathol Lab Med 1992;116:138–42.

48. Busuttil A. Ectopic adrenal within the gallbladder wall. J Pathol 1974;113:231–3.

49. Christensen AH, Ishak KG. Benign tumors and pseudotumors of the gallbladder. Arch Pathol 1970;90:423–32.

50. Curtis LE, Sheahan DG. Heterotopic tissues in the gallbladder. Arch Pathol 1969;88:677–83.

51. Elfving G. Heterotopic pancreatic tissue in the gallbladder wall. Acta Chir Scand 1959;118:32–6.

52. Gitlitz AJ. Peptic ulcer in gallbladder diverticulum. J Mt Sinai Hosp 1957;24:875-87.

53. Gunter E, Ell C, Heyder N, Hahn EG, Giedl J, Scheele J. Ectopic tissue as polypoid lesion of the gallbladder. Dtsch Med Wochenschr 1989;114:1984.

54. Jarvi O, Meurman L. Heterotopic gastric mucosa and pancreas in the gallbladder with reference to the question of heterotopias in general. Ann Acad Sci Fenn Biol 1964;106:221–42.

55. Kalman PG, Stone RM, Phillips MJ. Heterotopic gastric tissue of the bile duct. Surgery 1981;89:384–6.

56. Larsen EH, Diederich PJ, Sorensen FB. Peptic ulcer in the gallbladder. A case report. Acta Chir Scand 1985;151:575–6.

57. Martinez-Urrutia MJ, Vazquez Estevez J, Larrauri J, Diez Pardo JA. Gastric heterotopy of the biliary tract. J Pediatr Surg 1990;25:356–7.

58. Mooney B, O'Malley E, Dempsey J. Gastric heterotopia in a gallbladder. Ir J Med Sci 1979;148:50–3.

59. Pradines P, Brauner M, Legrand I, Sibony M, Garin B. Heterotopic gastric mucosa in the gallbladder [Letter]. AJR Am J Roenterol 1989;152:432.

60. Qizilbash AH. Acute pancreatitis occurring in heterotopic pancreatic tissue in the gallbladder. Can J Surg 1976;19:413–4.

61. Runge PM, Schwartz JN, Seigler HF, Woodard BH, Shelburne JD. Gallbladder with ectopic mucosa. Arch Pathol Lab Med 1978;102:209–11.

62. Tejada E, Danielson C. Ectopic or heterotopic liver (choristoma) associated with the gallbladder. Arch Pathol Lab Med 1989;113:950–2.

63. Thorsness ET. The relationship of "true Luschka ducts," adenomas, and aberrant liver tissue in the wall of the human gallbladder. Am J Clin Pathol 1941;11:878–81.

64. Vallera DU, Dawson PJ. Gastric heterotopia in the gallbladder. Case report and review of literature. Path Res Pract 1992;188:49–52.

65. Vidgoff IJ, Lewis A. Acute hemorrhage from aberrant pancreatic tissue in gallbladder. Calif Med 1961;94:317–9.

66. Williams MJ, Humm JJ. Heterotopia composed of gastric epithelium and smooth muscle in the wall of the gallbladder. Surgery 1953;34:133–9.

67. Yamamoto M, Murakami H, Ito M, Nakajo S, Tahara E. Ectopic gastric mucosa of the gallbladder: comparison with metaplastic polyp of the gallbladder. Am J Gastroenterol 1989;84:1423–6.

Cholesterol and Inflammatory Polyps

68. Christensen AH, Ishak KG. Benign tumors and pseudo-tumors of the gallbladder. Arch Pathol 1970;90:423–32.
68a.Price RJ, Stewart TE, Foley D, Dodds WJ. Sonography of polypoid cholesterolosis. Am J Radiol 1982;139:1197–8.

69. Ruhe AH, Zachman JP, Mulder BD, Rime AE. Choles-terol polyps of the gallbladder: ultrasound demonstra-tion. J Comput Ultrasound 1979;7:386–8.
70. Ukai K, Akita Y, Mizuno S, et al. Cholesterol polyp of the gallbladder showing rapid growth and atypical changes. A case report. Hepatogastroenterology 1992;39:371–3.

Xanthogranulomatous Cholecystitis

71. Amazon K, Rywlin AM. Ceroid granulomas of the gall-bladder. Am J Clin Pathol 1980;73:123–7.
72. Benbow EW, Taylor PM. Simultaneous xanthogran-ulomatous cholecystitis and primary adenocarcinoma of gallbladder. Histopathology 1988;12:672–5.
73. Charpentier P, Prade M, Bognel C, Gadenne C, Duvillard P. Malacoplakia of the gallbladder. Hum Pathol 1983;14:827–8.
74. Duber C, Storkel S, Wagner PK, Muller J. Xanthogran-ulomatous cholecystitis mimicking carcinoma of the gallbladder: CT findings. J Comput Assist Tomogr 1984;8:1195–8.
75. Goodman ZD, Ishak KG. Xanthogranulomatous chole-cystitis. Am J Surg Pathol 1981;5:653–9.

76. Guo KJ, Yamaguchi K, Izumi Y, Enjoji M. Xanthogran-ulomatous cholecystitis: a clinicopathologic study of 68 cases. Surg Pathol 1988;1:241–8.
77. Lopez JI, Elizalde JM, Calvo MA. Xanthogranulomat-ous cholecystitis associated with gallbladder adenocar-cinoma. A clinicopathologic study of 5 cases. Tumori 1991;77:358–60.
78. Roberts KM, Parsons MA. Xanthogranulomatous cho-lecystitis: clinicopathological study of 13 cases. J Clin Pathol 1987;40:412–7.
79. Yoshida J, Chijiiwa K, Shimura H, et al. Xanthogran-ulomatous cholecystitis versus gallbladder cancer: clini-cal differentiating factors. Am Surg 1997;63:367–71.

Chronic Cholecystitis with Lymphoid Hyperplasia (Pseudolymphoma)

80. Albores-Saavedra J, Gould E, Manivel-Rodriguez C, Angeles-Angeles A, Henson DE. Chronic cholecystitis with lymphoid hyperplasia. La Rev Invest Clin (Mex) 1989;41:159–64.
81. Hatae Y, Kikuchi M. Lymph follicular cholecystitis. Acta Pathol Jpn 1979;29:67–71.
82. Helwig EB, Hansen J. Lymphoid polyps (benign lym-phoma) and malignant lymphoma of the rectum and anus. Surg Gynecol Obstet 1951;92:233–9.

83. Hussain SA, English WE, Lytle LH, Thomas DW Jr. Pseudolymphoma of the gallbladder. Am J Gas-troenterol 1976;65:152–5.
84. Yamaguchi K, Enjoji M. Gallbladder polyps: inflamma-tory, hyperplastic and neoplastic types. Surg Pathol 1988;1:203–13.
84a.Yoshida J, Chijiiwa K, Shimura H, et al. Xanthogran-ulomatous cholecystitis versus gallbladder cancer: clini-cal differentiating factors. Am Surg 1997;63:367–71.

Myofibroblastic Proliferations

85. Albores-Saavedra J, Manivel JC, Essenfeld H, et al. Pseudosarcomatous myofibroblastic proliferations in the urinary bladder of children. Cancer 1990;66:1234–41.
86. Arber DA, Kamel OW, Van de Riju M, et al. Frequent presence of the Epstein-Barr virus in inflammatory pseudotumor. Hum Pathol 1995;26:1093–8.

87. Ikeda H, Oka T, Imafuku I, et al. A case of inflammatory pseudotumor of the gallbladder and bile duct. Am J Gastroenterol 1990;85:203–6.

11

BENIGN EPITHELIAL TUMORS AND PAPILLOMATOSIS
OF THE EXTRAHEPATIC BILE DUCTS

BENIGN EPITHELIAL TUMORS

Adenoma

Adenomas of the extrahepatic bile ducts are benign, polypoid, epithelial neoplasms composed of papillary, tubular, or both kinds of structures, lined by dysplastic epithelium. According to their cell phenotype, these adenomas can be subclassified as intestinal and biliary types (1). However, the incidence of these tumors is difficult to determine because cystadenomas, ampullary adenomas that extend into the common channel, papillomatosis, and tumor-like lesions were often included as extrahepatic bile duct adenomas in older publications (2,4,5). If these lesions are excluded, then adenomas of the extrahepatic bile ducts become extremely rare (3,9,11). Therefore, it is not surprising that most of our information is based on case reports. Based on our limited experience with six cases, and a review of the literature, intestinal type adenoma is perhaps the only type found in this location. The pyloric type of adenoma, which is the most common form of adenoma in the gallbladder, has not been reported in the extrahepatic bile ducts. This may be due in part to the low incidence of pyloric gland metaplasia in the extrahepatic bile ducts as compared to the gallbladder. Most likely, pyloric gland metaplasia is the precursor of pyloric gland adenoma. Likewise, adenomas composed entirely of biliary type epithelium have not been documented in the extrahepatic bile ducts. In contrast to gallbladder adenomas, those of the extrahepatic bile ducts are not associated with lithiasis. Most adenomas are found in the common bile duct, followed by the common hepatic duct, the cystic duct, and the hepatic ducts.

Clinical Features. Adenomas usually obstruct the extrahepatic bile ducts, leading to jaundice and requiring surgical intervention (3,4,11). Rarely are they resected endoscopically (18). The jaundice usually has an insidious onset and can be intermittent or persistent. Adenomas that arise in the cystic duct can cause distention of the gallbladder and pain (14). Differentiation of adenomas from malignant tumors is often difficult prior to biopsy. However, the correct diagnosis can sometimes be suspected on the basis of cholangiography, endoscopic ultrasonography, and selective angiography.

A few examples of symptomatic tubular adenomas, intestinal type, of the distal common bile duct have been reported in patients with familial polyposis/Gardner's syndrome (7,17). The simultaneous occurrence of tubular adenomas of the common bile duct and carcinoma in situ of the ampulla and main pancreatic duct has been documented in another patient with Gardner's syndrome (12). A patient with familial adenomatous polyposis coli had a tubular adenoma of the common bile duct and an infiltrating adenocarcinoma of the duodenum (10).

A patient with Peutz-Jeghers' syndrome had a solitary hamartomatous polyp of the distal common bile duct (16). However, the photomicrograph of the polyp did not show the distinctive histologic features of the hamartomatous lesion which are characteristic of the syndrome and did not correspond to a tubular or a papillary adenoma.

Microscopic Findings. Tubular adenomas have an intestinal phenotype and consist of varying sized tubular glands. These glands are lined by columnar cells with elongated, hyperchromatic and pseudostratified nuclei (figs. 11-1, 11-2). Goblet cells and endocrine cells are admixed with the columnar cells. The endocrine cells are immunoreactive for chromogranin and serotonin (fig. 11-3). Less frequently, they are reactive for the peptide hormones. Paneth cells are rarely found in adenomas.

Papillary adenomas also show intestinal differentiation. They are composed of finger-like projections or papillary structures that are lined by columnar cells that often contain mucin (fig. 11-4). The nuclei are hyperchromatic, ovoid, or elongated and pseudostratified (fig. 11-5). Goblet cells and endocrine cells are found among the columnar cells (fig. 11-6). Paneth cells are uncommon.

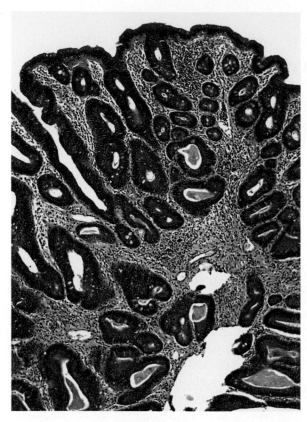

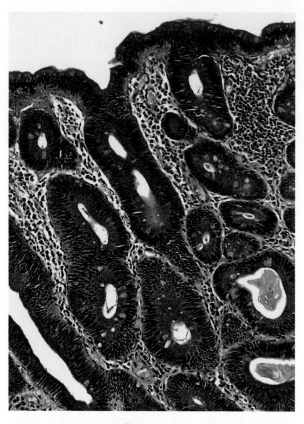

Figure 11-1
TUBULAR ADENOMA, INTESTINAL TYPE,
OF COMMON BILE DUCT

This tumor, which is composed of tubular glands, is indistinguishable from tubular adenoma of the small and large intestines.

Figure 11-2
TUBULAR ADENOMA, INTESTINAL TYPE,
OF COMMON BILE DUCT

Higher magnification of tumor shown in figure 11-1. The tubular glands are lined by columnar cells with elongated hyperchromatic nuclei.

Figure 11-3
ENDOCRINE CELLS
IN TUBULAR ADENOMA

Numerous chromogranin-positive cells are admixed with the columnar cells.

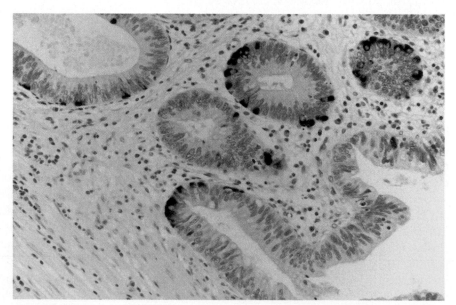

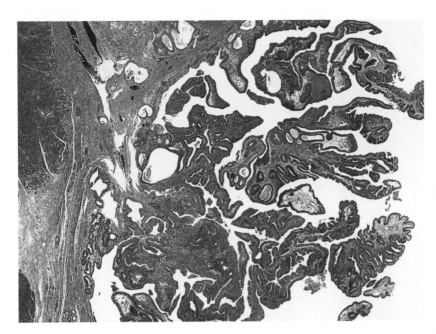

Figure 11-4
PAPILLARY ADENOMA,
INTESTINAL TYPE,
OF COMMON BILE DUCT
Low-power view of papillary ade-
noma that arose from the intrapan-
creatic portion of the common bile duct.

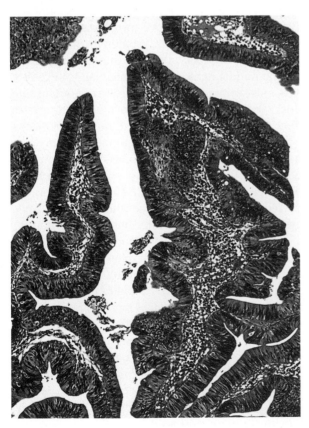

Figure 11-5
PAPILLARY ADENOMA, INTESTINAL TYPE,
OF COMMON BILE DUCT
The papillary structures are lined by pseudostratified
columnar epithelium.

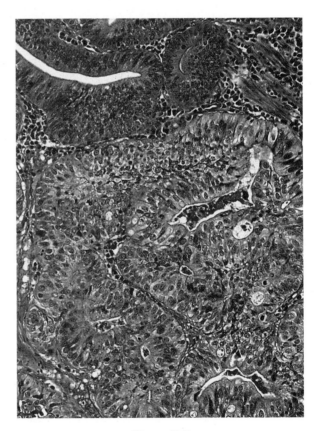

Figure 11-6
PAPILLARY ADENOMA, INTESTINAL TYPE,
OF COMMON BILE DUCT
Focus of carcinoma in situ in the papillary adenoma
shown in figure 11-5. Closely packed tubular glands are lined
by highly dysplastic epithelium.

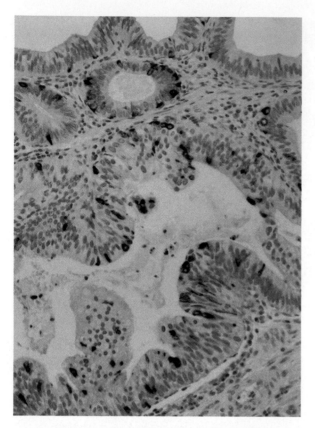

Figure 11-7
ENDOCRINE CELLS IN PAPILLARY ADENOMA,
INTESTINAL TYPE
Many chromogranin-positive cells are seen in a minor tubular component of the tumor.

Despite varying degrees of dysplasia and the occasional foci of carcinoma in situ in these adenomas, we, as well as others (6,8,13,19), believe that adenomas are not the precursors of most carcinomas of the extrahepatic bile ducts (fig. 11-7). In our experience, only a small proportion of adenomas progress to carcinoma. This is in contrast with adenomas of the ampulla of Vater which often transform into carcinoma. The arguments against the adenoma-carcinoma sequence can be summarize as follows: 1) adenomas are much less common than carcinomas of the extrahepatic bile ducts; 2) most carcinomas of the extrahepatic bile ducts do not show evidence of a residual adenoma. In our series of 143 cases, only 4 had foci of preexisting adenomas; and 3) the mucosa adjacent to most carcinomas shows flat dysplasia and carcinoma in situ which are considered the cancer precursors (6,8,13,19). Some carcinomas are

associated with ulcerative colitis and primary sclerosing cholangitis which late in their course are often complicated with flat and papillary dysplasia but not with adenomas (8,15).

Cystadenoma

Cystadenoma of the extrahepatic bile ducts is a benign, multiloculated neoplasm lined by cuboidal or columnar epithelial cells closely resembling biliary or gastric foveolar cells. The subepithelial stroma is densely cellular and resembles ovarian stroma. This rare but distinctive neoplasm belongs to a family of mucinous cystic tumors that can arise within the liver (20,22–24,29), in the extrahepatic biliary tree (21,22,24,26–28,34,35), in the pancreas, or even in the retroperitoneum unattached to any organ (21). Of 52 biliary cystadenomas, 43 were located within the liver, 8 in the extrahepatic bile ducts, and 1 in the gallbladder (22). Cystadenomas of the liver and pancreas may coexist in the same patient (25). Likewise, cystadenomas of the liver may extend into the extrahepatic bile ducts. Cystadenomas of the extrahepatic bile ducts are seen almost exclusively among middle-aged females (mean age, 45 years). The most common locations are the common bile duct, the common hepatic duct, and the cystic duct. Often larger than noncystic adenomas, cystadenomas are usually symptomatic. Many are palpable on physical examination and may be painful. Others may lead to obstructive jaundice. Elevated serum levels of CA19-9 have been reported in patients with these tumors (31). Rarely, cystadenomas are incidental findings at autopsy.

Gross Findings. Cystadenomas are multilocular or unilocular, well-demarcated cystic masses that contain carcinoembryonic antigen (CEA)-rich serous or mucinous fluid. Their size varies from 1.5 to 20 cm. The fibrous wall is smooth and of variable thickness. The inner surface can be smooth, finely granular, or trabeculated. In some cystadenomas, small polypoid structures project into the lumen of the locules. We have seen a biliary cystadenoma that appeared as a polypoid, microcystic, yellow mass that seemed to have arisen within the liver and extended into the common hepatic duct (fig. 11-8).

Microscopic Findings. The locules of most cystadenomas have a characteristic three layer structure (fig. 11-9): a columnar epithelial lining,

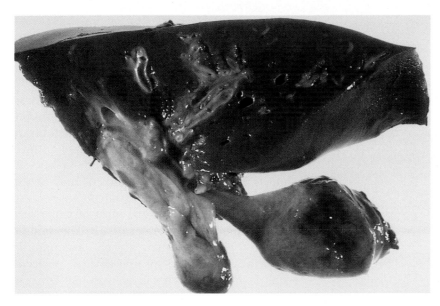

Figure 11-8
POLYPOID BILIARY
CYSTADENOMA
Polypoid biliary cystadenoma
that involved both the intrahepatic
and extrahepatic bile ducts. This
gross appearance is most unusual in
biliary cystadenoma.

a cellular ovarian-like stroma, and an outer layer of hyalinized fibrous tissue (figs. 11-10, 11-11). Ten to 15 percent of the tumors lack the ovarian-like stroma (22). The surface-lining epithelial cells are cuboidal or columnar and closely resemble biliary or gastric foveolar cells. Goblet and Paneth cells are present in 20 percent of the tumors. One third of cystadenomas contain scattered endocrine cells that are argyrophilic. These three cell types reflect intestinal metaplasia. Around 13 percent of the cystadenomas show dysplastic changes, suggesting that some may progress to carcinoma (22). Underlying the epithelial lining there is a cellular band composed of spindle cells reminiscent of ovarian stroma which is supported by an outer layer of hyalinized fibrous tissue. Inflammatory changes occur in some cases. Foamy histiocytes, multinucleated giant cells, hemosiderin laden macrophages, areas of hemorrhage, and cholesterol clefts efface the ovarian-like stroma and the characteristic three-layer structure.

Histogenesis. It has been suggested that biliary cystadenomas arise from displaced embryonic tissue destined to form the gallbladder (30). However, this hypothesis fails to explain: 1) the almost exclusive occurrence of cystadenomas among adult women; 2) the presence of an ovarian-like stroma in mucinous cystic tumors of the pancreas; 3) the existence of tumors similar to biliary

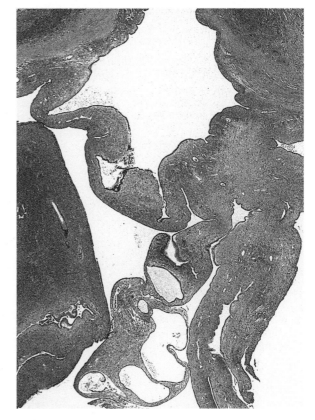

Figure 11-9
BILIARY CYSTADENOMA
Low-power view of a cystadenoma showing multiple locules of different sizes.

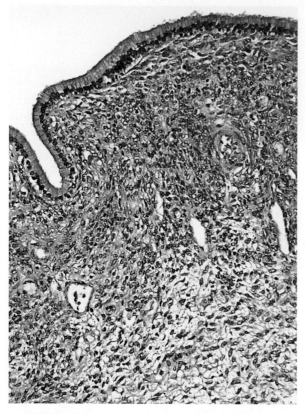

Figure 11-10
CYSTADENOMA OF THE COMMON BILE DUCT

The cyst wall is lined by a single layer of columnar mucin-secreting cells. The cellular stroma beneath the epithelium resembles ovarian stroma and contains numerous small blood vessels.

cystadenomas in the retroperitoneum unattached to any organ; and 4) the fact that estrogen and progesterone receptors have been demonstrated in the mesenchymal stromal cells of cystadenomas, but not in the stroma of the fetal gallbladder.

Immunohistochemical Findings. The epithelial component of cystadenomas is immunoreactive for cytokeratin, epithelial membrane antigen, CEA, and the tumor-associated antigen CA19-9 (31). Focal or diffuse reactivity to lysozyme is seen in the epithelium of half of the tumors. About one third of cystadenomas contain chromogranin-positive cells, most of which are also immunoreactive for serotonin. The spindle cells of the ovarian-like stroma are usually vimentin and muscle-specific antigen positive. Focal desmin positivity is seen in one third of tumors. This immunohistochemical profile is consistent with fibroblastic and myofibroblastic differentiation. The spindle cells of the ovarian-like stroma are usually positive for estrogen and progesterone receptors (fig. 11-12) (32).

We have examined two cystadenomas by electron microscopy. Three cell types were identified in the stroma: undifferentiated mesenchymal cells, fibroblasts, and myofibroblasts. The lining epithelial cells were columnar and joined by desmosomes. Short apical microvilli and mucin droplets of different sizes were present in many cells.

Differential Diagnosis. Cystadenomas should be distinguished from choledochal cysts,

Figure 11-11
CYSTADENOMA OF THE COMMON HEPATIC DUCT

The epithelial lining is cuboidal and contains no mucin. The cellular ovarian-like stroma is seen beneath the biliary epithelium.

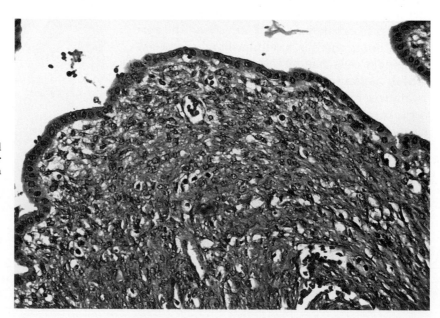

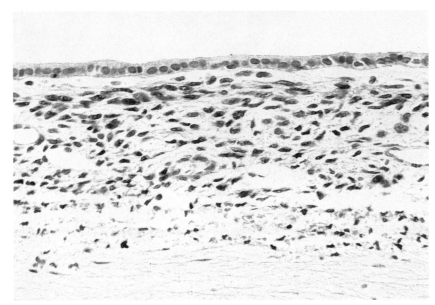

Figure 11-12
CYSTADENOMA
Most nuclei of the spindle cells from the ovarian-like stroma are immunoreactive for estrogen receptors.

the most common congenital anomaly of the extrahepatic biliary tree. Choledochal cysts, however, are not multiloculated. Their wall consists of dense fibrous tissue which may be lined by normal biliary epithelium or may be devoid of an epithelial lining. The mesenchymal stroma characteristic of cystadenoma is lacking in choledochal cysts. Retention cysts of periductal gland origin can be confused with cystadenomas. These retention cysts are usually multiple, asymptomatic, and smaller than cystadenomas. Their wall lacks mesenchymal stroma and may contain inflammatory cells (28,33).

Treatment and Prognosis. Cystadenomas of the extrahepatic bile ducts usually recur following incomplete excision (22). Despite the foci of dysplasia present in 13 percent of cystadenomas, malignant transformation has not been reported in tumors of the extrahepatic bile ducts. Biliary cystadenocarcinomas have been documented in the gallbladder and within the liver.

PAPILLOMATOSIS

This rare clinicopathologic entity is characterized by multifocal papillary tumors prone to local recurrence (36–40). These tumors usually involve extensive areas of the extrahepatic bile ducts, occasionally extending into the intrahepatic bile ducts, gallbladder, and main pancreatic duct (40,42,43). In some cases the papillary lesions

are confined to the intrahepatic bile ducts (44,48,49). Twenty-seven cases have been reported (40); we have seen three additional cases.

The disease affects both sexes equally. Most patients are adults between 50 and 60 years of age who present with biliary obstruction. Percutaneous transhepatic cholangiography or endoscopic retrograde cholangiography usually reveals multiple filling defects or mural irregularities along the biliary tree (43).

Histologically, multiple complex papillary lesions as well as gland-like structures are recognized (figs. 11-13, 11-14). The lining epithelial cells are cuboidal or columnar, and contain a variable amount of cytoplasmic mucin. The nuclei are round, ovoid, or elongated and contain small nucleoli (fig. 11-15). Cytologic atypia and mitotic figures are uncommon although obvious carcinomatous changes can be identified in some cases (47).

Because of the high incidence of local recurrence and extensive involvement of the biliary tree, the question of papillary carcinoma often arises with these lesions. Traditionally, the lack of invasion into the wall, absence of mitotic figures, and minimal nuclear atypia was considered helpful in excluding papillary carcinoma. However, it should be noted that hepatic metastases were found in one patient (42) and in one of our cases carcinoma had metastasized to the regional lymph nodes and liver. The metastatic deposits contained both the benign-appearing or

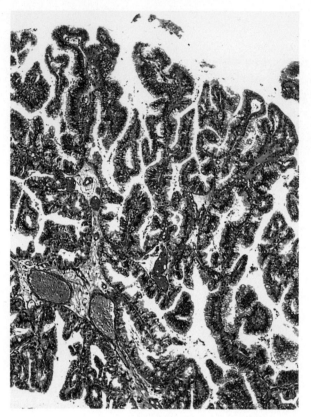

Figure 11-13
PAPILLOMATOSIS
Numerous, long, slender and complex papillary structures lined by columnar epithelium project into the lumen of the common duct.

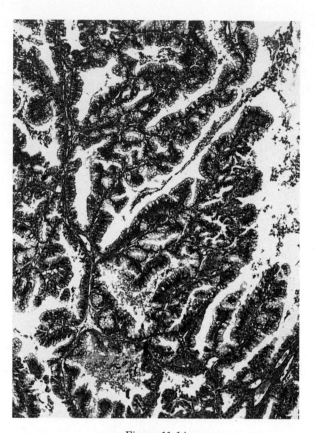

Figure 11-14
PAPILLOMATOSIS
Another area of tumor shown in figure 11-13 depicting multiple branching papillary structures.

Figure 11-15
PAPILLOMATOSIS
Higher magnification of papillary structures shown in figure 11-14. The columnar cells are pseudostratified, exhibit mild dysplastic changes, and contain mucin.

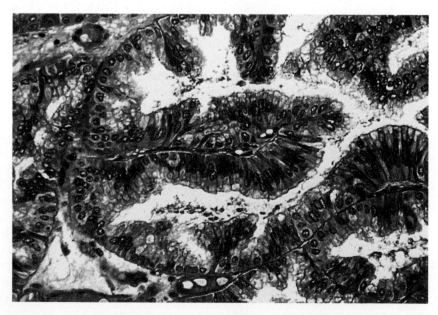

less atypical epithelial cells as well as the obvious carcinomatous elements. Therefore, we now believe that papillomatosis is a form of intraductal papillary carcinoma with a broad morphologic spectrum rather than a benign papillary lesion that may become malignant. More studies are needed to confirm these observations. In many respects, papillomatosis of the extrahepatic biliary tree is similar to those papillary lesions of the main pancreatic duct (intraductal papillary mucinous neoplasms) that are now regarded as multifocal, mucin-producing, intraductal papillary carcinomas (45,46,50). Recent experimental work supports this view. Papillary lesions, including papillary carcinomas, similar to the human tumors, have been induced in the main pancreatic duct and in the gallbladder of hamsters treated with N-nitroso(2-hydroxypropyl) (2-oxopropyl)amine. The incidence of these tumors increases when orotic acid is added to the diet (41).

A point mutation at codon 12 of the K-*ras* oncogene, similar to the mutations reported in extrahepatic bile duct carcinomas, was found in a case of biliary papillomatosis that arose in a congenital choledochal cyst (48). This genetic abnormality was considered as support for the concept that biliary papillomatosis is a premalignant or malignant lesion. However, a K-*ras* mutation is not a marker for malignancy, since it has been detected in hyperplastic and metaplastic lesions as well as in histologically normal tissues (51).

Complete excision of the lesions is very difficult or impossible with conservative surgery such as local excision or curettage. Therefore, local recurrence eventually occurs in most cases (40).

The prognosis is poor. The mean survival period for 13 patients for whom adequate follow-up was available was 3 years. Five patients (38 percent) survived for more than 5 years. Two patients lived for 6 years following curettage and external drainage. However, almost half of the patients died within 3 years after diagnosis (40).

REFERENCES

Adenoma

1. Albores-Saavedra J, Vardaman C, Vuitch F. Non-neoplastic polypoid lesions and adenomas of the gallbladder. Pathol Ann 1993;28:145–77.
2. Baggenstoss AH. Major duodenal papilla. Variations of pathologic interest and lesions of the mucosa. Arch Pathol 1938;26:853–68.
3. Buckley JG, Salimi Z. Villous adenoma of the common bile duct. Abdom Imaging 1993;18:245–6.
4. Burhans R, Myers RT. Benign neoplasms of the extrahepatic biliary ducts. Am Surg 1971;37:161–6.
5. Chu PT. Benign neoplasms of the extrahepatic biliary ducts. Arch Pathol 1950;50:84–97.
6. Davis RI, Sloan JM, Hood JM, Maxwell P. Carcinoma of the extrahepatic biliary tract: a clinicopathological and immunohistochemical study. Histopathology 1988;12:623–31.
7. Erwald R. Gardner's syndrome with adenoma of the common bile duct, a case report. Acta Chir Scand 1984;520:63–8.
8. Haworth AC, Manley PN, Groll A, Pace R. Bile duct carcinoma and biliary tract dysplasia in chronic ulcerative colitis. Arch Pathol Lab Med 1989;113:434–6.
9. Hulten J, Johansson H, Olding L. Adenomas of the gallbladder and extrahepatic bile ducts. Acta Chir Scand 1970;136:203–7.
10. Jarvinen H, Nyberg M, Peltokallio P. Biliary involvement in familial adenomatosis coli. Dis Colon Rectum 1983;26:525–8.
11. Jennings PE, Rode J, Coral A, Dowsett J, Lees WR. Villous adenoma of the common hepatic duct: the role of ultrasound in management. Gut 1990;31:558–60.
12. Komorowski RA, Tresp MG, Wilson SD. Pancreatobiliary involvement in familial polyposis coli/Gardner's syndrome. Dis Colon Rectum 1986;29:55–8.
13. Laitio M. Carcinoma of extrahepatic bile ducts: a histopathological study. Pathol Res Pract 1983;178:67–72.
14. Loh A, Kamar S, Dickson GH. Solitary benign papilloma (papillary adenoma) of the cystic duct: a rare cause of biliary colic. Br J Clin Pract 1994;48:167–8.
15. Ludwig J, Wahlstrom HE, Batts KP, Weisner RH. Papillary bile duct dysplasia in primary sclerosing cholangitis. Gastroenterology 1992;102:2134–8.
16. Parker MC, Knight M. Peutz-Jeghers syndrome causing obstructive jaundice due to polyp in common bile duct. J Roy Soc Med 1983;76:701–3.
17. Spigelman AD, Farmer KC, James M, Richman PI, Phillips RK. Tumours of the liver, bile ducts, pancreas and duodenum in a single patient with familial adenomatous polyposis. Br J Surg 1991;78:979–80.
18. Sturgis T, Fromkes JJ, Marsh W. Adenoma of the common bile duct: endoscopic diagnosis and resection. Gastrointest Endosc 1992;38:504–5.
19. Suzuki M, Takahashi T, Ouchi K, Matsuno S. The development and extension of hepatohilar bile duct carcinoma. A three-dimensional tumor mapping in the intrahepatic biliary tree visualized with the aid of a graphics computer system. Cancer 1989;64:658–66.

Cystadenoma

20. Akwari OE, Tucker A, Siegler HF, Itani KM. Hepatobiliary cystadenoma with mesenchymal stroma. Ann Surg 1990;211:18–27.
21. Albores-Saavedra J, Vardaman CJ, Vuitch F. Non-neoplastic polypoid lesions and adenomas of the gallbladder. Pathol Ann 1993;28:145–77.
22. Devaney K, Goodman ZD, Ishak KG. Hepatobiliary cystadenoma and cystadenocarcinoma. A light microscopic and immunohistochemical study of 70 patients. Am J Surg Pathol 1994;18:1078–91.
23. Gourley WK, Kumar D, Bouton MS, Fish JC, Nealon W. Cystadenoma and cystadenocarcinoma with mesenchymal stroma of the liver: immunohistochemical analysis. Arch Pathol Lab Med 1992;116:1047–50.
24. Ishak KG, Willis GW, Cummins SD, Bullock AA. Biliary cystadenoma and cystadenocarcinoma. Report of 14 cases and review of the literature. Cancer 1977;38:322–38.
25. Keech MK. Cystadenomata of the pancreas and intrahepatic bile ducts. Gastroenterology 1951;19:568–74.
26. Marsh JL, Dahms B, Longmire WG, Jr. Cystadenoma and cystadenocarcinoma of the biliary system. Arch Surg 1974;109:41–3.
27. Nakajima T, Sugano I, Matsuzaki O, et al. Biliary cystadenocarcinoma of the liver. A clinicopathologic and histochemical analysis of nine cases. Cancer 1992;69:2426–32.
28. Nakanuma Y, Kurumaya H, Ohta G. Multiple cysts in the hepatic hilum and their pathogenesis. A suggestion

29. of periductal gland origin. Virchows Arch [A] 1984;404:341–50.
29. Short WF, Nedwich A, Levy HA, Howard JM. Biliary cystadenoma. Report of a case and review of the literature. Arch Surg 1971;102:78–80.
30. Subramony C, Herrera GA, Turbat-Herrera E. Hepatobiliary cystadenoma. A study of five cases with reference to histogenesis. Arch Pathol Lab Med 1993;117:1036–42.
31. Thomas JA, Scriven MW, Puntis MC, Jasani B, Williams GT. Elevated serum CA 19-9 levels in hepatobiliary cystadenoma with mesenchymal stroma: two case reports with immunohistochemical confirmation. Cancer 1992;70:1841–6.
32. Vuitch F, Battifora H, Albores-Saavedra J. Demonstration of steroid hormone receptors in pancreato-biliary mucinous cystic neoplasms [Abstract]. Lab Invest 1993;68:114A.
33. Wanless IR, Zahradnik J, Heathcote EJ. Hepatic cysts of periductal gland origin presenting as obstructing jaundice. Gastroenterology 1987;93:894–8.
34. Wheeler DA, Edmondson HA. Cystadenoma with mesenchymal stroma (CMS) in the liver and bile ducts. A clinicopathologic study of 17 cases, 4 with malignant change. Cancer 1985;56:1434–45.
35. Woods GL. Biliary cystadenocarcinoma: case report of hepatic malignancy originating in benign cystadenoma. Cancer 1981;47:2936–40.

Papillomatosis

36. Albores-Saavedra J, Henson DE. Tumors of the gallbladder and extrahepatic bile ducts. Atlas of Tumor Pathology, 2nd Series, Fascicle 22. Washington, D.C.: Armed Forces of Institutes of Pathology, 1986.
37. Albores-Saavedra J, Vardaman C, Vuitch F. Non-neoplastic polypoid lesions and adenomas of the gallbladder. Pathol Ann 1993;28:145–77.
38. Böttger TK, Sorger E, Junzinger T. Progressive papillomatosis of the intrahepatic and extrahepatic bile ducts. Acta Chir Scand 1989;155:125–9.
39. Eiss S, Dimaio D, Caedo JP. Multiple papillomas of the entire biliary tract: case report. Ann Surg 1960;152:320–4.
40. Hubens G, Delvaux G, Willems G, Bourgain C, Klöppel G. Papillomatosis of the intra- and extrahepatic bile ducts with involvement of the pancreatic duct. Hepatogastroenterology 1991;38:413–8.
41. Kokkinakis DM, Albores-Saavedra J. Orotic acid enhancement of preneoplastic and neoplastic lesions induced in the pancreas and liver of hamsters by N-Nitroso(2-hydroxypropyl) (2-oxopropyl)amine. Cancer Res 1994;54:5324–32.
42. Madden JJ, Smith GW. Multiple biliary papillomatosis. Cancer 1974;34:1316–20.
43. Marchal G, Vernette M, Roustan J, Henry G. Papillomatose biliaire cancerisee avec atteinte de l'ampoule de Vater et du canal de Wirsung. J Chir (Paris) 1974;107:555–78.

44. Mercadier M, Bodard M, Fungerhut A, Chigot JP. Papillomatosis of the intrahepatic bile ducts. World J Surg 1984;8:30–5.
45. Milchgrub S, Campuzano M, Casillas J, Albores-Saavedra J. Intraductal carcinoma of the pancreas. A report of four cases. Cancer 1992;69:651–6.
46. Morohoshi T, Kanda M, Asanuma K, Klöppel G. Intraductal papillary neoplasms of the pancreas. A clinico-pathologic study of six patients. Cancer 1989;64:1329–35.
47. Neumann RD, LiVolsi VA, Rosenthal NS, Burrell M, Ball TJ. Adenocarcinoma in biliary papillomatosis. Gastroenterology 1976;70:779–82.
48. Ohta H, Yamaguchi Y, Yamakawa O, et al. Biliary papillomatosis with the point mutation of K-ras gene arising in congenital choledochal cyst. Gastroenterology 1993;105:1209–12.
49. Okulski EG, Dohn BJ, Kandawalla NM. Intrahepatic biliary papillomatosis. Arch Pathol Lab Med 1979;103:647–9.
50. Sessa F, Solcia E, Capella C, et al. Intraductal papillary-mucinous tumours represent a distinct group of pancreatic neoplasms: an investigation of tumour cell differentiation and K-ras, p53 and c-erbB-2 abnormalities in 26 patients. Virchows Arch [A] 1994;425:357-67.
51. Sugio K, Molberg K, Albores-Saavedra J, Virmani AK, Kishimoto Y, Gazdar AF. K-ras mutations and allelic loss at 5q and 18q in the development of human pancreatic cancers. Int J Pancreatol 1997;21:205–17.

12

MALIGNANT EPITHELIAL TUMORS
OF THE EXTRAHEPATIC BILE DUCTS

Malignant tumors of the extrahepatic bile ducts are relatively rare, yet they are the third most common cause of extrahepatic bile duct obstruction in the United States. Histologically, these tumors are similar to and, therefore, classified the same as those occurring in the gallbladder. However, their incidence, sex distribution, clinical features, association with lithiasis, frequency of histologic types, molecular pathology, and treatment are different (Table 12-1). Malignant tumors can arise in any part of the extrahepatic bile ducts, although the majority seem to arise near the origin of the cystic duct. For the pathologist, these tumors often present diagnostic problems because of small biopsy specimens, confusion with sclerosing cholangitis, or hyperplasia of intramural glands which occurs in both inflammatory conditions and benign tumors.

Table 12-1

COMPARISON OF GALLBLADDER AND EXTRAHEPATIC BILE DUCT CARCINOMAS

	Gall-bladder	Extra-hepatic Bile Ducts
Geographic variation in incidence	Yes	No
More common in certain ethnic groups	Yes	No
Female predominance	Yes	No
Associated with stones	Yes	No
Increased incidence with ulcerative colitis and primary sclerosing cholangitis	Insignificant	Yes
Biliary obstruction is usually the initial sign	No	Yes
Cholangiography essential for diagnosis	No	Yes
Adenocarcinoma, the most common histologic type	Yes	Yes
Elevated serum CEA	Yes	Yes
Most common genetic abnormality	P53 (LOH)	K-*ras* mutation
Poor prognosis	Yes	Yes

EPIDEMIOLOGY

Cancers of the extrahepatic bile ducts are less common than malignant tumors of the gallbladder. According to the Surveillance, Epidemiology, and End Results (SEER) Program of the National Cancer Institute, 2,893 cases of gallbladder cancer and 1,330 cases of extrahepatic bile duct cancer were recorded from 1981 through 1991. Among 1,808 cases of extrahepatic biliary tract cancer reported from California, there were 1,629 cases of gallbladder cancer, but only 179 of the extrahepatic bile ducts (2). Among 56,000 autopsies performed at Los Angeles County Hospital, there were 203 gallbladder cancers and 29 malignant tumors of the extrahepatic ducts (1).

Incidence. In the United States the incidence of cancer of the extrahepatic ducts is 0.54 cases per 100,000 population, which is less than half the rate for malignant tumors of the gallbladder.

Age Distribution. Cancer of the extrahepatic bile ducts is a disease of older age groups. The average age is 68.4 years for men and 72.7 years for women. Age-specific rates for 1981 to 1991 are shown in figure 12-1. For all age groups, the rates were higher in males.

Sex Distribution. Carcinomas of the extrahepatic ducts are more common in men. For the years 1981 to 1991, the age-adjusted rates were 0.68 cases for every 100,000 males and 0.42 cases for every 100,000 females, which accounted for 0.16 percent of all invasive cancers in males and 0.15 percent in females.

Race. In contrast to gallbladder cancer, which is more common in whites, the rates for extrahepatic bile duct cancer are essentially the same in blacks and whites, 0.46 and 0.51 percent, respectively.

ETIOLOGY

Except for its frequent association with ulcerative colitis, primary sclerosing cholangitis, and choledochal cysts, the causes of extrahepatic bile duct cancer are unknown. The following risk factors have been considered.

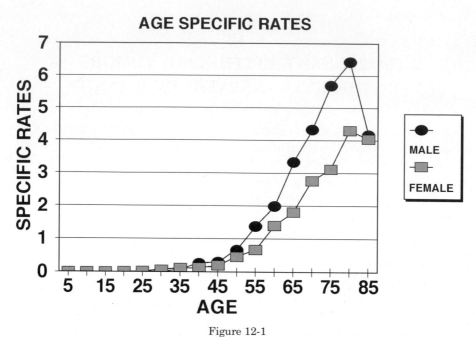

Figure 12-1

EXTRAHEPATIC BILE DUCT CANCER: AGE-SPECIFIC RATES

Age-specific rates for males and females for cancers of the extrahepatic bile ducts for the years 1981-1991. Rates are expressed per 100,000 population. Data from the National Cancer Institute.

Ulcerative Colitis and Sclerosing Cholangitis. The association of bile duct carcinoma with ulcerative colitis was first reported in 1954 as an incidental finding (30). This association shares a common pathogenesis for there is evidence that the extrahepatic bile ducts are also involved in some patients with ulcerative colitis (36). Such involvement is known as sclerosing cholangitis, especially after the signs and symptoms of bile duct disease appear (see page 239). Indeed, it has been suggested that sclerosing cholangitis is a prerequisite for the development of bile duct carcinoma in patients with ulcerative colitis (37), a relative risk of 31.2 percent (25). Conversely, in patients with carcinoma of the extrahepatic bile ducts the incidence of ulcerative colitis is higher than that observed in patients without carcinoma (35).

As a group, patients who develop bile duct carcinoma as a complication of ulcerative colitis are younger (mean age, 42 years [25]), than those who have spontaneous cancer of the extrahepatic tree (mean age, 70 years) and usually do not have gallstones (26,35). Furthermore, they often have a long history of colitis (mean duration, 15 to 20 years with medical treatment) and extensive involvement of the colon. As for the pathogenesis, it seems reasonable to conclude that similar inflammatory processes occur in the bile ducts as the

colon (15). Most likely, biliary epithelium as a result of the chronic inflammation and immune response (which may lead to sclerosing cholangitis clinically) becomes more susceptible to malignant transformation, just as colonic mucosa becomes more susceptible in ulcerative colitis. Histologically, dysplastic changes have been found along the extrahepatic biliary tree in patients with ulcerative colitis (15).

In patients with extrahepatic bile duct cancer associated with ulcerative colitis, there is no difference in the histologic appearance, sites of origin, or clinical course compared to patients with spontaneous bile duct cancer. Carcinoma can develop years after protocolectomy, which suggests that the disease process continues in the biliary passages even after the affected colon is removed.

Crohn's Disease. Carcinoma of the extrahepatic bile ducts (3,4,7) can complicate Crohn's disease. Nonetheless, this relation is infrequent and not well documented since many investigators have failed to find an increased risk of biliary cancer in these patients. Sclerosing cholangitis is less commonly associated with Crohn's disease than it is with ulcerative colitis. In reported cases, the cancer has tended to occur in younger patients, a tendency also seen with carcinomas of the extrahepatic bile ducts associated with ulcerative colitis. Reported cases have been tabulated (7).

Abnormal Choledochopancreatic Junction. Reports, largely from Japan, indicate that an abnormal choledochopancreatic junction may predispose to carcinoma of the common bile duct (17,19,36). The abnormal junction is defined as the union of the pancreatic duct with the common bile duct outside the wall of the duodenum and beyond the influence of the sphincter of Oddi. Normally the union occurs within the sphincter, which governs the pressure within the two ductal systems. As a result of the anomaly, the common channel, that is the pancreaticobiliary duct, is unusually long and no longer under the control of the sphincter. Cancer may be the result of reflux of pancreatic juice into the common bile duct or into choledochal cysts. Abnormal junctions should rightfully be considered a predisposing condition for carcinomas of the extrahepatic biliary tract. However, the frequency of this congenital anomaly is unknown in many countries, including the United States.

Malignant tumors have been associated with a variety of congenital anomalies of the extrahepatic tree. In most cases, the association is probably coincidental. There are at least three reports of extrahepatic bile duct carcinoma occurring in patients with congenital absence of the gallbladder (14,32,34).

Familial Adenomatous Polyposis Coli. Carcinoma of the extrahepatic bile ducts has been described in patients with familial adenomatous polyposis coli (11,18,22,23,38,39). Often these tumors in the bile ducts coexist with additional benign or malignant tumors in the upper gastrointestinal tract. Lesions occurring in the upper gastrointestinal tract or in the extrahepatic biliary system probably represent an expression of the underlying genetic abnormality that occurs in familial adenomatous polyposis.

Carcinoma of the biliary tract has also been associated with hereditary nonpolyposis colorectal cancer, the HNPCC syndrome (24).

von Recklinghausen's Disease. Occasionally, carcinomas arising in the gallbladder or in the ampulla of Vater are associated with von Recklinghausen s disease (6,8,29). More common, however, is the association of this disease with carcinoid tumors, especially somatostatinomas.

Choledochal Cysts. A condition that predisposes to extrahepatic bile duct carcinoma is congenital cystic dilatation or choledochal cyst (12, 13,40). Most often, cystic dilatation affects the extrahepatic bile ducts alone, but occasionally the intrahepatic ducts are also involved. Although these cysts are relatively rare, carcinoma as a complication has been well described. The incidence of carcinoma varies with age. In patients less than 10 years, the incidence is less than 1 percent; in those between 10 and 20 years, the incidence is 6.8 percent; and in those more than 20 years of age, it rises to 15 percent (21, 42). Adenocarcinomas are usually found in these cysts, although cases of squamous cell carcinoma, sarcoma botryoides, and carcinoid tumors have been reported (31,41). Papillomatosis has also been described (28). Carcinoma can develop anywhere along the biliary tract in addition to originating in the cyst.

A mixture of bile and pancreatic secretions may promote the development of carcinoma, since 90 percent of choledochal cysts are associated with abnormal choledochal pancreatic junctions (21). Choledochal cysts are further discussed on page 231.

Carcinomas rarely, if ever, arise in a choledochocele (type III choledochal cyst) which is an infrequent anomaly of the terminal biliary tree. A choledochocele may be the result of a congenital duplication of the duodenum that occurs near the ampulla of Vater and may not be a true choledochal cyst (43).

In all excised cysts, the pathologist should carefully exclude the presence of carcinoma.

Infections. Infestation with the liver flukes *Clonorchis sinensis* (also known as *Opisthorchis sinensis*) or *Opisthorchis viverrine* has long been associated with carcinoma of both the extrahepatic and intrahepatic bile ducts. In the Orient, infestation is the most frequently cited cause of carcinoma of the biliary tree (5,20,27). Initially the mucosa is edematous but the bile duct epithelium is intact. With persistent infection the epithelium becomes hyperplastic and undergoes mucinous metaplasia. Dysplastic changes and carcinoma occur in longstanding infections.

Chronic carriers of *Salmonella typhi* seem to be at risk for bile duct cancer. In Egypt, 39 percent of patients with carcinoma of the bile ducts were salmonella carriers compared to only

2 percent of healthy controls (10). Thirty-four percent of patients with non-neoplastic bile duct obstruction were also salmonella carriers. In California, hepatobiliary cancer accounted for 5.2 percent of the deaths in chronic salmonella carriers (33). Case observations indicate that chronic carriers can develop sclerosing cholangitis that progresses to carcinoma (33).

Cholelithiasis. Stones do not appear to play a role in the etiology, although cholelithiasis has been proposed as a risk factor. From 20 to 30 percent of patients with carcinoma of the extrahepatic bile ducts have gallstones. Interestingly, cholecystectomy for cholelithiasis is associated with a reduced risk of extrahepatic bile duct cancer beginning 10 years after surgery (9). Less than 20 percent of extrahepatic bile duct carcinomas are associated with choledocholithiasis.

Enterobiliary Anastomosis. Isolated case reports indicate that patients with enterobiliary anastomosis may be at risk for cancer of the extrahepatic bile ducts, although this remains to be substantiated (16).

CLINICAL MANIFESTATIONS

Malignant tumors of the extrahepatic bile ducts usually cause early obstruction that results in jaundice, which can rapidly progress or fluctuate. Jaundice usually appears while the tumor is relatively small, before widespread dissemination has occurred (44,46). Other symptoms include right upper quadrant pain, malaise, weight loss, pruritus, anorexia, nausea, and vomiting (45). If cholangitis develops, chills and fever appear. A palpable mass or ascites usually indicates advanced disease which precludes complete resection of the tumor. As a rule, the liver is enlarged, and if the patient survives long enough, it may become nodular because of secondary biliary cirrhosis or metastases. In patients with carcinoma of the proximal bile ducts (right and left hepatic ducts, common hepatic duct) the gallbladder is not palpable and the common duct often collapses. Patients with carcinoma in the common or cystic ducts have a distended and palpable gallbladder as well as a markedly dilated proximal duct system. Carcinoma of the bile ducts has presented as acanthosis nigricans (47).

We have seen a patient with carcinoma of the cystic duct stump 9 years following cholecystectomy. The stump was markedly dilated, resembling a small gallbladder, and, in addition to the carcinoma, contained a single stone.

Laboratory Findings. Laboratory findings are usually consistent with extrahepatic bile duct obstruction. They include hyperbilirubinemia, bilirubinuria, and a moderate rise in serum alkaline phosphatase and glutamic transferase activity.

In bile the levels of CEA increase. However, CEA should be separated from nonspecific cross-reacting antigen (NCA) and biliary glycoprotein 1 (BGP1) that are also found in bile (48). Elevation of these cross-reacting antigens may give a false impression of an elevated CEA level.

Circulating Tumor Markers. Although CEA and CA19-9 may increase in the serum of patients with extrahepatic bile duct cancer, these markers are not reliable for diagnostic purposes because they lack specificity. Moreover, an increase occurs with extrahepatic obstruction from any cause. Therefore, caution should be used in the interpretation of elevated serum levels of tumor markers in the presence of cholestasis (44).

DIAGNOSIS

Although the presence of cancer can often be suspected from laboratory and radiologic studies, microscopic confirmation is essential for the appropriate management of extrahepatic bile duct lesions.

Imaging Studies. Ultrasound examination, especially endoscopic ultrasonography, is a reliable procedure in the preoperative diagnosis and staging of these tumors. In 25 patients with biliary tract carcinoma, the malignant obstruction was demonstrated in all patients by endoscopic ultrasonography as well as by endoscopic retrograde cholangiopancreatography (ERCP) while with ultrasound alone this was possible in only 17 of the 25 patients (49). Endoscopic ultrasonography is also useful for assessing tumor infiltration in the hepatoduodenal ligament (52). Computed tomography may not reveal a discrete mass. However, an abrupt change in the caliber of the bile duct from dilated to normal is highly suggestive of carcinoma (51). Cholangiography performed transhepatically or endoscopically is an essential procedure that usually reveals the

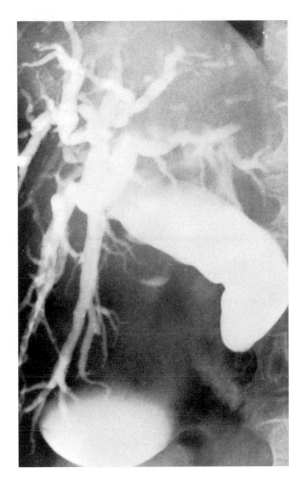

Figure 12-2
TRANSHEPATIC CHOLANGIOGRAM
Transhepatic cholangiogram shows obstruction and dilatation of the common bile duct that was caused by a well-differentiated adenocarcinoma of the distal common bile duct. The fundus of the gallbladder is also distended. (Fig. 165 from Fascicle 22, 2nd Series.)

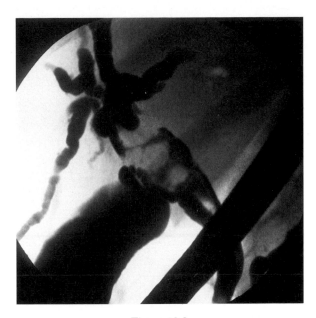

Figure 12-3
ERCP OF ADENOSQUAMOUS CARCINOMA
ERCP shows a multilobulated filling defect extending from the left hepatic duct into the dilated common hepatic duct.

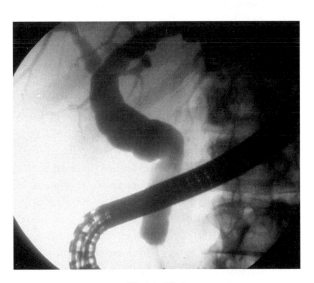

Figure 12-4
ERCP OF ADENOSQUAMOUS CARCINOMA
OF DISTAL COMMON BILE DUCT
The ERCP reveals a tight, irregular, distal common bile duct stricture caused by a well-differentiated adenocarcinoma.

site of obstruction and occasionally the extent of the lesion (figs. 12-2–12-5) (50,51).

Brush Cytology. Cytologic examination of brushings obtained during ERCP is a safe and useful procedure for the diagnosis of extrahepatic bile duct tumors (53–62). A limitation of this procedure is the small amount of tissue obtained for examination which may result in hypocellular or acellular smears. Furthermore, many bile duct tumors are small and grow beneath the mucosa, therefore, representative material for cytology may not be obtained. Inflammatory lesions of the extrahepatic bile ducts, especially primary or secondary sclerosing cholangitis, on occasion give rise to a false-positive diagnosis due

to the presence of reactive atypical epithelial cells or large endothelial cells which can be confused with malignant cells. Although false-positive diagnoses are not mentioned in most series, in others they reach 1 percent (58). The sensitivity

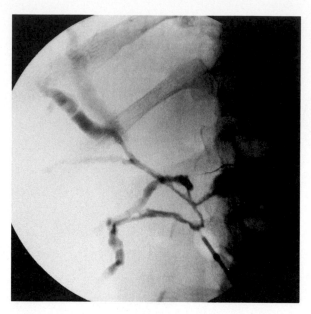

Figure 12-5
ERCP OF ADENOSQUAMOUS CARCINOMA
OF DISTAL COMMON HEPATIC DUCT
The ERCP reveals an extensive infiltrating adenocarcinoma involving the common hepatic duct and both the right and left hepatic ducts which also invaded the intrahepatic bile ducts.

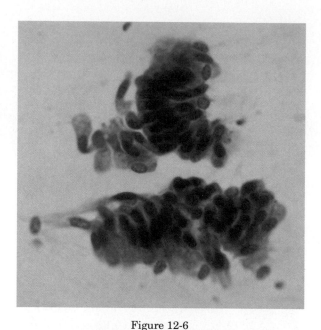

Figure 12-6
BILE DUCT BRUSHINGS
A group of normal columnar biliary type cells. The normal polarity of the cells is maintained.

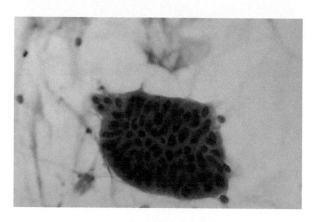

Figure 12-7
BILE DUCT BRUSHINGS
Tangential view of a fragment of cohesive normal columnar cells.

of ERCP brushings has reportedly varied from 40 to 70 percent and the specificity between 70 and 100 percent (58a). If a diagnosis of bile duct carcinoma is clinically suspected and the cytologic brushings are negative, the procedure should be repeated. The sensitivity of brush cytology increases with repeated brushings (59). Normal biliary epithelium is often present in the smears and is useful because it can be compared with the malignant cells (figs. 12-6–12-8). Malignant cells show enlarged nuclei, an increased nuclear:cytoplasmic ratio, chromatin clumping, nuclear molding, irregular nuclear contours, prominent nucleoli, and cytoplasmic vacuoles (fig. 12-9). Malignant cells are often arranged in disordered cords and sheets (figs. 12-10, 12-11). If sufficient material is available, cell blocks should be prepared. Experienced endoscopists may also take small biopsies during ERCP. Although the biopsies are small (1 to 2 mm) they are usually diagnostic (fig. 12-12) (58).

Image analysis has also been employed in the diagnosis of malignant epithelial tumors of the extrahepatic bile ducts. The nuclear DNA content and the percentage of proliferating cells permit distinction of normal and inflammatory cells from malignant epithelium with 95 percent sensitivity and 100 percent specificity (63). Unfortunately, this technique requires special instrumentation that is not available in most cytology laboratories.

In recent years the diagnostic value of K-*ras* mutational analysis in endobiliary brush cytology has been assessed. The test is considered a

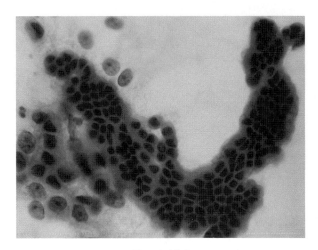

Figure 12-8
BILE DUCT BRUSHINGS
A group of normal biliary type cells and adjacent discohesive malignant cells with large nuclei and small nucleoli.

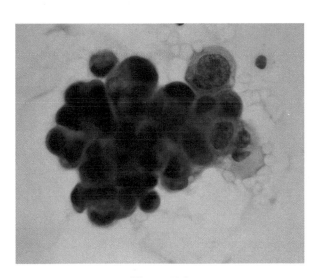

Figure 12-9
BILE DUCT BRUSHINGS
A group of malignant epithelial cells. Note the variation in size and shape of nuclei, the granular chromatin, prominent nucleoli, and small cytoplasmic vacuoles.

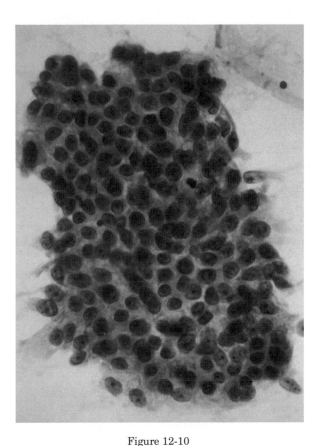

Figure 12-10
BILE DUCT BRUSHINGS
A sheet of malignant epithelial cells, most of which have round or ovoid nuclei with small nucleoli.

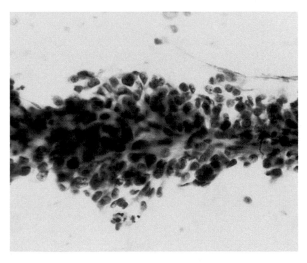

Figure 12-11
BILE DUCT BRUSHINGS
The neoplastic cells in this papillary carcinoma of common bile duct show considerable variation in size and shape of the nuclei. The cells are arranged around a blood vessel.

valuable diagnostic adjunct to conventional light microscopy of biliary brush cytology specimens because it increases the sensitivity for detecting malignancy (61a). It should be stressed, however, that K-*ras* mutations are not specific for carcinoma and can be seen in hyperplastic ductal lesions, especially from the pancreas.

Biopsy. Techniques available for biopsy of the biliary tract include percutaneous transluminal biopsy under fluoroscopic control (65); percutaneous fine needle aspiration biopsy under ultrasound, computed tomography, or fluoroscopy guidance; and endoscopic transpapillary biopsy (64). Use of the percutaneous fine needle aspiration biopsy technique guided by selective angiography or transhepatic cholangiography permits a correct diagnosis of bile duct carcinomas in 50 percent of cases (66). All these procedures require a high degree of skill by the endoscopist or radiologist. Moreover, some tumors are not accessible by this type of approach. Consequently, brush cytology is now considered to be the preferred preoperative diagnostic procedure for extrahepatic bile duct carcinoma (67).

Delay in Diagnosis. About 10 percent of patients with carcinoma of the extrahepatic ducts have had previous surgery without a definitive diagnosis. Unfortunately, additional surgery is often necessary to reach a final diagnosis. In some patients a small carcinoma is overlooked during laparotomy. This is especially true for tumors in the proximal bile ducts, since they are difficult to observe and palpate unless the hilum of the liver is dissected. Sometimes the biopsy is not representative and a diagnosis of sclerosing cholangitis is made. On occasion, when a cholecystectomy is performed for lithiasis, a neoplasm in the extrahepatic ducts is mistaken for a fibrous scar and a biopsy is not obtained. In summary, a diagnosis is often established late and

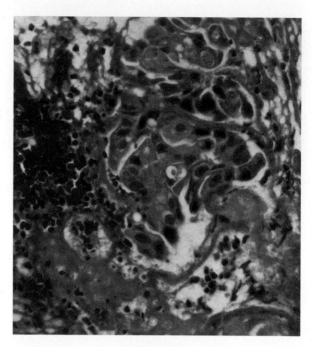

Figure 12-12
ADENOCARCINOMA OF
DISTAL COMMON BILE DUCT
This endoscopic biopsy shows nests of malignant epithelial cells with mucin vacuoles, diagnostic of adenocarcinoma.

usually during laparotomy. Reasons for the delay include lack of an obvious tumor or confusion with lithiasis, fibrous stricture, or sclerosing cholangitis (68).

REFERENCES

Epidemiology

1. Edmondson HA. Tumors of the gallbladder and extrahepatic bile ducts. Atlas of Tumor Pathology, 1st Series, Fascicle 26. Washington, D.C.: Armed Forces Institute of Pathology, 1967.

2. Krain LS. Gallbladder and extrahepatic bile duct carcinoma. Analysis of 1,808 cases. Geriatrics 1972;27:111–7.

Etiology

3. Altaee MY, Johnson PJ, Farrant JM, Williams R. Etiologic and clinical characteristics of peripheral and hilar cholangiocarcinoma. Cancer 1991;68:2051–5.

4. Berman MD, Falchuk KR, Trey C. Carcinoma of the biliary tree complicating Crohn s disease. Dig Dis Sci 1980;25:795–7.

5. Chen MF, Jan YY, Wang CS, Jeng LB, Hwang TL, Chen SC. Intrahepatic stones associated with cholangiocarcinoma. Am J Gastroenterol 1989;84:391–5.

6. Ching CK, Greer AJ. Metachronous biliary tract cancers in a patient with von Recklinghausen's disease. Am J Gastroenterol 1993;88:1124–5.

7. Choi PM, Nugent FW, Zelig MP, Munson JL, Schoetz DJ Jr. Cholangiocarcinoma and Crohn s disease. Dig Disc Sci 1994;39:667–70.

8. Colarian J, Pietruk ST, Lafave L, Calzada R. Adenocarcinoma of the ampulla of Vater associated with neurofibromatosis. J Clin Gastroenterol 1990;12:118–9.

9. Ekbom A, Hsieh CC, Yuen J, et al. Risk of extrahepatic bile duct cancer after cholecystectomy. Lancet 1993;342:1262–5.
10. El-Zayadi A, Ghoneim M, Kabil SM, El Tawil A, Sherif A, Selim O. Bile duct carcinoma in Egypt: possible etiological factors. Hepatogastroenterology 1991;38:337–40.
11. Erwald R. Gardner's syndrome with adenoma of the common bile duct. A case report. Acta Chir Scand 1984;520 (Suppl):63–8.
12. Flanigan DP. Biliary cysts. Ann Surg 1975;182:635–43.
13. Flanigan DP. Biliary carcinoma associated with biliary cysts. Cancer 1977;40:880–3.
14. Gurll N. Small-bowel metastasis from bile duct carcinoma with coincidental congenital absence of gallbladder. Postgrad Med 1976;59:229–31.
15. Haworth AC, Manley PN, Groll A, Pace R. Bile duct carcinoma and biliary tract dysplasia in chronic ulcerative colitis. Arch Pathol Lab Med 1989;113:434–6.
16. Herba MJ, Casola G, Bret PM, Lough J, Hampson LG. Cholangiocarcinoma as a late complication of choledochoenteric anastomoses. Am J Radiol 1986;147:513–5.
17. Ikoma A, Nakamura N, Miyazaki T, Maeda M. Double cancer of the gallbladder and common bile duct associated with anomalous junction of pancreaticobiliary ductal system. Surgery 1992;111:595–600.
18. Jarvinen H, Nyberg M, Peltokallio P. Biliary involvement in familial adenomatosis coli. Dis Colon Rectum 1983;26:525–8.
19. Kimura W, Shimada H, Kuroda A, Morioka Y. Carcinoma of the gallbladder and extrahepatic bile ducts in autopsy cases of the aged, with special reference to its relationship to gallstones. Am J Gastroenterol 1989;84:386–90.
20. Koga A, Ichimiya H, Yamaguchi K, Miyazaki K, Nakayama F. Hepatolithiasis associated with cholangiocarcinoma. Possible etiologic significance. Cancer 1985;55:2826–9.
21. Komi N, Tamura T, Miyoshi Y, Kunitomo K, Udaka H, Takehara H. Nationwide survey of cases of choledochal cyst. Analysis of coexistent anomalies, complications and surgical treatment in 645 cases. Surg Gastroenterol 1984;3:69–72.
22. Komorowski RA, Tresp MG, Wilson SD. Pancreaticobiliary involvement in familial polyposis coli/Gardner's syndrome. Dis Colon Rectum 1986;29:55–8.
23. Lees CD, Hermann RE. Familial polyposis coli associated with bile duct cancer. Am J Surg 1981;141:378–80.
24. Mecklin JP, Jarvinen HE, Virolainen M. The association between cholangiocarcinoma and hereditary nonpolyposis colorectal carcinoma. Cancer 1992;69:1112–4.
25. Mir-Madjlessi SH, Farmer RG, Sivak MV Jr. Bile duct carcinoma in patients with ulcerative colitis. Relationship to sclerosing cholangitis: report of six cases and review of the literature. Dig Dis Sci 1987;32:145–54.
26. Morowitz DA, Glagov S, Dordal E, Kirsner JB. Carcinoma of the biliary tract complicating chronic ulcerative colitis. Cancer 1971;27:356–61.

27. Nakanuma Y, Terada T, Tanaka Y, et al. Are hepatolithiasis and cholangiocarcinoma aetiologically related? A morphological study of 12 cases of hepatolithiasis associated with cholangiocarcinoma. Virchows Arch [A] 1985;406:45–58.
28. Ohta H, Yamaguchi Y, Yamakawa O, et al. Biliary papillomatosis with the point mutation of K-ras gene arising in congenital choledochal cyst. Gastroenterology 1993;105:1209–12.
29. Paraf F, Poynard T, Bedossa P, et al. Adenocarcinoma of the Vater's ampulla and von Recklinghausen's disease. Ann Intern Med 1987;107:785.
30. Parker RG, Kendall EJ. The liver in ulcerative colitis. Br Med J 1954;2:1030–2.
31. Patil KK, Omojola MF, Khurana P, Iyengar JK. Embryonal rhabdomyosarcoma within a choledochal cyst. Can Assoc Radiol J 1992;43:145–8.
32. Richards RN. Congenital absence of the gallbladder and cystic duct associated with primary carcinoma of the common bile duct. Can Med Assoc J 1966;94:859–60.
33. Robbins S, Chuang VP, Hersh T. The development of hepatobiliary cancer in a carrier of Salmonella typhus. Am J Gastroenterol 1988;83:675–8.
34. Robertson HF, Robertson WE, Bower JO. Congenital absence of the gallbladder with primary carcinoma of the common duct and carcinoma of the liver. JAMA 1940;114:1514–7.
35. Ross AP, Braasch JW. Ulcerative colitis and carcinoma of the proximal bile ducts. Gut 1973;14:94–7.
36. Sameshima Y, Uchimura M, Muto Y, Maeda J, Tsuchiyama H. Coexistent carcinoma in congenital dilatation of the bile duct and anomalous arrangement of the pancreatico-bile duct. Cancer 1987;60:1883–90.
37. Schrumpf E, Elgjo K, Fausa O, et al. Sclerosing cholangitis in ulcerative colitis. Scand J Gastroenterol 1980;15:689–97.
38. Smith MD, Robbins PD, Cullingford GL, Levitt MD. Cholangiocarcinoma and familial adenomatous polyposis. Aust N Z J Surg 1993;63:24–7.
39. Spigelman AD, Farmer KC, James M, Richman PI, Phillips RK. Tumours of the liver, bile ducts, pancreas and duodenum in a single patient with familial adenomatous polyposis. Br J Surg 1991;78:979–80.
40. Todani T, Tabuchi K, Watanabe Y, Kobayashi T. Carcinoma arising in the wall of congenital bile duct cysts. Cancer 1979;44:1134–41.
41. Tsuchiya R, Harada N, Ito T, Furukawa M, Yoshihiro I. Malignant tumours in choledochal cysts. Ann Surg 1977;186:22–8.
42. Voyles CR, Smadja C, Shands C, Blumgart LH. Carcinoma in choledochal cysts: age related incidence. Arch Surg 1983;118:986–8.
43. Wearn F, Wiot J. Choledochocele: not a form of choledochal cyst. Can Assoc Radiol J 1982;33:110–2.

Clinical Manifestations

44. Basso D, Meggiato T, Fabris C, et al. Extra-hepatic cholestasis determines a reversible increase of glycoprotein tumour markers in benign and malignant diseases. Eur J Clin Invest 1992;22:800–4.

45. Bedikian AY, Valdivieso M, DeLaCruz A, et al. Cancer of the extrahepatic bile ducts. Med Pediatr Oncol 1988;8:53–61.
46. Braasch JW, Warren KW, Kune GA. Malignant neoplasms of the bile ducts. Surg Clin N Am 1967;47:627–38.

47. Ravnborg L, Thomsen K. Acanthosis nigricans and bile duct malignancy. Acta Derm Venereol (Stockh) 1993;73:378–9

48. Uchino R, Kanemitsu K, Obayashi H, Hiraoka T, Miyauchi Y. Carcinoembryonic antigen (CEA) and CEA-related substances in the bile of patients with biliary diseases. Am J Surg 1994;167:306–8.

Diagnosis

49. Dancygier H, Nattermann C. The role of endoscopic ultrasonography in biliary tract disease: obstructive jaundice. Endoscopy 1994;26:800–2.

50. Okuda K, Kubo Y, Okazaki N, Arishima T, Hashimoto M. Clinical aspects of intrahepatic bile duct carcinoma including hilar carcinoma: a study of 57 autopsy-proven cases. Cancer 1977;39:232–46.

51. Saini S. Imaging of the hepatobiliary tract. N Engl J Med 1997;336:1889–94.

52. Tamada K, Ido K, Ueno N, Kimura K, Ichiyama M, Tomiyama T. Preoperative staging of extrahepatic bile duct cancer with intraductal ultrasonography. Am J Gastroenterol 1995;90:239–46.

Brush Cytology

53. Cohen MB, Wittchow RJ, Johlin FC, Bottles K, Raab SS. Brush cytology of the extrahepatic biliary tract: comparison of cytologic features of adenocarcinoma and benign biliary strictures. Modern Pathol 1995;8:498–502.

54. Foutch PG, Harlan JR, Kerr D, Sanowski RA. Wire-guided brush cytology: a new endoscopic method for diagnosis of bile duct cancer. Gastrointest Endosc 1989;35:243–7.

55. Foutch PG, Kerr DM, Harlan JR, Kummet TD. A prospective, controlled analysis of endoscopic cytotechniques for diagnosis of malignant biliary strictures. Am J Gastroenterol 1991;86:577–80.

56. Foutch PG, Kerr DM, Harlan JR, Manne RK, Kummet TD, Sanowski RA. Endoscopic retrograde wire-guided brush cytology for diagnosis of patients with malignant obstruction of the bile duct. Am J Gastroenterol 1990;85:791–5.

57. Howell LP, Chow HS, Russell LA. Cytodiagnosis of extrahepatic biliary duct tumors from specimens obtained during cholangiography. Diagn Cytopathol 1988;4:328–34.

58. Kurzawinski T, Deery A, Davidson BR. Diagnostic value of cytology for biliary stricture. Br J Surg 1993;80:414–21.

58a. Ponchon T, Gagnon P, Berger F, et al. Value of endobiliary brush cytology and biopsies for the diagnosis of malignant bile duct stenosis. Gastrointest Endosc 1995;42:565–72.

59. Rabinovitz M, Zajko AB, Hassanein T, et al. Diagnostic value of brush cytology in the diagnosis of bile duct carcinoma: a study of 65 patients with bile duct strictures. Hepatology 1990;12:747–52.

60. Ryan ME. Cytologic brushings of ductal lesions during ERCP. Gastrointest Endosc 1991;37:139–42.

61. Scudera PL, Koizumi J, Jacobson IM. Brush cytology evaluation of lesions encountered during ERCP. Gastrointest Endosc 1990;36:281–4.

61a. Sturm PD, Rauws EA, Hruban RH, et al. The clinical value of K-ras codon 12 analysis and endobiliary brush cytology for the diagnosis of malignant extrahepatic biliary stenosis. Clin Cancer Res 1999;5:629–35.

62. Venu RP, Greenen JE, Kini M, et al. Endoscopic retrograde brush cytology. A new technique. Gastroenterology 1990;99:1475–9.

63. Yeaton P, Kiss R, Deviere J, et al. Use of cell image analysis in the detection of cancer from specimens obtained during endoscopic retrograde cholangiopancreatography. Am J Clin Pathol 1993;100:497–501.

Biopsy

64. Dancygier H. Endoscopic transpapillary biopsy (ETPB) of human extrahepatic bile ducts—light and electron microscopic findings, clinical significance. Endoscopy 1989;21:312–20.

65. Donald JJ, Fache JS, Burhenne HJ. Percutaneous transluminal biopsy of the biliary tract. Can Assoc Radiol J 1993;44:185–8.

66. Evander A, Ihse I, Lunderquist A, Tylen U, Ackerman M. Percutaneous cytodiagnosis of carcinoma of the pancreas and bile duct. Ann Surg 1978;188:90–2.

67. Fortner JY, Kallum BO, Kim DK. Surgical management of carcinoma of the junction of the main hepatic ducts. Ann Surg 1976;184:68–73.

68. Wanebo HJ, Grimes OF. Cancer of the bile duct: the occult malignancy. Am J Surg 1975;130:262–8.

❖❖❖

13

DYSPLASIA, CARCINOMA IN SITU, AND
INVASIVE CARCINOMA OF THE EXTRAHEPATIC BILE DUCTS

DYSPLASIA AND
CARCINOMA IN SITU

During the last decade a number of studies have shown that flat dysplasia and carcinoma in situ occur adjacent to invasive carcinomas of the extrahepatic bile ducts. The foci of dysplasia and carcinoma in situ are multicentric in most cases, a finding which probably has therapeutic implications and explains the high incidence of local recurrence. As a result, it has been suggested that the dysplasia-carcinoma sequence is the usual pathway for the development of invasive carcinoma of the extrahepatic bile ducts (1,4,6).

The morphologic criteria for dysplasia and carcinoma in situ in the extrahepatic bile ducts are the same as those for the gallbladder. Briefly, dysplasia is characterized by large, cuboidal or columnar cells with nuclear atypia, loss of polarity, and pseudostratification. According to the extent of nuclear atypia and loss of polarity, dysplasia is graded into mild, moderate, or severe. The terms low-grade and high-grade dysplasia are also used. Dysplastic cells may extend into the sacculi of Beale or into the metaplastic pyloric glands and should not be confused with invasive adenocarcinoma (figs. 13-1, 13-2). In carcinoma in situ, the cells are indistinguishable from those of invasive carcinoma, but are confined to the surface epithelium (figs. 13-3, 13-4). However, in situ carcinoma may also extend to the sacculi of Beale, to the metaplastic pyloric type glands, or to the intramural glands, mimicking invasion.

As in other organs, separation between high-grade dysplasia and carcinoma in situ is subjective and difficult. Moreover, few surgical pathologists have accumulated experience with these uncommon lesions that frequently need to be recognized in small biopsy samples. As a result, there is considerable interobserver disagreement in the classification of these two lesions. This is further complicated by the lack of established morphologic criteria for high-grade dysplasia and carcinoma in situ, and their frequent confusion with reactive epithelial atypia.

In a retrospective study, Albores-Saavedra and Henson (1) described dysplasia and carcinoma in situ adjacent to 6 of 61 (10 percent) extrahepatic bile duct carcinomas. However, because of the large size of the cancers, the majority probably had obliterated the precursor lesions. Moreover, in some cases the mucosa adjacent to the carcinomas was ulcerated or not sampled. Laitio (4) found severe dysplastic changes in 45 percent of invasive carcinomas. Davis et al. (2) were able to detect dysplastic changes in one third of extrahepatic bile duct carcinomas. Suzuki et al. (6) studied 12 cases of hepatohilar bile duct carcinoma with the use of computer-assisted three-dimensional reconstruction of the biliary tree. They found high-grade dysplasia in 75 percent and carcinoma in situ in 42 percent of invasive carcinomas. Based on these findings, it seems reasonable to conclude that carcinomas of the extrahepatic bile ducts evolve through a dysplasia-carcinoma sequence. Despite these data, the natural history of dysplasia and carcinoma in situ remains unknown.

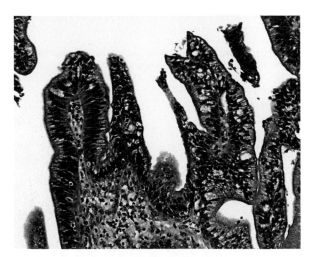

Figure 13-1
HIGH-GRADE DYSPLASIA
High-grade dysplasia of common bile duct is adjacent to a well-differentiated adenocarcinoma. The columnar cells are pseudostratified and show elongated hyperchromatic nuclei. Some cells show clear cytoplasm.

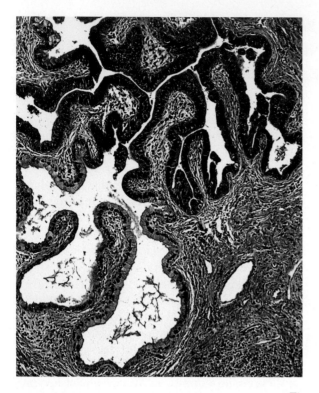
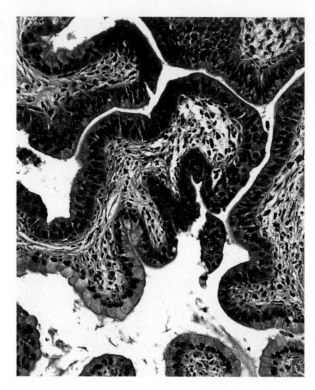

Figure 13-2
DYSPLASIA

Left: Low-power view of dysplastic cells extending into the sacculi of Beale.

Right: Higher magnification showing detail of dysplastic columnar cells which are hyperchromatic and pseudostratified. The lower part of the sacculi are lined by nondysplastic cells.

Figure 13-3
CARCINOMA IN SITU OF COMMON HEPATIC DUCT

Below: The neoplastic epithelium forms micropapillary structures and does not infiltrate the stroma.

Right: Higher magnification shows that the degree of cytologic atypia justifies a diagnosis of carcinoma in situ.

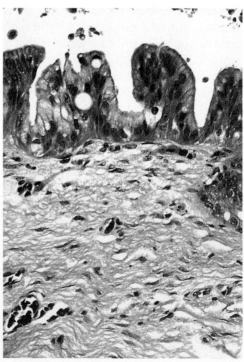

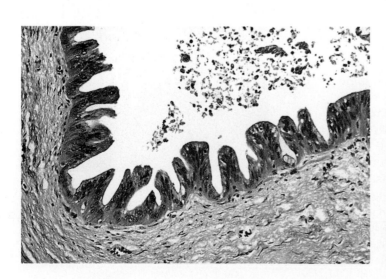

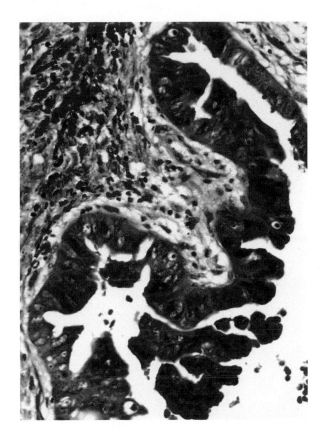
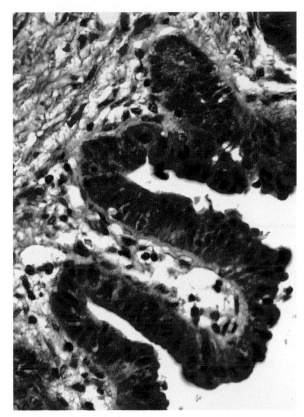

Figure 13-4
CARCINOMA IN SITU

Left: Carcinoma in situ with a micropapillary pattern of right hepatic duct found adjacent to a well-differentiated adenocarcinoma.

Right: Carcinoma in situ found adjacent to an invasive carcinoma of the cystic duct. The neoplastic cell population is homogenous and shows pseudostratification.

Dysplasia and carcinoma in situ can arise in a background of metaplasia. Metaplastic changes have been described in the extrahepatic bile ducts, although the pathologic stimulus that triggers the process is unknown. Pyloric gland metaplasia is more common than intestinal metaplasia and some of the dysplastic changes and foci of carcinoma in situ arise in a background of pyloric gland metaplasia (fig. 13-5). Dysplasia of the extrahepatic bile ducts has been associated with ulcerative colitis and primary sclerosing cholangitis (3,5,7). There is now considerable circumstantial evidence that in these inflammatory conditions, dysplasia and carcinoma in situ are late complications of the underlying non-neoplastic disease.

In conclusion, carcinomas of the extrahepatic bile ducts essentially follow the same histogenetic

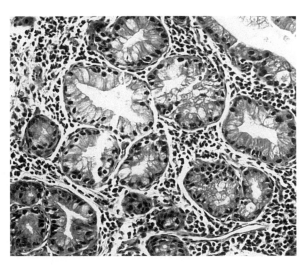

Figure 13-5
METAPLASTIC PYLORIC TYPE GLANDS
A chronic inflammatory infiltrate is seen between the glands.

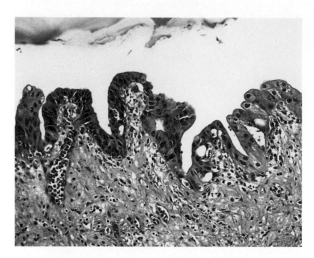

Figure 13-6
REACTIVE EPITHELIAL ATYPIA
A cystic duct is lined by a heterogeneous population of reactive cells. Note the large basophilic cells with hyperchromatic nuclei adjacent to cells with pale cytoplasm and bland nuclei.

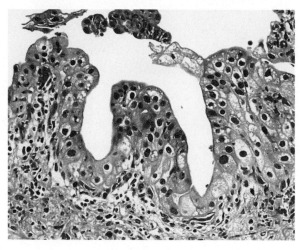

Figure 13-7
REACTIVE EPITHELIAL ATYPIA
Atypical cuboidal cells with clear cytoplasm and round nuclei predominate in this cystic duct. Some cells have prominent nucleoli.

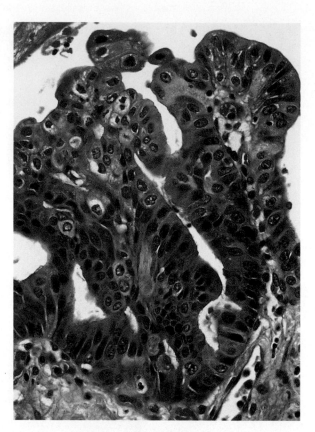

Figure 13-8
REACTIVE EPITHELIAL ATYPIA
A micropapillary architecture with nuclear pseudo-stratification is seen in this cystic duct. Most cells have large vesicular or hyperchromatic nuclei and prominent nucleoli. Intraepithelial inflammatory cells are also seen.

pathway as carcinomas of the gallbladder. This in turn explains the close histologic similarity between both.

Dysplasia and carcinoma in situ should be distinguished from reactive atypia which occurs in a number of situations. If, for instance, a stent has been left in the common bile duct for longer than 2 weeks, reactive atypia is often prominent. Inflammatory diseases, such as primary and secondary sclerosing cholangitis, may also cause atypical reactive changes in the epithelium. Impacted stones are another cause of reactive atypia. In contrast to dysplasia and carcinoma in situ, atypical reactive cells are heterogenous; they may be cuboidal or columnar and have a clear or basophilic cytoplasm (figs. 13-6, 13-7). The nuclei are usually vesicular and contain prominent nucleoli. Pseudostratification and even pseudo-cribriform structures are common (fig. 13-8). A variable number of normal mitotic figures are present. More importantly, atypical reactive cells may extend into the intramural glands which can cause confusion with invasive cancer. It is advisable to avoid a diagnosis of dysplasia or carcinoma in situ in areas with extensive inflammatory changes; in small endoscopic biopsies, the distinction may be impossible.

INVASIVE CARCINOMAS

Distribution of Histologic Types

Table 13-1 shows the distribution of histologic types recorded in the Surveillance, Epidemiology, and End Results (SEER) Program of the National Cancer Institute. The Table represents all cases of cancer of the extrahepatic bile ducts reported in 10 percent of the population for the years 1981 to 1990. Table 13-2 shows the histologic types in a series of 143 cases that one of us (JA-S) examined during the last 20 years. Well and moderately differentiated adenocarcinomas are the most common. The differences in distribution of the histologic types in the two series most likely reflect variations in histologic criteria as well as the use of different terminology.

Table 13-1

HISTOLOGIC DISTRIBUTION FOR CANCERS OF THE EXTRAHEPATIC BILE DUCTS, 1982–1991*

Histologic Types	Number of Patients	Percent of Total	Males	Percent of Total	Females	Percent of Total
Carcinoma in situ	9	0.68	6	0.84	3	0.48
Adenocarcinoma, NOS	1042	78.35	549	77.22	493	79.64
Papillary adenocarcinoma	79	5.94	44	6.19	35	5.65
Adenocarcinoma, intestinal type	0	0	0	0	0	0
Mucinous adenocarcinoma	51	3.83	34	4.78	17	2.75
Clear cell carcinoma	1	0.08	1	0.14	0	0
Signet ring cell carcinoma	5	0.38	3	0.42	2	0.32
Adenosquamous carcinoma	9	0.68	5	0.7	4	0.65
Squamous cell carcinoma	0	0	0	0	0	0
Small cell carcinoma	5	0.38	3	0.42	2	0.32
Adenocarcinoma in villous adenoma	6	0.45	3	0.42	3	0.48
Cholangiocarcinoma	59	4.44	36	5.06	23	3.72
Infiltrating duct carcinoma	36	2.71	15	2.11	21	3.39
Undifferentiated carcinoma	5	0.38	2	0.28	3	0.48
Total	**1307**	**98.27**	**701**	**98.59**	**606**	**97.9**
Carcinoid tumors	3	0.23	0	0	3	0.48
Mixed carcinoid-adenocarcinoma	1	0.08	1	0.14	0	0
Total	**4**	**0.3**	**1**	**0.14**	**3**	**0.48**
Sarcoma, NOS	0	0	0	0	0	0
Rhabdomyosarcoma	3	0.23	3	0.42	0	0
Kaposi's sarcoma	0	0	0	0	0	0
Leiomyosarcoma	0	0	0	0	0	0
Malignant fibrous histiocytoma	0	0	0	0	0	0
Angiosarcoma	0	0	0	0	0	0
Total	**3**	**0.23**	**3**	**0.42**	**0**	**0**
Carcinosarcoma	0	0	0	0	0	0
Malignant melanoma	0	0	0	0	0	0
Malignant lymphoma	3	0.23	2	0.28	1	0.16
Others, NOS	13	0.98	4	0.56	9	1.45
Total Invasive	**1321**	**99.32**	**705**	**99.16**	**616**	**99.52**
Total Invasive and In Situ	**1330**	**100**	**711**	**100**	**619**	**100**

*Data from the Surveillance, Epidemiology, and End Results Program, National Cancer Institute.

Table 13-2

HISTOLOGIC TYPES IN 143 CASES OF EXTRAHEPATIC BILE DUCT CARCINOMAS*†

Histologic Type	Number of Patients	Percent
Adenocarcinoma, well to moderately differentiated	108	76
Adenosquamous carcinoma	8	5.5
Papillary adenocarcinoma	6	4.1
Undifferentiated carcinoma	6	4.1
Adenocarcinoma, intestinal type	4	2.7
Adenocarcinoma, clear cell type	4	2.7
Small cell carcinoma	3	2
Mucinous carcinoma	2	1.3
Signet ring cell carcinoma	1	0.7
Adenocarcinoma, foveolar type	1	0.7
Total	**143**	**100**

*Cases obtained from the General Hospital of Mexico City, Jackson Memorial Hospital, Miami, FL, University of Texas Southwestern Medical Center, and personal consultation files (JA-S).
†Table 1 from Albores-Saavedra J, Delgado R, Henson DE. Well differentiated adenocarcinoma, gastric foveolar type, of the extrahepatic bile ducts: a previously unrecognized and distinctive morphologic variant of bile duct carcinoma. Ann Diagn Pathol 1999;3:75–80.

Anatomic Distribution

For prognostic and therapeutic purposes it has been useful to divide the extrahepatic ductal system into three parts: upper, middle, and lower thirds. Over 50 percent of all carcinomas are located in the upper third, 18 percent in the middle third, and 22 percent in the lower third (19). In less than 10 percent of cases, it is not possible to specify the origin because of diffuse involvement of the bile ducts (fig. 13-9). More recent studies, however, indicate that most carcinomas arise within 5 mm of the junction of the cystic duct or within the cystic duct (16). Furthermore, it has been proposed that the extrahepatic system be divided into five regions which can account for the variations in the anatomic location of the cystic duct junction (16). Precise location of the primary tumor can now be accomplished by diagnostic imaging. However, with diffusely infiltrating tumors, it is often difficult or impossible to ascertain the site of origin.

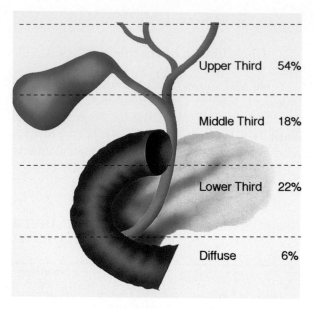

Figure 13-9
ANATOMIC DISTRIBUTION OF 143 MALIGNANT EPITHELIAL TUMORS IN THE EXTRAHEPATIC BILE DUCTS

Gross Features

Carcinomas of the extrahepatic bile ducts usually appear as diffusely infiltrating, nodular and constricting lesions or as polypoid indurated masses (figs. 13-10–13-12). A combination of these two features is often seen. On occasion, there is minimal thickening or induration of the bile duct which, when opened longitudinally, reveals only a roughened and granular mucosa (fig. 13-13). These changes can be overlooked easily on macroscopic examination even by experienced surgeons and pathologists. Invariably, mucosal ulceration and obstruction occur (fig. 13-14).

Most bile duct carcinomas are gray-white, firm, and not well defined (fig. 13-15). A few are friable and necrotic, especially pleomorphic giant cell and small cell carcinomas. Mucinous carcinomas have a gelatinous appearance. Extensive necrosis, however, is not common. Despite the small size of most tumors, by the time of diagnosis they have usually spread to adjacent tissues and about one third have metastasized to regional lymph nodes. If the tumor has spread along the entire biliary ductal system, it may not be possible to determine its origin.

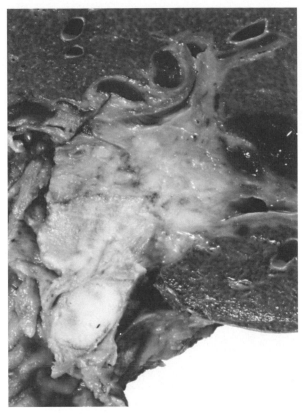

Figure 13-10
CARCINOMA OF THE COMMON HEPATIC DUCT
The tumor, which arose in the common hepatic duct, has extended along the right and left hepatic ducts into the hilum of the liver. A lymph node replaced by metastatic carcinoma is visible. (Fig. 166 from Fascicle 22, 2nd Series.)

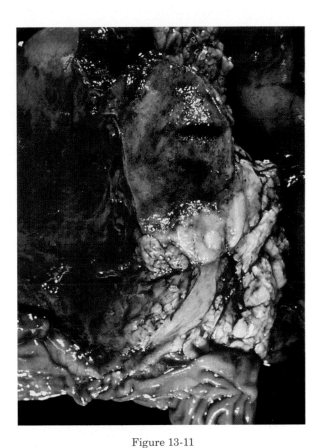

Figure 13-11
CARCINOMA OF COMMON BILE DUCT
This moderately differentiated adenocarcinoma appears as a gray-white, nodular mass that obstructed the common bile duct. The proximal portion of the common duct is greatly dilated.

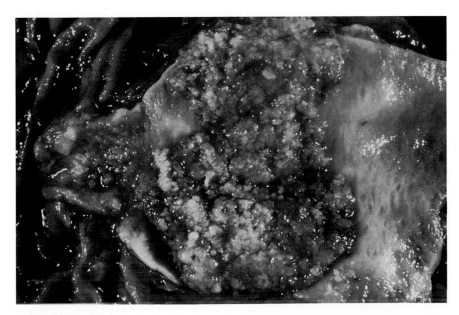

Figure 13-12
PAPILLARY CARCINOMA OF THE COMMON BILE DUCT
This large (4 cm) papillary carcinoma of the distal portion of the common bile duct had a single focus of superficial infiltration into the wall.

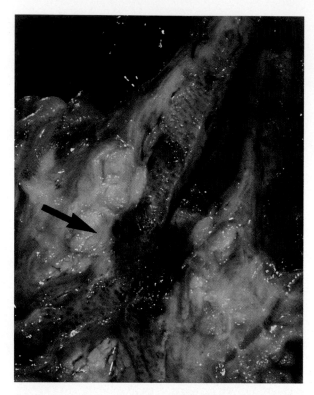

Figure 13-13
CARCINOMA OF
THE COMMON BILE DUCT

The common bile duct has been opened and bisected. The hemorrhagic granular and ulcerated lesion represents a diffusely infiltrating carcinoma (arrow).

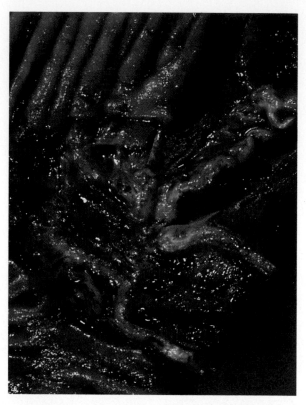

Figure 13-14
CARCINOMA OF THE COMMON BILE DUCT

Carcinoma of the common bile duct appears as a stricture near the cystic duct. The proximal portion of the common bile duct is dilated.

Carcinomas of the extrahepatic bile ducts have been divided into polypoid, nodular, scirrhous constricting, and diffusely infiltrating types (18). This separation is important for the surgeon because it often provides a guide to the operative procedure, extent of resection, and prognosis. However, except for the polypoid tumors, this separation is rarely possible in practice because of overlapping gross features. As with the gallbladder, patients with polypoid tumors, which usually prove to be papillary carcinomas histologically, have the best prognosis (fig. 13-16). The nodular and scirrhous types tend to infiltrate surrounding tissues and are difficult to resect (figs. 13-17, 13-18). The diffusely infiltrating types tend to spread linearly along the ducts.

Microscopic Features

The microscopic features of these tumors do not differ from those found in the gallbladder and for

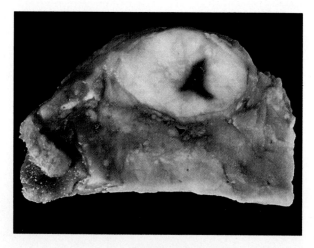

Figure 13-15
ADENOSQUAMOUS CARCINOMA
OF THE INTRAPANCREATIC SEGMENT
OF THE COMMON BILE DUCT

Cross section of the common bile duct shows that its entire circumference is infiltrated by a gray-white mass that obstructs the lumen.

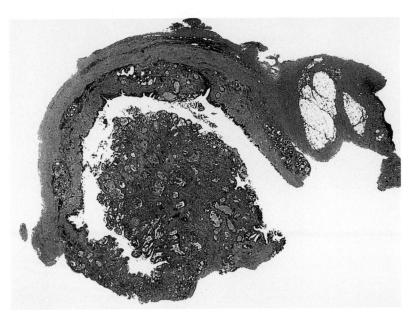

Figure 13-16
POLYPOID ADENOCARCINOMA
OF THE COMMON BILE DUCT
This small polypoid adenocarcinoma of the common bile duct projects into the lumen and shows minimal superficial invasion of the wall. Lobules of hyperplastic intramural glands are seen scattered throughout.

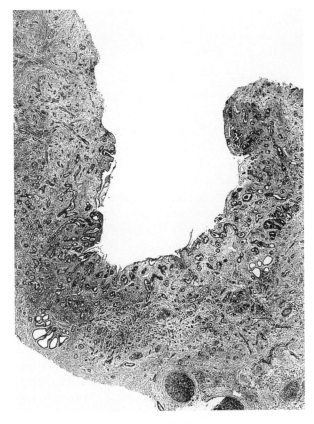

Figure 13-17
DIFFUSELY INFILTRATING
WELL-DIFFERENTIATED ADENOCARCINOMA
OF THE COMMON BILE DUCT
Two lobules of hyperplastic and dilated intramural glands can be easily distinguished from neoplastic glands.

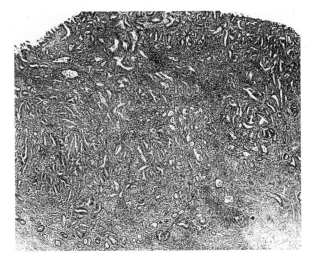

Figure 13-18
NODULAR ADENOCARCINOMA
OF THE COMMON BILE DUCT
Low-power view of a well-differentiated adenocarcinoma that displays a nodular growth pattern.

this reason will not be described in detail (8a). However, some similarities and differences should be noted. In the SEER Program and in our 143 cases, the proportion of well- to moderately differentiated adenocarcinomas was essentially the same: 76 to 78 percent of patients had this type of tumor. Surrounded by a desmoplastic stroma, a variable proportion of short and long

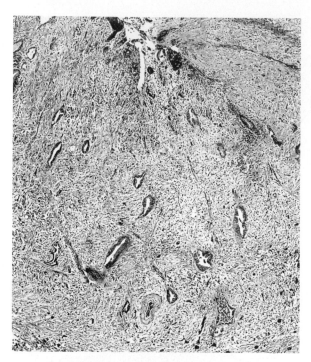

Figure 13-19
WELL-DIFFERENTIATED ADENOCARCINOMA
OF RIGHT HEPATIC DUCT
Randomly distributed, short tubular glands lie in an abundant fibrous stroma.

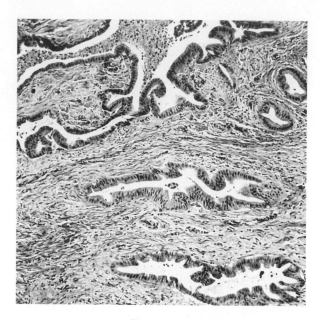

Figure 13-20
WELL-DIFFERENTIATED
ADENOCARCINOMA OF THE LEFT HEPATIC DUCT
Branching long tubular glands in a well-differentiated adenocarcinoma of the left hepatic duct.

tubular glands are found in most adenocarcinomas. The glands are lined by either tall columnar, cuboidal, or flat cells similar to those described in gallbladder carcinomas (figs. 13-19–13-21A–C). Occasionally, scattered goblet and endocrine cells are present among the cuboidal and tall columnar cells (22). Foveolar type cells predominate in a few very well-differentiated tumors, which in superficial biopsies can be confused with adenomas (fig. 13-21D,E) (8). However, adenomas composed predominantly of foveolar type cells have not been reported in the extrahepatic bile ducts. Also, the deep portion of these tumors are less well differentiated and may show perineural invasion which facilitates the diagnosis. Rarely, adenocarcinomas may show focal cribriform features (fig. 13-22A), but cribriform carcinomas such as those described in the gallbladder have not been reported in the extrahepatic bile ducts. Likewise, moderately differentiated adenocarcinomas of the extrahepatic bile ducts rarely show focal pseudoangiosarcomatous features as described in carcinomas of the gallbladder (fig. 13-22B,C).

As in the gallbladder, papillary carcinomas are usually well to moderately differentiated and grow into the lumen before they invade the wall. Histologically, they exhibit a complex papillary architecture, varying degrees of cytologic atypia, and can be of intestinal or biliary type (fig. 13-23). Moderately differentiated papillary adenocarcinomas usually contain a greater number of mitotic figures than well-differentiated tumors. Because noninvasive papillary carcinomas are associated with a better outcome (15), extensive sampling is advisable to exclude invasion (9a). Intestinal type adenocarcinomas, mucinous carcinomas, and clear cell adenocarcinomas also occur in the extrahepatic bile ducts. Most of the intestinal type adenocarcinomas are similar to adenocarcinomas of the colon (fig. 13-24) (9). The only goblet cell type of intestinal adenocarcinoma included in our series occurred in a patient with ulcerative colitis. Although the predominant component of clear cell carcinoma is glandular, some have a prominent nesting and trabecular pattern that is maintained in metastatic deposits, where they can be confused with metastatic renal cell carcinomas (figs. 13-25, 13-26) (20). A positive stain for mucin and reactivity for carcinoembryonic

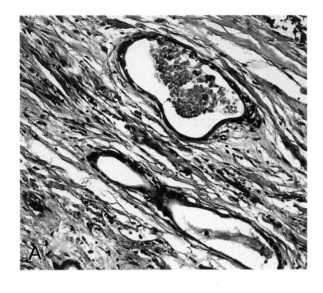

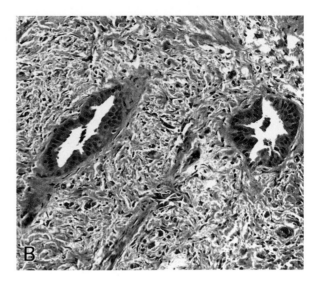

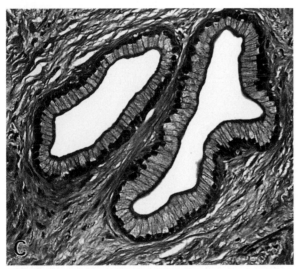

Figure 13-21
VARIATIONS IN THE NEOPLASTIC LINING
EPITHELIUM OF ADENOCARCINOMAS
OF THE EXTRAHEPATIC BILE DUCTS

A: A single layer of low cuboidal and flat epithelial cells.

B: Pseudostratified cuboidal epithelium.

C: A single layer of tall, slender, columnar, mucin-secreting cells resembling gastric foveolar cells line two glands.

D: Polypoid well-differentiated adenocarcinoma of foveolar type in common hepatic duct. Closely packed glands of different sizes are seen in the lamina propria.

E: Higher magnification of glands lined by gastric foveolar type epithelium with basal nuclei showing minimal atypia.

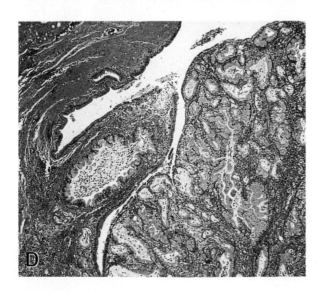

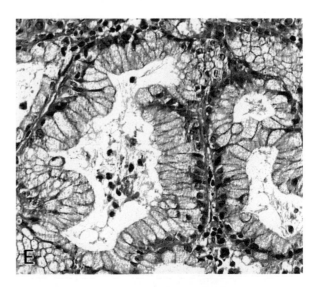

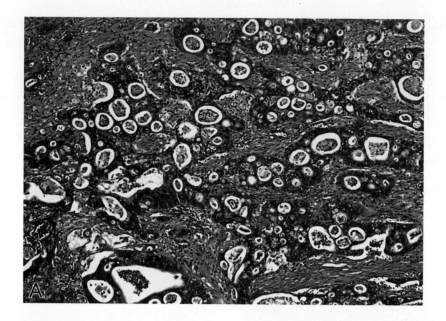

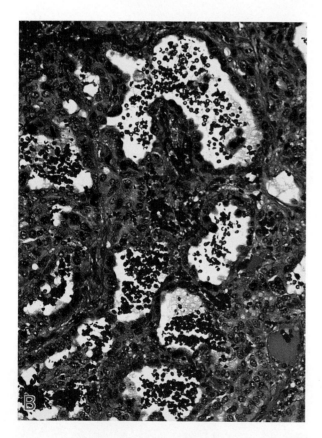
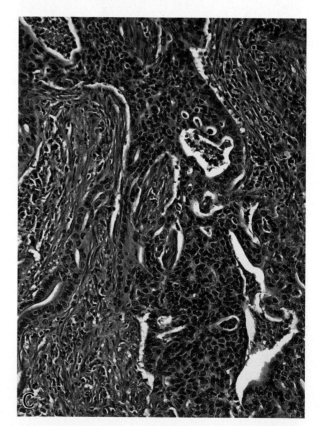

Figure 13-22
DIFFERENT HISTOLOGIC PATTERNS OF ADENOCARCINOMAS

A: Focal cribriform pattern in a moderately differentiated adenocarcinoma of the common bile duct.

B: Adenocarcinoma of the common hepatic duct with pseudoangiosarcomatous features. The vascular-like spaces contain red blood cells, but are lined by cuboidal epithelial cells that were cytokeratin positive and negative for endothelial markers.

C: Solid component in a moderately differentiated adenocarcinoma of the common bile duct.

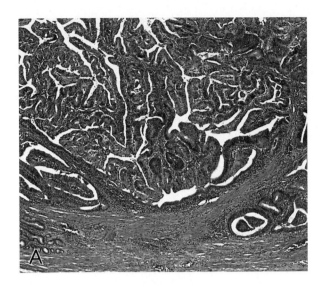

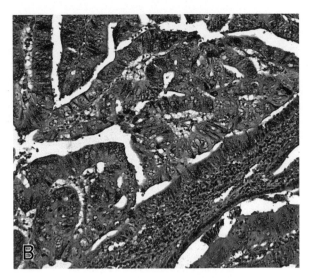

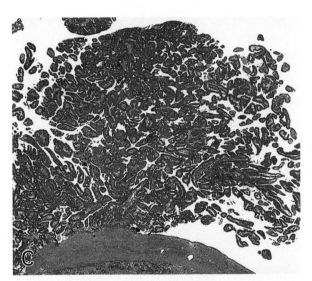

Figure 13-23
PAPILLARY CARCINOMAS

A: This intestinal type papillary carcinoma which has grown into the lumen of the common bile duct shows several foci of invasion.

B: Higher magnification of the complex papillary structures lined by tall columnar neoplastic cells.

C: Low-power view of a noninvasive papillary carcinoma of common bile duct.

D: Detail of neoplastic columnar cells showing a biliary phenotype.

E: Invasive moderately differentiated papillary carcinoma shows greater cytologic atypia than that seen in the tumor shown in D.

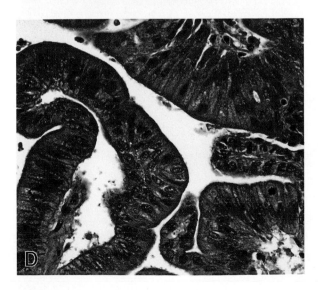

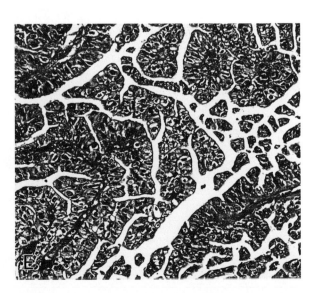

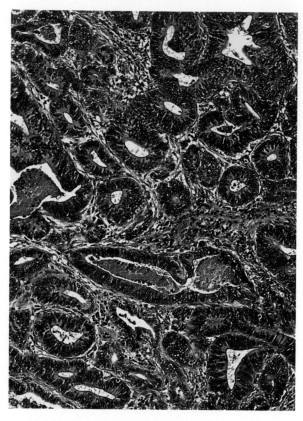

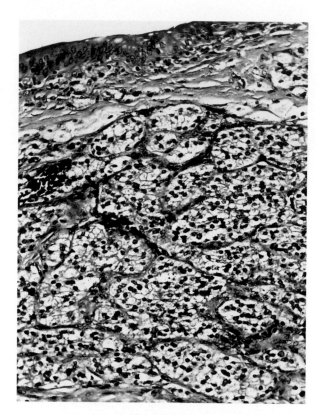

Figure 13-24
INTESTINAL TYPE ADENOCARCINOMA
OF CYSTIC DUCT
The tumor closely resembles adenocarcinomas of the colon.

Figure 13-25
CLEAR CELL CARCINOMA
OF THE RIGHT HEPATIC DUCT
Clear cell carcinoma of the right hepatic duct showing a prominent nesting pattern. The overlying biliary epithelium is normal. (Fig. 2 from Vardaman C, Albores-Saavedra J. Clear cell carcinomas of the gallbladder and extrahepatic bile ducts. Am J Surg Pathol 1995;19:91–9.)

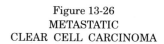

Figure 13-26
METASTATIC
CLEAR CELL CARCINOMA
Metastasis in a porta hepatis lymph node from tumor shown in figure 13-25 closely resembles renal cell carcinoma. (Fig. 9 from Vardaman C, Albores-Saavedra J. Clear cell carcinomas of the gallbladder and extrahepatic bile ducts. Am J Surg Pathol 1995;19:91–9.)

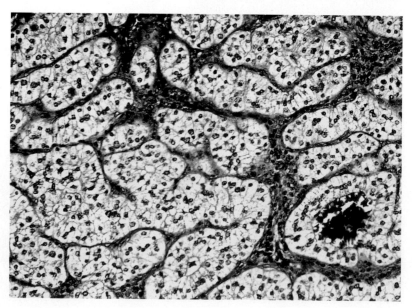

antigen (CEA) favor a primary tumor in the extrahepatic bile ducts.

The squamous component of adenosquamous carcinoma often shows intercellular bridges and keratinization (fig. 13-27). However, in poorly differentiated tumors these features are focal and found only after extensive sampling. Anaplastic areas, which consist of sheets of large polygonal cells and fascicles of spindle cells, predominate in some poorly differentiated examples.

A few squamous cell carcinomas have been reported in the proximal segment of the extrahepatic biliary tree (10). Extensive sampling is required to exclude a glandular component which may not be present in small biopsy specimens. The frequency of small cell carcinomas and undifferentiated carcinomas, spindle and giant cell type, is lower in the bile ducts than in the gallbladder. Both the pure and combined forms of small cell carcinoma have been described in the extrahepatic bile ducts (fig. 13-28, left) (14). Undifferentiated carcinomas, spindle and giant cell type, often show a minor component of well- to moderately differentiated adenocarcinoma, but are highly aggressive and rapidly extend to adjacent structures. We have seen a single example of signet ring cell carcinoma, although several more cases have been recorded in the SEER Program (fig. 13-28, right).

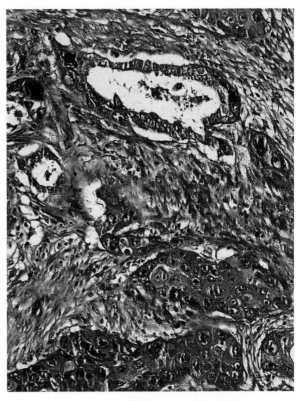

Figure 13-27
ADENOSQUAMOUS CARCINOMA
OF THE COMMON BILE DUCT
The glandular and squamous components are separated by fibrous stroma.

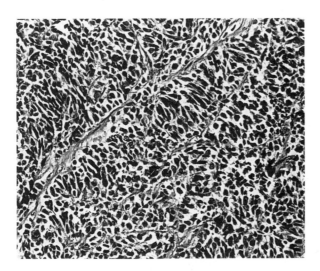
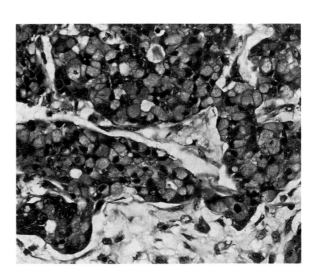

Figure 13-28
SMALL CELL AND SIGNET RING CELL CARCINOMAS
Left: Small cell carcinoma of the common bile duct. Cords of fusiform and round cells with hyperchromatic nuclei, no visible nucleoli, and scant cytoplasm are illustrated.
Right: Signet ring cell carcinoma. Trabeculae of signet ring cells infiltrate the wall of the common bile duct.

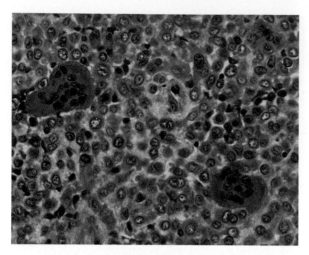

Figure 13-29
UNDIFFERENTIATED CARCINOMA
MIMICKING GIANT CELL TUMOR OF BONE
Multinucleated osteoclast-like giant cells are admixed with ovoid or round mononuclear cells. (Figures 13-29 and 13-30 are from the same patient.)

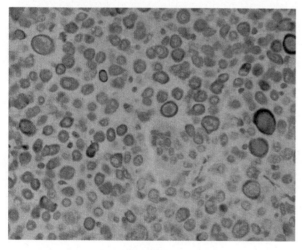

Figure 13-30
UNDIFFERENTIATED CARCINOMA
MIMICKING GIANT CELL TUMOR OF BONE
Nearly all mononuclear cells are epithelial membrane antigen positive whereas the multinucleated osteoclast-like giant cells are negative.

A case of adenocarcinoma with a spindle cell component and containing multinucleated osteoclast-like giant cells has been reported involving the bile ducts of the hilum of the liver (12). Because of their immunoreactivity for histiocytic markers and lack of immunostaining with cytokeratins, the suggestion has been made that

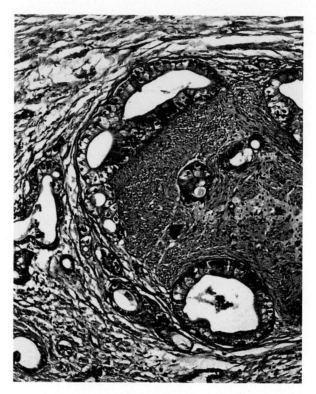

Figure 13-31
PERINEURAL AND INTRANEURAL
INVASION IN ADENOCARCINOMA OF
COMMON BILE DUCT, CLEAR CELL TYPE

the osteoclast-like multinucleated giant cells might be reactive rather than neoplastic. We recently studied two neoplasms from the common bile duct with similar histologic features but without the glandular component. They were composed of sheets of ovoid cells and fascicles of spindle cells as well as numerous osteoclast-like giant cells. The pattern of growth and the cytologic features closely resembled a giant cell tumor of bone (fig. 13-29). However, the ovoid and spindle cells were epithelial membrane antigen positive whereas the osteoclast-like giant cells were positive for CD68 and negative for epithelial markers, supporting the view that these tumors are indeed undifferentiated carcinomas (fig. 13-30).

Perineural invasion is seen in 75 to 80 percent of the cases that are adequately sampled and should be specifically evaluated, since it allows separation from primary sclerosing cholangitis and because of its prognostic implications (fig. 13-31). The incidence of perineural invasion is higher in carcinomas of the extrahepatic bile ducts than in those arising in the ampulla, but is similar to that of carcinomas of the gallbladder (13). Likewise, lymphatic invasion is more common than blood vessel invasion in extrahepatic bile duct carcinomas.

As a group, tumors arising in the proximal segment of the extrahepatic bile ducts tend to be better differentiated. The stroma is more sclerotic and usually contains chronic inflammatory cells. Consequently, these tumors are more apt to be confused with sclerosing cholangitis than the less-differentiated tumors that arise more distally. To our knowledge, undifferentiated carcinomas, spindle and giant cell type, and small cell carcinomas have not been reported in this proximal location. In fact, in our material, these two types were found only in the common duct.

Immunohistochemistry

Approximately one third of well- to moderately differentiated adenocarcinomas contain endocrine cells that are immunoreactive for the general neuroendocrine markers, such as neuron-specific enolase, synaptophysin, and chromogranin (fig. 13-32) (26). Serotonin and peptide hormones, including somatostatin, pancreatic polypeptide, and gastrin, have been detected in these cells by immunohistochemistry. The number of endocrine cells varies from tumor to tumor and even in different areas of the same tumor. These endocrine cells are similar to those found in many carcinomas of the gastrointestinal tract including those of the colon, pancreas, and stomach. Their clinical significance, however, is unknown. We have not seen systemic manifestations in association with carcinomas of the extrahepatic bile ducts that contain endocrine cells. In our experience, the presence of endocrine cells does not correlate with the stage of disease or biologic behavior.

Approximately 65 percent of extrahepatic bile duct carcinomas stain for p53 protein (25). However, it is not known whether the p53 nuclear reactivity correlates with genetic mutation.

The human nm23-H1 gene belongs to the family of genes nm23 with antimetastatic activity. The immunohistochemical expression of the nm23-H1 protein has been shown to be reduced in a variety of human carcinomas (24). However, all adenocarcinomas of the extrahepatic bile ducts have shown moderate to strong nm23-H1 pro-

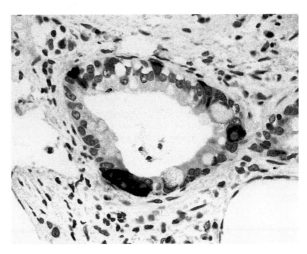

Figure 13-32
ENDOCRINE CELLS IN
ADENOCARCINOMA OF INTESTINAL TYPE
Chromogranin-positive cells admixed with goblet and columnar cells in an intestinal type of adenocarcinoma of the common hepatic duct.

tein immunoreactivity, indicating no relationship to metastatic ability (24). Most carcinomas that have been studied by immunocytochemistry contain CEA (11,23). This antigen is also found in dysplastic lesions and in carcinomas in situ. In normal bile duct epithelium, polyclonal CEA is seen only along the apical cytoplasm of epithelial cells. Although CEA is not needed for diagnosis it may help to highlight the extent of tumor infiltration and to discriminate between hyperplastic intramural glands and neoplastic elements (11).

Molecular Pathology

In recent years a number of studies have suggested that K-*ras* mutations are important in the pathogenesis of extrahepatic bile duct carcinoma (27–29). The incidence of these mutations has varied from 0 to 100 percent (31). The differences reported may be due to the variation in the sensitivity of the methods employed for detection of the mutations. Another possible explanation is the inclusion of pancreatic carcinomas invading the wall of the common bile duct as primary extrahepatic bile duct tumors. Most studies have found a higher incidence of K-*ras* codon 12 mutations in extrahepatic bile duct carcinomas than in gallbladder carcinomas. In one study K-*ras* codon 12 mutations were found to be an

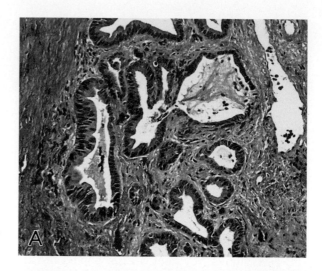

Figure 13-33
REACTIVE ATYPIA

A: Reactive atypia of intramural glands of common bile duct. A lobule composed of glands of different sizes is seen.

B: Higher magnification of the glands shows low cuboidal and columnar pseudostratified cells with mild nuclear atypia. These changes are characteristic of reactive atypia.

C: A neoplastic gland separates two lobules of small hyperplastic intramural glands. Note the marked nuclear atypia in the neoplastic gland. A long ductal structure lined by mucin-containing cells is seen in one of the lobules.

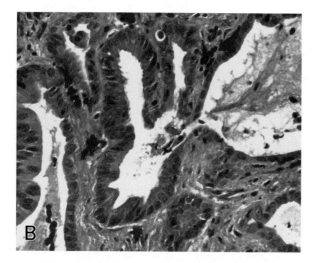

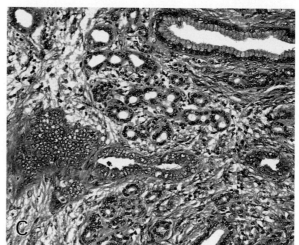

independent prognostic indicator in patients with extrahepatic bile duct carcinomas (30).

Differential Diagnosis

One of the most important diagnostic problems for the pathologist relates to the small size of the biopsy specimen which is usually obtained through endoscopic retrograde cholangiopancreatography. In inflammatory strictures, in addition to the inflammation and fibrosis, there is reactive atypia of the surface epithelium as well as hyperplasia and atypia of the intramural glands (fig. 13-33A). Reactive atypia of the surface epithelium usually occurs in association with acute or chronic inflammation, and the columnar cells are mixed with low cuboidal cells, and are, as a rule, less atypical than those seen in carcinoma.

Preservation of the lobular arrangement of the glands strongly favors a benign process. Moreover, the intramural glands are often lined by both low cuboidal and tall columnar cells showing pseudostratification, nuclear enlargement, small nucleoli, and occasional mitotic figures (fig. 13-33B,C). Perineural invasion, a common finding in carcinomas, has not been reported in cases of hyperplasia of intramural glands or in reactive epithelial atypia.

Another problem in the differential diagnosis results from local extension of the tumor and obliteration of its primary site. Carcinomas of the extrahepatic bile ducts can extend to the liver, pancreas, ampulla, duodenum, or gallbladder. Since all of these organs give rise to malignant epithelial neoplasms similar to those originating in the extrahepatic ducts, identification of the exact origin may be difficult, especially with large cancers. Microscopic examination alone is often of minimal help unless carcinoma in situ or severe dysplasia is found in the mucosa adjacent to the bile duct carcinoma. In our material, which consisted of relatively large tumors, this was not helpful, since we found these precursor lesions in only 10 percent of patients. However, other authors have described high-grade dysplasia and carcinoma in situ in the majority of cases. Rarely, synchronous noninvasive and invasive carcinomas of the extrahepatic bile ducts, ampulla of Vater, and pancreas complicate the differential diagnosis even more (36a). In many patients, the diagnosis can be reached only after careful clinicopathologic correlation, including a review of the radiographic and operative findings. Also, the pathologist should recall that the clinical presentation and biologic behavior vary according to the site of origin of the tumor. Carcinomas of the pancreas, for example, tend to metastasize more widely than carcinomas of the bile ducts or ampulla. Grossly, the bulk of the tumor is found at the site of origin. Nevertheless, in some cases it may not be possible to specify with certainty the site of origin of the tumor. This uncertainty has led to the use of nonspecific terms such as carcinoma of the periampullary region (33) or hilar carcinoma of the liver (32), which reflect the difficulties involved in locating the primary site. Even at autopsy, it is often difficult to identify the origin of the primary tumor.

The differential diagnosis between extrahepatic bile duct carcinoma and sclerosing cholangitis is discussed on page 239.

Spread

Malignant tumors of the extrahepatic bile ducts usually spread early by direct extension to adjacent tissue which includes the portal vein, hepatic artery, liver parenchyma surrounding the hilum, and pancreas. Local spread through the wall of the bile ducts into the periductal connective tissue is common and the ducts are often transformed into rigid tubes. Specifically, carcinomas arising in the left or right hepatic ducts may either extend proximal to the intrahepatic ducts, largely following an extramucosal route, or distal to the common hepatic duct (35). Neoplasms from the

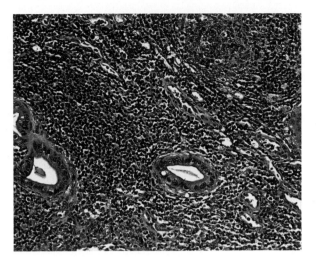

Figure 13-34
METASTATIC ADENOCARCINOMA IN LYMPH NODE
Lymph node metastasis of a well-differentiated adenocarcinoma of common bile duct.

cystic duct tend to invade the neck of the gallbladder or common bile duct. Carcinomas arising in the distal third of the common bile duct usually extend to the pancreas, colon, or duodenum, but rarely to the stomach.

Tumors can also spread along blood vessels and lymphatic channels and along small nerves. Perineural invasion should be reported, since it has an adverse effect on survival (34). It is least likely to occur with papillary carcinomas. Because tumors that originate in the hepatic ducts are often well differentiated, they are usually characterized by a slow rate of growth and a low propensity for metastasis.

Despite the well-differentiated character of most tumors, a character maintained in metastatic deposits, lymph nodes are frequently involved (fig. 13-34). In patients with carcinoma arising in the distal common bile duct the frequency of nodal involvement is 69 percent (36), with the most commonly involved nodes including the posterior-superior pancreaticoduodenal (52 percent), pericholedochal (28 percent), and those around the superior mesenteric artery (22 percent) (36). The frequency of lymph node involvement increases with the depth of tumor invasion, or, in the case of tumors arising in the distal common bile duct, deeper infiltration into the head of the pancreas (36,39).

Distant metastases have been reported in 30 to 70 percent of cases. Hematogenous spread is uncommon and usually occurs late. Diffuse peritoneal seeding is also a late manifestation that often results from local recurrence.

Local Recurrence. A major cause of death, local recurrence results from residual tumor located in the proximal or distal surgical margins of the bile duct or from tumor located along the dissected transverse margin in the portal area (37). For this reason, it is important for the pathologist to evaluate carefully all surgical margins, including an assessment of vascular and perineural invasion. Malignant tumors of the extrahepatic bile ducts often originate from multiple separate foci (38). Therefore, microscopic foci may be found at the margin even though the main tumor mass has been completely resected. In some cases it may be difficult to evaluate margins on frozen section because of inflammation or reactive atypia of the surface epithelium, or hyperplastic intramural mucous glands. Local recurrence, usually at the surgical margins, is most common with carcinomas arising in the hepatic ducts.

Since five percent of patients with bile duct carcinoma have synchronous carcinomas of the gallbladder, careful examination of the entire surgical specimen including the gallbladder is advised.

Prognosis

Although most of these tumors are usually small, well differentiated, and tend to remain localized, the results of surgical treatment have been disappointing. According to the National Cancer Institute, the 2-year relative survival rate for patients with all stages combined is 23 percent and the 5-year rate is 10 percent (55). The 5-year survival rates for those with tumors occurring in the upper middle and lower segments of the extrahepatic bile ducts vary among different series (40,41a,51).

Patients with lesions in the proximal ductal system are the most difficult to treat and often require major hepatic resections (44). In a series of 80 hilar carcinomas, only 4 could be resected (41). Of 47 patients with carcinomas of the upper third of the extrahepatic ductal system treated surgically, none survived 5 years (50). However, recent reports document higher resection and cure rates in a selected group of patients with carcinomas of the proximal ductal system (47a, 48). When these slow-growing malignant tumors are considered unresectable, palliative treatment that reestablishes biliary flow is usually indicated. Some patients have survived several years following such a procedure (45). Death often results from bile duct obstruction, liver failure, and ascending cholangitis.

The best results are observed in patients with tumors located in the distal third of the common bile duct in whom a pancreatoduodenectomy is possible (47). In this group the 5-year survival rate is 28 percent (48,51). Tumors of the middle part of the common bile duct are usually treated by local excision with anastomosis of the proximal duct to the intestine. Of 24 patients with tumors in this region, only 3 (12.5 percent) survived 5 years (48). For 103 patients whose tumors were not resected, the 2-year survival rate was 19 percent (42).

Early reports indicated that postoperative radiotherapy reduces local recurrence and increases survival (46). However, recent studies have shown no long-term benefits from adjuvant irradiation (43,47a,49). Moreover, a significant number of biliary complications associated with irradiation have been described (49). Liver transplantation has also been tried in the treatment of extrahepatic bile duct carcinomas but with no success.

Prognostic Factors

Several prognostic factors based on the characteristics of the primary tumor have been reported for carcinomas of the extrahepatic bile ducts (55,58).

Histologic Type. Papillary carcinomas that grow outward into the lumen have the most favorable prognosis and for this reason should be correctly reported (55,58,60). According to the National Cancer Institute, the 5-year relative survival rate for patients with papillary carcinoma is 22 percent compared to 8 percent for those with conventional adenocarcinoma (fig. 13-35).

Histologic Grade. There is a correlation between grade and outcome (fig. 13-36). Extrahepatic bile duct carcinomas are graded as well, moderately, and poorly differentiated, and undifferentiated using the same criteria as for gallbladder carcinomas. Well-differentiated

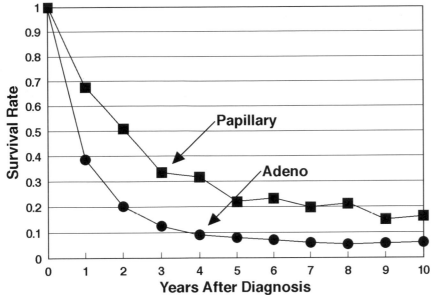

Figure 13-35
RELATIVE SURVIVAL RATES
FOR TWO COMMON
HISTOLOGIC TYPES OF
EXTRAHEPATIC
BILE DUCT CANCER
There were 1168 cases of adenocarcinoma (adeno) and 85 cases of papillary carcinoma (papillary). Adenocarcinomas include cases reported as adenocarcinoma and as cholangiocarcinoma. All stages and grades are combined. Data from the Surveillance, Epidemiology, and End Results Program, National Cancer Institute.

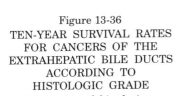

Figure 13-36
TEN-YEAR SURVIVAL RATES
FOR CANCERS OF THE
EXTRAHEPATIC BILE DUCTS
ACCORDING TO
HISTOLOGIC GRADE
All stages and histologic types are combined. Data taken from the Surveillance, Epidemiology, and End Results Program, National Cancer Institute, for the years 1981 to 1990. Number of cases for grade 1 was 239; grade 2, 305; grade 3, 205; and grade 4, 10.

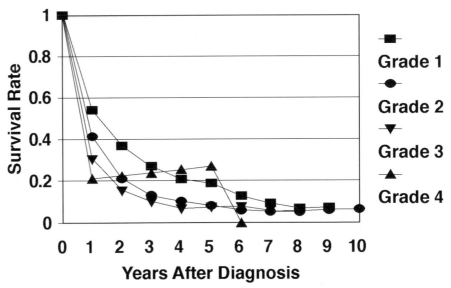

carcinomas show gland formation in 95 percent of the tumor, moderately differentiated carcinomas in 40 to 94 percent of the tumor, and poorly differentiated carcinomas in 6 to 39 percent of the tumor. If greater than 95 percent of the tumor exhibits a solid or cord pattern of growth the carcinoma is classified as undifferentiated.

Perineural Invasion. In some studies, perineural invasion has correlated with a decreased survival rate (53,57).

Vascular Invasion. Vascular invasion indicates a less favorable outcome (58). Blood vessel or lymphatic involvement should be reported.

Extent of Disease. From a prognostic point of view, resection of a malignant bile duct tumor must be accompanied by reliable information on the extent of disease. For classifying extent, we advocate using the TNM staging system (Table 13-3) that has been published by the American Joint Committee on Cancer and the International Union

Table 13-3

DEFINITION OF TNM

T - Primary Tumor

TX Primary tumor cannot be assessed
T0 No evidence of primary tumor
Tis Carcinoma in situ
T1 Tumor invades subepithelial connective tissue or fibromuscular layer
    T1a Tumor invades subepithelial connective tissue
    T1b Tumor invades fibromuscular layer
T2 Tumor invades perifibromuscular connective tissue
T3 Tumor invades adjacent structures: liver, pancreas, duodenum, gallbladder, colon, stomach

N - Regional Lymph Nodes

NX Regional lymph nodes cannot be assessed
N0 No regional lymph node metastasis
N1 Metastasis in cystic duct, pericholedochal, and/or hilar lymph nodes (i.e., in the hepatoduodenal ligament)
N2 Metastasis in peripancreatic (head only), periduodenal, periportal, coeliac, superior mesenteric, posterior mesenteric, posterior pancreaticoduodenal lymph nodes

M - Distant Metastasis

MX Distant metastasis cannot be assessed
M0 No distant metastasis
M1 Distant metastasis

Stage Grouping

Stage 0	Tis	N0	M0
Stage I	T	N0	M0
Stage II	T2	N0	M0
Stage III	T1	N1, N2	M0
	T2	N1, N2	M0
Stage IVA	T3	Any N	M0
Stage IVB	Any T	Any N	M1

Against Cancer (52,59). Since lymph nodes are one of the most important components of radical resection, the assessment of nodal status is critical for evaluating prognosis. The 10-year relative survival rates according to the stage of disease are shown in figure 13-37. For patients with tumors confined to the bile duct, the 10-year survival rate is 19 percent; for patients with regional and distant disease, the survival rates are 9 and 1 percent, respectively. Invasion of the pancreas is a poor prognostic finding (54).

Other Factors. Data indicate that mutations in codon 12 of the Ki-*ras* gene are associated with reduced survival (56).

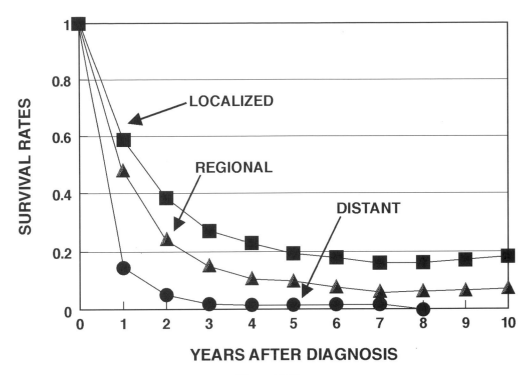

Figure 13-37
TEN-YEAR RELATIVE SURVIVAL RATES ACCORDING TO STAGE
OF DISEASE FOR CANCERS OF THE EXTRAHEPATIC BILE DUCTS
There were 335 cases with localized, 558 with regional, and 348 with distant disease. The 10-year relative rates were 19 percent for localized, 9 percent for regional, and 1 percent for distant. Data include all histologic types. Data from the Surveillance, Epidemiology, and End Results Program, National Cancer Institute.

REFERENCES

Dysplasia and Carcinoma In Situ

1. Albores-Saavedra J, Henson DE. Tumors of the gallbladder and extrahepatic bile ducts. Atlas of Tumor Pathology, 2nd Series, Fascicle 22. Washington, D.C.: Armed Forces Institute of Pathology, 1986:44–53.
2. Davis RI, Sloan JM, Hood JM, Maxwell P. Carcinoma of the extrahepatic biliary tract: a clinicopathological and immunohistochemical study. Histopathology 1988;12:623–31.
3. Haworth AC, Manley PN, Groll A, Pace R. Bile duct carcinoma and biliary tract dysplasia in chronic ulcerative colitis. Arch Pathol Lab Med 1989;113:434–6.
4. Laitio M. Carcinoma of extrahepatic bile ducts. A histopathological study. Pathol Res Pract 1983;178:67–72.
5. Ludwig J, Wahlstrom HE, Batts KP, Wiesner RH. Papillary bile duct dysplasia in primary sclerosing cholangitis. Gastroenterology 1992;102:2134–8.
6. Suzuki M, Takahashi T, Ouchi K, Matsuno S. The development and extension of hepatohilar bile duct carcinoma. A three-dimensional tumor mapping in the intrahepatic biliary tree visualized with the aid of a graphics computer system. Cancer 1989;64:658-66.
7. Wee A, Ludwig J, Coffey RJ Jr, LaRusso NF, Wiesner RH. Hepatobiliary carcinoma associated with primary sclerosing cholangitis and chronic ulcerative colitis. Hum Pathol 1985;16:719–26.

Anatomic Distribution, Gross and Microscopic Features

8. Albores-Saavedra J, Delgado R, Henson DE. Well differentiated adenocarcinoma, gastric foveolar type, of the extrahepatic bile ducts: a previously unrecognized and distinctive morphologic variant of bile duct carcinoma. Ann Diagn Pathol 1999;3:75–80.
8a. Albores-Saavedra J, Henson DE, Sobin LH. Histological typing of tumours of the gallbladder and extrahepatic bile ducts. World Health Organization, Springer-Verlag, Berlin, 1991.
9. Albores-Saavedra J, Henson DE. Tumors of the gallbladder and extrahepatic bile ducts. Atlas of Tumor Pathology, 2nd Series. Fascicle 22, Washington, DC: Armed Forces Institute of Pathology, 1986.

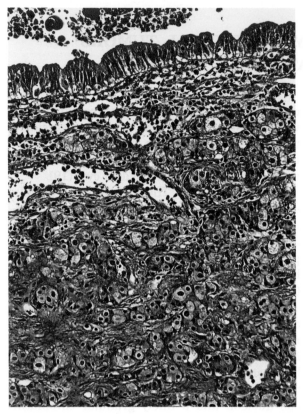

Figure 14-1
CARCINOID TUMOR
This carcinoid tumor is composed of round and polygonal cells arranged in cords separated by scant fibrous stroma containing dilated blood vessels. The overlying epithelium is normal.

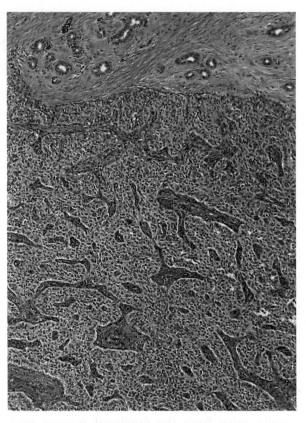

Figure 14-2
CARCINOID TUMOR SHOWING
A TRABECULAR ARCHITECTURE
The small intramural glands are compressed but not infiltrated by tumor.

Figure 14-3
CARCINOID TUMOR
Thin cords of round and polygonal cells with clear cytoplasm are separated by abundant fibrous stroma.

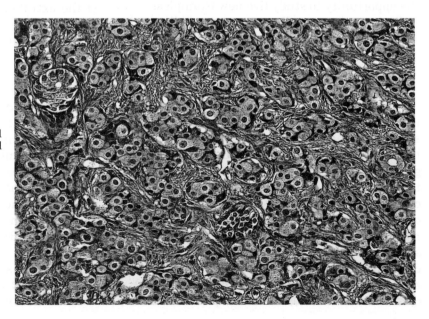

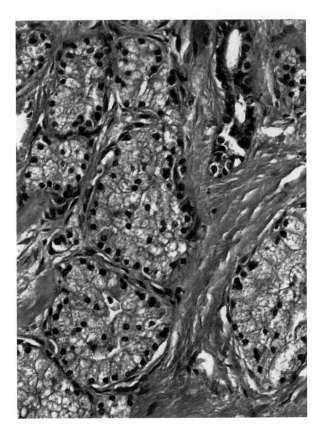 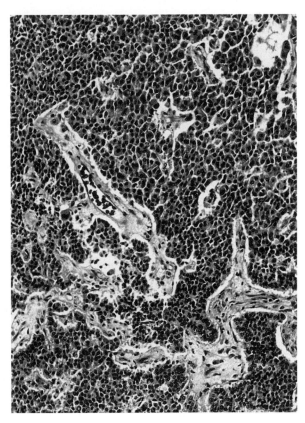

Figure 14-4
CARCINOID TUMOR

Left: A nesting pattern is seen in this somatostatin-producing clear cell carcinoid tumor of the cystic duct. (Courtesy of Dr. Z. Goodman, Washington, D.C.)

Right: Anastomosing trabecular structures characterize this gastrin-producing carcinoid of the common bile duct.

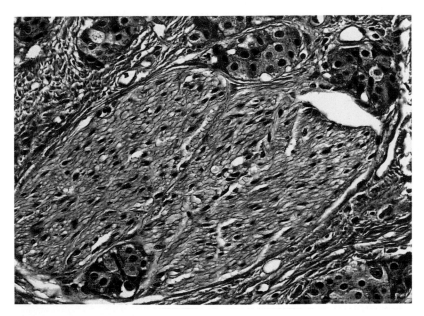

Figure 14-5
CARCINOID TUMOR OF
THE COMMON BILE DUCT
Perineural and intraneural invasion by a carcinoid are seen.

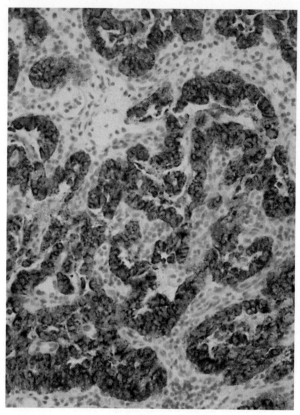

Figure 14-6
CARCINOID TUMOR OF
THE COMMON BILE DUCT

Anastomosing cords of chromogranin-positive cells are seen.

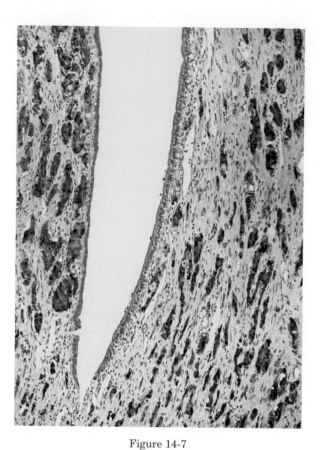

Figure 14-7
CARCINOID TUMOR OF
THE COMMON BILE DUCT

Low-power view of a carcinoid tumor of the common bile duct. Nearly all cells are immunoreactive for serotonin.

Figure 14-8
CARCINOID TUMOR

Many cells of this carcinoid tumor are immunoreactive for gastrin. A few pancreatic polypeptide and somatostatin-producing cells were also identified.

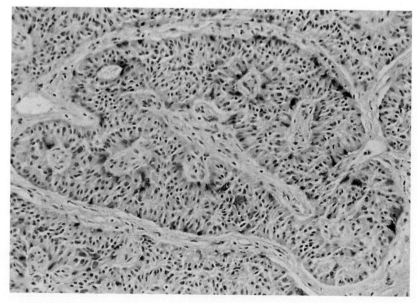

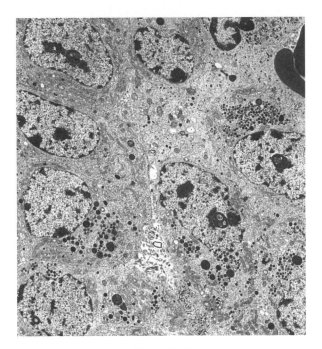

Figure 14-9
ULTRASTRUCTURE OF A CARCINOID TUMOR
The cells have round or ovoid nuclei and contain cytoplasmic granules. Microvilli are seen in some of the cells. (Courtesy of Dr. J. Kennedy, Atlanta, GA.)

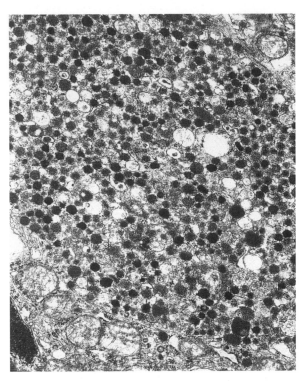

Figure 14-10
ULTRASTRUCTURE OF A CARCINOID TUMOR
Numerous, round, membrane-bound neurosecretory granules are seen in the cytoplasm of a cell. (Courtesy of Dr. J. Kennedy, Atlanta, GA.)

including gastrin, cholecystokinin, pancreatic polypeptide, and somatostatin (9,12).

Electron microscopy has shown many cells with numerous round and pleomorphic neurosecretory granules of variable density, measuring from 200 to 600 nm (figs. 14-9, 14-10).

Histogenesis. Since the normal mucosa of the extrahepatic bile ducts lacks enterochromaffin and argyrophil cells, it has been suggested that carcinoid tumors arise from metaplastic pyloric glands or from foci of intestinal metaplasia which contain those types of endocrine cells (2). Somatostatin-producing cells have been found in the extrahepatic bile ducts (8), and therefore could be the source of somatostatinomas (12).

Differential Diagnosis. Some small cell carcinomas, especially those with numerous festoons or trabeculae, simulate carcinoid tumors. A diffuse chromatin pattern, numerous mitoses, and foci of necrosis favor a diagnosis of small cell carcinoma. The presence of many chromogranin-positive or serotonin-containing cells points to a carcinoid tumor.

Prognosis. These are low-grade malignant tumors that eventually metastasize to the regional lymph nodes and liver. Unfortunately, long-term follow-up is available in only a few of the reported patients with carcinoid tumors of the extrahepatic bile ducts (19). Therefore, the natural history of these tumors is unknown. However, some patients have died as a direct result of the tumor (2).

TUMORS OF PARAGANGLIA

Paraganglioma

A single example of a paraganglioma involving the right and left hepatic ducts has been reported (23). The tumor, which caused obstruction, was successfully removed. It probably arose from the small paraganglia located in the hilum of the liver. We recently examined a paraganglioma of the common bile duct that caused biliary obstruction (figs. 14-11, 14-12).

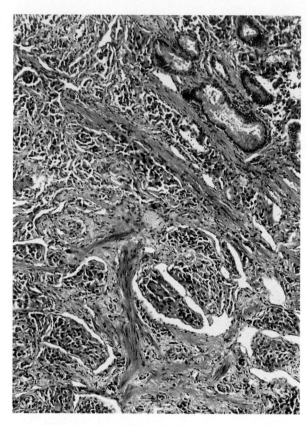

Figure 14-11
PARAGANGLIOMA OF THE COMMON BILE DUCT
Low-power view of a paraganglioma of the common bile duct. Intramural glands are seen in the right upper corner.

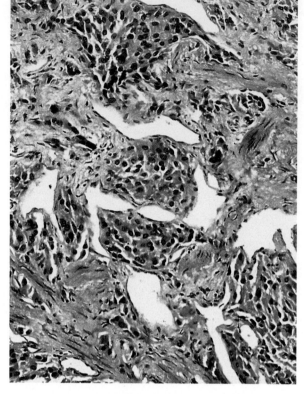

Figure 14-12
PARAGANGLIOMA OF THE COMMON BILE DUCT
Higher magnification of tumor shown in figure 14-11. The characteristic nesting pattern and dilated vascular channels are illustrated.

BENIGN NONEPITHELIAL TUMORS OF THE EXTRAHEPATIC BILE DUCTS

Benign nonepithelial tumors of the extrahepatic bile ducts are exceptional. Fibromas, lipomas, leiomyomas, and neurilemomas have been described (24,25).

Granular Cell Tumor

Granular cell tumors of the extrahepatic bile ducts are histologically distinctive neoplasms of uncertain histogenesis that have engendered considerable interest among clinicians and pathologists. They occur most commonly in the common bile duct (50 percent), cystic duct (38 percent), and hepatic ducts (12 percent) (37). Ninety percent of the patients are young adult females (mean age, 34 years) and 65 percent are blacks (26–28,37). Children and adolescents are

rarely affected, only three cases having been reported (29,36,40).

Signs and symptoms depend on the location of the tumor. Jaundice and abdominal pain are the characteristic manifestations of common bile duct tumors (31,38); cystic duct tumors usually give rise to cholecystitis-like symptoms (27,29, 36). The gallbladder may be distended and palpable. A mucocele or a hydropic gallbladder can be caused by granular cell tumors of the cystic duct (36,39). Cholangiography and ultrasound usually reveal the site of obstruction which is often confused with carcinoma. Since the symptoms and radiologic findings lack specificity it is impossible to diagnose these tumors prior to biopsy or surgical excision.

Occasionally, granular cell tumors of the extrahepatic bile ducts are multicentric and coexist with granular cell tumors in other sites, such as

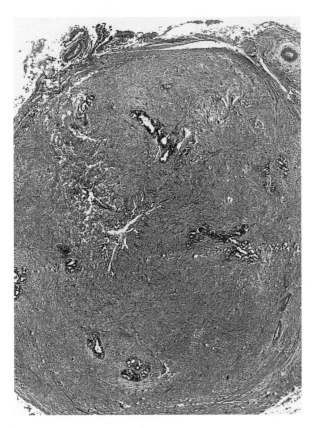

Figure 14-13
GRANULAR CELL TUMOR OF THE CYSTIC DUCT
Low-power view of a granular cell tumor of the cystic duct. The lumen is almost obliterated by the tumor that has infiltrated the full thickness of the wall. Lobules of hyperplastic intramural glands are also seen.

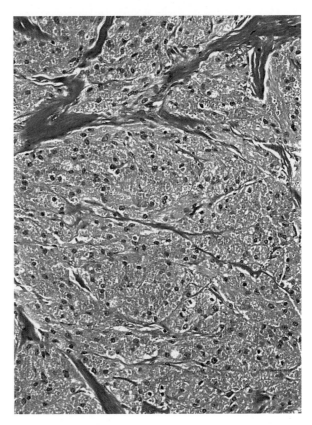

Figure 14-14
GRANULAR CELL TUMOR OF
THE COMMON HEPATIC DUCT
There are nests of cells with abundant granular cytoplasm and small, round, hyperchromatic nuclei.

in the gallbladder, skin, esophagus, stomach, or omentum (26,31,32).

Gross Findings. Granular cell tumors are poorly circumscribed, firm, yellow-tan, and usually no greater than 2 cm in diameter.

Microscopic Findings. Sheets or clusters of large ovoid, round, or polygonal granular cells infiltrate the wall of the bile ducts, eventually obliterating the lumen (fig. 14-13). Rarely, fascicles of spindle cells are a prominent feature. The cells have abundant eosinophilic and granular periodic acid–Schiff (PAS)-positive cytoplasm. Large cytoplasmic hyaline globules are found in some tumors. Nuclei are small, round, centrally placed, and often hyperchromatic (figs. 14-14, 14-15). A mild degree of nuclear pleomorphism occurs in a few cases, but mitotic figures are not seen. Features that may raise concern for malignancy are extension into the periductal fibroadi-

pose tissue, perineural invasion, and direct extension into lymph nodes (figs. 14-16, 14-17). We have seen all three features in benign granular cell tumors of the extrahepatic bile ducts (fig. 14-18). We are not aware of any malignant granular cell tumor reported in this location. Granular cell tumors that arise at the hepatic confluence can extend into the liver, simulating malignant behavior and requiring major surgical resections (37). Hyperplasia of the overlying epithelium and of the intramural glands occurs with some of these tumors and has been confused with carcinoma (29). The lobular arrangement of the gland-like structures and the recognition of reactive atypia should prevent this mistake (fig. 14-18).

Immunohistochemical and Ultrastructural Findings. Granular cell tumors of the extrahepatic bile ducts are immunoreactive to S-100 protein, neuron-specific enolase, myelin

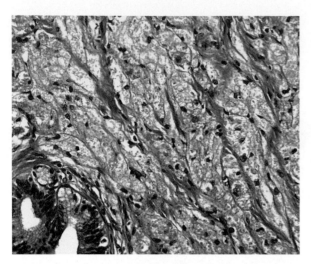

Figure 14-15
GRANULAR CELL TUMOR OF THE CYSTIC DUCT
A cord pattern is seen.

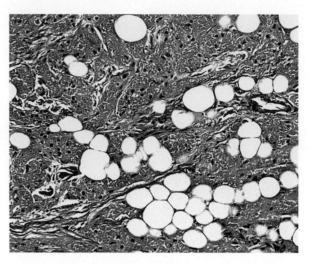

Figure 14-16
GRANULAR CELL TUMOR OF
THE COMMON HEPATIC DUCT
The tumor infiltrates periductal adipose tissue.

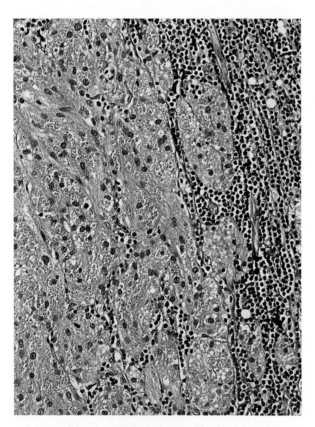

Figure 14-17
GRANULAR CELL TUMOR OF
THE COMMON HEPATIC DUCT
Direct extension of a granular cell tumor of the common hepatic duct into a lymph node.

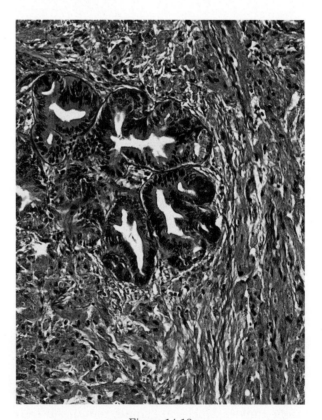

Figure 14-18
LOBULE OF REACTIVE INTRAMURAL GLANDS
SURROUNDED BY A GRANULAR CELL TUMOR
OF THE COMMON BILE DUCT
These atypical reactive glands have been confused with adenocarcinoma.

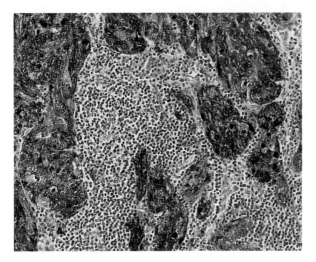

Figure 14-19
GRANULAR CELL TUMOR
S-100 protein-positive granular cell tumor extends into a lymph node.

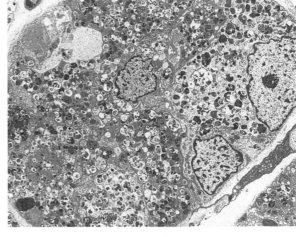

Figure 14-20
ULTRASTRUCTURE OF GRANULAR CELL TUMOR
OF COMMON HEPATIC DUCT
The cells contain numerous autophagic lysosomes with myelin-like figures.

basic protein, Leu-7, cathepsin β, and vimentin (fig. 14-19) (30,33–35). Electron microscopy shows cells arranged in small clusters surrounded by a well-developed basal lamina. Numerous autophagic lysosomes with myelin-like figures and degenerated mitochondria are seen in the cytoplasm of granular cells (fig. 14-20)

(30). Both the immunohistochemical profile and the ultrastructural features are characteristic and suggest a Schwann cell derivation, but are of no diagnostic value since granular cell tumors are histologically distinctive neoplasms that can be recognized by light microscopy with conventional stains.

REFERENCES

Carcinoid Tumor

1. Angeles-Angeles A, Quintanilla L, Larriva-Sahd J. Primary carcinoid of the common bile duct. Immunohistochemical characterization of a case and review of the literature. Am J Clin Pathol 1991;96:341–4.
2. Barron-Rodriguez L, Manivel JC, Mendez-Sanchez N, Jessurun J. Carcinoid tumor of the common bile duct: evidence for its origin in metaplastic endocrine cells. Am J Gastroenterol 1991;86:1073–6.
3. Bergdahl L. Carcinoid tumors of the biliary tract. Aust NZ J Surg 1976;46:136–8.
4. Bickerstaff DR, Ross WB. Carcinoid of the biliary tree: a case report and review of the literature. J R Coll Surg Edinb 1987;32:48–51.
5. Brown WM, Henderson JM, Kennedy JC. Carcinoid tumor of the bile duct: a case report and literature review. Am Surg 1990;56:343–6.
6. Burke AP, Sobin LH, Federspiel BH, et al. Carcinoid tumors of the duodenum. A clinicopathologic study of 99 cases. Arch Pathol Lab Med 1990;114:700–4.
7. Chittal SM, Ra PM. Carcinoid of the cystic duct. Histopathology 1989;15:643–6.
8. Dancygier H, Klein U, Hubner K, Classen M. Somatostatin-containing cells in the extrahepatic biliary tract of humans. Gastroenterology 1984;86:892–?.
9. Fellows IW, Leach IH, Smith PG, et al. Carcinoid tumor of the common bile duct—a novel complication of von Hippel-Lindau syndrome. Gut 1990;31:728–9.
10. Gembala RB, Arsuaga JE, Friedman AC, et al. Carcinoid of the intrahepatic ducts. Abdom Imaging 1993;18:242–4.
11. Gerlock AJ Jr, Muhletaler CA. Primary common bile duct carcinoid. Gastrointest Radiol 1979;4:263–4.

12. Goodman ZD, Albores-Saavedra J, Lundblad DM. Somatostatinoma of the cystic duct. Cancer 1984;53:498–502.
13. Judge DM, Dickman PS, Trapukdi S. Nonfunctioning argyrophilic tumor (APUDoma) of the hepatic duct: simplified methods of detecting biogenic amines in tissue. Am J Clin Pathol 1976;66:40–5.
14. Jutte DL, Bell RH, Penn IM, Powers J, Kilinjivadi J. Carcinoid tumor of the biliary system. Dig Dis Sci 1986;32:763–9.
15. Mandujano-Vera G, Angeles-Angeles A, Cruz-Hernandez J, Sansores-Perez M, Larriva-Sahd J. Gastrinoma of the common bile duct: immunohistochemical and ultrastructural study of a case. J Clin Gastroenterol 1995;20:321–4.
16. Nicolescu PG, Popescu AL. Carcinoid tumor of the cystic duct. Morphol Embryol (Bucur) 1986;32:275–7.
17. Rugge M, Sonego F, Militello C, Guido M, Ninfo V. Primary carcinoid tumor of the cystic and common bile ducts. Am J Surg Pathol 1992;16:802–7.
18. Sobol RE, Memoli V, Deftos LJ. Hormone negative, chromogranin A-positive endocrine tumors. N Engl J Med 1989;320:444–7.
19. Neyama T, Ding J, Hashimoto H, Tsunesohi M, Enjoji M. Carcinoid tumor arising in the wall of a congenital bile duct cyst. Arch Pathol Lab Med 1992;116:291–3.
20. Van Steengerben W, Fevery J, Venstapel MJ, et al. Case report: fourteen-year follow-up of an apudoma of the bile ducts in the hilum of the liver. Gastroenterology 1983;84:1585–91.
21. Vitaux J, Salmon RJ, Laguille O, Buffet C, Martin E, Chaput JC. Carcinoid tumor of the common bile duct. Am J Gastroenterol 1981;76:360–2.
22. Wrazidlo W, Gamroth A, Hofmann WJ, Koch K. Primäres Karzinoid des ductus choledochus. Radiologe 1989;29:191–4.

Paraganglioma

23. Sarma DE, Rodriguez FH Jr, Hoffmann EO. Paraganglioma of the hepatic duct. South Med J 1980;1677–8.

Benign Nonepithelial Tumors

24. Archambault H, Archambault R. Leiomyoma of the common bile duct. Arch Surg 1952;64:531–4.
25. Chu PT. Benign neoplasms of the extrahepatic biliary ducts. Arch Pathol 1950;50:84–97.

Granular Cell Tumor

26. Aisner SC, Khaneja S, Ramirez O. Multiple granular cell tumors of the gallbladder and biliary tree. Report of a case. Arch Pathol Lab Med 1982;106:470–1.
27. Barber CJ. Granular cell tumour of the cystic duct. A cause of cholecystitis. J R Col Surg Edinb 1984;29:56–7.
28. Butterly LF, Schapiro RH, LaMuraglia GM. Biliary granular cell tumor: a little-known curable bile duct neoplasm of young people. Surgery 1988;103:328–4.
29. Eisen RN, Kirby WM, O'Quinn JL. Granular cell tumors of the biliary tree. A report of two cases and review of the literature. Am J Surg Pathol 1991;15:460–5.
30. Lafreniere R, Demetrick DJ, Benediktsson H. Granular cell neoplasm of the extrahepatic biliary tree: morphological, ultrastructural and immunohistochemical study of review of the literature. J Surg Oncol 1991;46:60–6.
31. Mackenzie DJ, Klapper E, Gordon LA, Silberman AW. Granular cell tumor of the biliary system. Med Pediatr Oncol 1994;23:50–6.
32. Mauro MA, Jaques PF. Granular cell tumors of the esophagus and common bile duct. J Can Assoc Radiol 1981;32:254–6.
33. Mazur MT, Shultz JJ, Myers JL. Granular cell tumor. Immunohistochemical analysis of 21 benign tumors and one malignant tumor. Arch Pathol Lab Med 1990;114:692–6.
34. Mukai M. Immunohistochemical localization of S-100 protein and peripheral nerve myelin proteins (P2 protein and P0 protein) in granular cell tumors. Am J Pathol 1983;112:139–46.
35. Nathrath WB, Remberger K. Immunohistochemical study of granular cell tumors. Demonstration of neuron specific enolase, S-100 protein, laminin, and alpha-one antichymotrypsin. Virchows Arch [A] 1986;408:421–34.
36. Reul GJ Jr, Rubio PA, Berkman NL. Granular cell myoblastoma of the cystic duct. A case associated with hydrops of the gallbladder. Am J Surg 1975;129:583–4.
37. Sanchez JA, Nauta RJ. Resection of a granular cell tumor at the hepatic confluence. A precarious location of a benign tumor. Am Surg 1991;57:446–50.
38. Whisnant DJ Jr, Bennett SE, Huffman SR, Weiss DL, Parker JC, Griffen WO Jr. Common bile duct obstruction by granular cell tumor (schwannoma). Am J Dig Dis 1974;.19:471–6.
39. Yamashina M, Stemmermann GN. Granular cell tumor: unusual cause for mucocele of gallbladder. Am J Gastroenterol 1984;79:701–3.
40. Zvargulis JE, Keating JP, Askin FB, Ternberg JL. Granular cell myoblastoma: a cause of biliary obstruction. Am J Dis Child 1978;132:68–70.

❖❖❖

15

MALIGNANT MESENCHYMAL AND MISCELLANEOUS TUMORS OF THE EXTRAHEPATIC BILE DUCTS

MALIGNANT MESENCHYMAL TUMORS

Malignant mesenchymal tumors of the extrahepatic ducts are extremely unusual, especially in adults. An analysis of 912 cases of extrahepatic bile duct cancer, collected by the Surveillance, Epidemiology, and End Results (SEER) Program of the National Cancer Institute, revealed only one example: a case of malignant fibrous histiocytoma. Because these tumors are unusual, very little information is available on treatment and prognosis. The most important member of this group is a type of rhabdomyosarcoma traditionally known as sarcoma botryoides.

Embryonal Rhabdomyosarcoma

Embryonal rhabdomyosarcoma *(sarcoma botryoides)* is the most common neoplasm of the biliary tree in childhood (2–4,12), but it represents less than 1 percent of all rhabdomyosarcomas (10). It may arise from any segment of the extrahepatic bile ducts, but the common bile duct is most often the site of origin. The tumor usually extends by submucosal growth along the remaining biliary tree, including the gallbladder and intrahepatic ducts, eventually causing obstruction (6).

Intermittent obstructive jaundice, with or without abdominal distention, fever, and loss of appetite, is the typical presentation. These symptoms are often attributed to hepatitis which results in delayed treatment (10). Ultrasound and cholangiography are valuable diagnostic procedures.

Grossly, embryonal rhabdomyosarcoma consists of soft and confluent polypoid structures that often have a characteristic grape-like appearance (fig. 15-1). Histologically, the polypoid structures are covered with a single layer of epithelial cells continuous with those of the bile ducts. Immediately beneath the epithelium is a concentration of primitive mesenchymal cells with hyperchromatic nuclei and little cytoplasm. This concentration is referred to as the cambium layer and is also found in embryonal rhabdomyosarcomas that arise in other hollow viscera (fig. 15-2). The central portion usually contains stellate cells loosely arranged in a myxomatous matrix (fig. 15-3). In some areas, but especially in the cambium layer, the tumor cells often have globular or elongated eosinophilic cytoplasm. These globular cells are malignant rhabdomyoblasts and may contain cross-striations that are best demonstrated by phosphotungstic acid hematoxylin (PTAH) or Masson trichrome stains (fig. 15-4). Although one third of these tumors have cells with cross-striations visible by light microscopy, these structures are not necessary to establish the diagnosis.

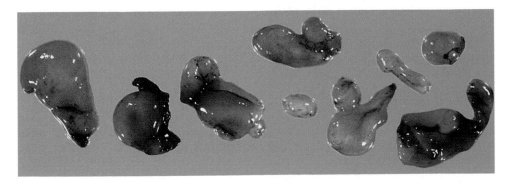

Figure 15-1

EMBRYONAL RHABDOMYOSARCOMA (SARCOMA BOTRYOIDES)

Multiple polypoid and grape-like masses mimicking nasal polyps are characteristic of embryonal rhabdomyosarcoma (sarcoma botryoides).

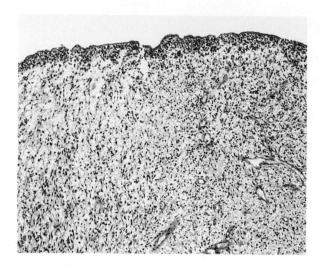

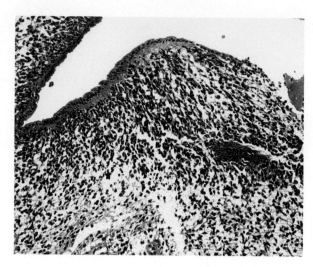

Figure 15-2
EMBRYONAL RHABDOMYOSARCOMA

Left: Embryonal rhabdomyosarcoma of common bile duct. The cambium layer appears as a concentration of small undifferentiated cells beneath the biliary epithelium. (Courtesy of Dr. A. Weinberg, Dallas, TX.)

Right: Higher magnification of cambium layer shows predominantly undifferentiated small cells with round hyperchromatic nuclei and scant cytoplasm.

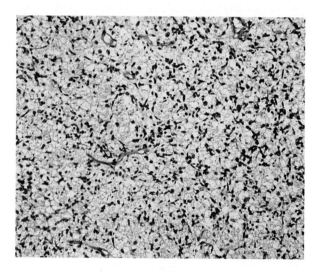

Figure 15-3
EMBRYONAL RHABDOMYOSARCOMA

Myxoid area contains undifferentiated stellate cells with hyperchromatic nuclei. (Courtesy of Dr. A. Weinberg, Dallas, TX.)

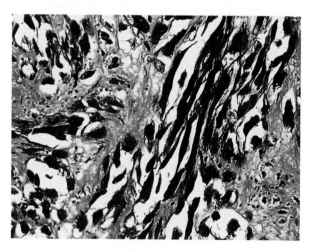

Figure 15-4
EMBRYONAL RHABDOMYOSARCOMA

Numerous rhabdomyoblasts with abundant elongated cytoplasm are present in the cambium layer of an embryonal rhabdomyosarcoma of the common bile duct (Masson trichrome stain). (Pl. IVC from Fascicle 22, 2nd Series.)

With immunohistochemical techniques, muscle-specific actin and desmin reactivity are usually detected in poorly differentiated rhabdomyosarcomas (figs. 15-5, 15-6) (9). Myoglobin reactivity on the other hand, is found in tumors containing well-differentiated rhabdomyoblasts (8). Therefore, staining for myoglobin is of limited diagnostic value, since these tumors can be identified with conventional stains. Genetic analysis of embryonal rhabdomyosarcoma has shown expression of the *MYOD1* gene and loss of heterozygosity at loci on chromosome 11 (11).

In cells without visible cross-striations light microscopically, electron microscopy frequently

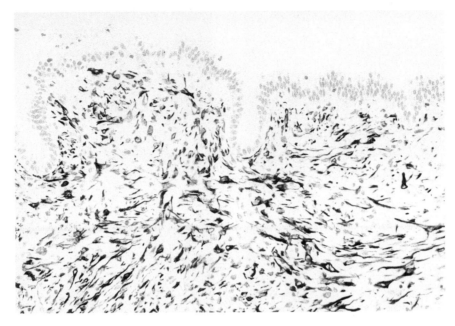

Figure 15-5
EMBRYONAL RHABDOMYOSARCOMA
Most spindle cells are desmin positive.

reveals thin and thick filaments often arranged in a sarcomere-like pattern (5). The prognosis of patients with embryonal rhabdomyosarcoma has improved with multidrug chemotherapy and irradiation, and correlates with stage of disease (1,7). Of 10 patients reviewed by the rhabdomyosarcoma study group, 4 survived disease-free 6 months to 6 1/2 years after diagnosis (10). In a more recent study from the same group, 95 percent of patients with embryonal rhabdomyosarcoma from all anatomic sites, including those arising in the extrahepatic biliary tree, survived 5 years (8).

Malignant Fibrous Histiocytoma

We were unable to find previously published cases of malignant fibrous histiocytomas of the extrahepatic bile ducts. However, we have seen one example that arose in the common bile duct of a 57-year-old man. The tumor, which infiltrated the full thickness of the wall, was composed of fibroblast type cells arranged in fascicular and storiform patterns, reminiscent of dermatofibrosarcoma protuberans (figs. 15-7, 15-8). Moderate nuclear atypia and occasional mitotic figures including abnormal ones were noted. Therefore, the tumor was considered to be

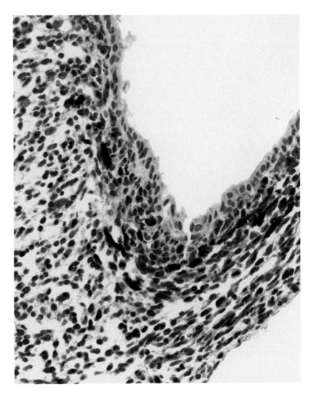

Figure 15-6
EMBRYONAL RHABDOMYOSARCOMA
Desmin-positive cells in the cambium layer.

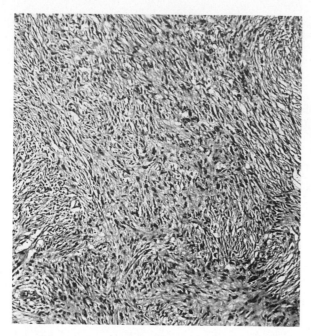

Figure 15-7
MALIGNANT FIBROUS HISTIOCYTOMA
OF COMMON BILE DUCT
The tumor, which is composed of spindle-shaped cells, shows fascicular and storiform patterns reminiscent of dermatofibrosarcoma protuberans.

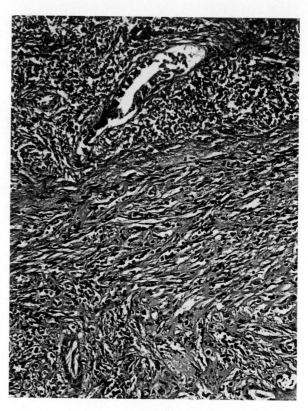

Figure 15-9
KAPOSI'S SARCOMA INVOLVING
THE LEFT HEPATIC DUCT
Part of the bile duct epithelium is still visible.

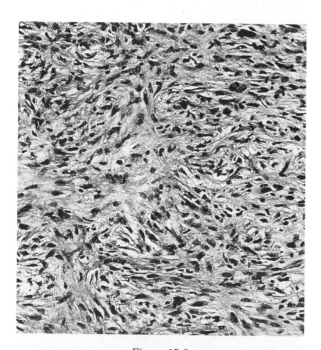

Figure 15-8
MALIGNANT FIBROUS HISTIOCYTOMA
OF COMMON BILE DUCT
Detail of storiform pattern. Most cells have ovoid or elongated hyperchromatic nuclei.

of low-grade malignancy. Neoplastic cells were immunoreactive only for vimentin and were negative for cytokeratins, epithelial membrane antigen, smooth muscle actin, desmin, and muscle-specific actin.

Leiomyosarcoma

Even though smooth muscle is normally present in the wall of the extrahepatic ducts, leiomyosarcomas are unusual in this location. We have been able to locate only three reported cases, one of which occurred in the ampulla (13,14).

Kaposi's Sarcoma

We have encountered two autopsy cases of Kaposi's sarcoma involving the extrahepatic bile ducts in patients with acquired immunodeficiency syndrome (AIDS) (fig. 15-9). Both patients also had hemorrhagic lesions of Kaposi's sarcoma in the liver.

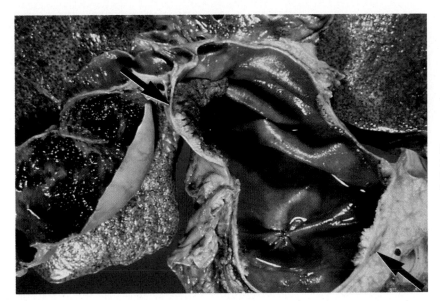

Figure 15-10
CARCINOMA IN
CHOLEDOCHAL CYST
Cystic dilatation of the common bile duct from which an adenocarcinoma arose involving only part of the cyst wall (arrows). (Courtesy of Dr. Jesus Aguirre, Mexico City, Mexico.)

MISCELLANEOUS TUMORS

Carcinosarcoma

Two carcinosarcomas have been reported in the extrahepatic bile ducts. They are histologically similar to those occurring in the gallbladder (15).

Malignant Lymphoma

Malignant lymphoma of the extrahepatic bile ducts is an exceedingly rare disease. Only four cases have been reported (16–19). These patients presented with obstructive jaundice. Sclerosing cholangitis or carcinoma was suspected in two patients preoperatively. The tumor involved the common bile duct in three patients, and the common hepatic duct and left and right hepatic ducts in another. Microscopically, the tumors were classified either as small lymphocytic, small cleaved, or high-grade B-cell lymphoma. One tumor contained many reactive T cells and was interpreted as a T-cell–rich B-cell lymphoma (16). Three patients developed disseminated lymphoma, one 5 months and two others 1 year after diagnosis.

Carcinoma In Choledochal Cyst

Choledochal cyst, or congenital cystic dilatation, is the second most common anomaly of the extrahepatic biliary tract. It can involve any part of the ductal system, including the intrahepatic

bile ducts as well as the intraduodenal segment of the common duct (20,23,25,26). These congenital cysts, which are found in all age groups, can become quite large, often reaching 15 cm in diameter. Most cases, however, are recognized in the first two decades of life, usually as a result of an abdominal mass, pain, and bile duct obstruction. The disease is most common in females and Orientals.

The etiology seems related to another anomaly of the extrahepatic biliary tree (28): the majority of patients with choledochal cysts also have an anomalous arrangement of the pancreaticobiliary ductal system in which the pancreatic duct enters the common duct outside the wall of the duodenum. This anomalous arrangement, which may be associated with partial obstruction, allows for reflux of pancreatic secretions into the common duct with secondary inflammation and dilatation of the bile ducts.

Five types of choledochal cysts have been described (29). Type I involves the hepatic or common bile ducts in a localized, segmental, or diffuse manner. It is the most common type and the one best known by surgeons and pathologists (fig. 15-10). Type II is a diverticulum type cyst located along any part of the extrahepatic bile ducts. Type III, which is a *choledochocele,* occurs in the intraduodenal segment of the common duct. It is often considered an *enterogenous cyst.* Type IV consists of multiple cysts along the extrahepatic or both the intrahepatic and

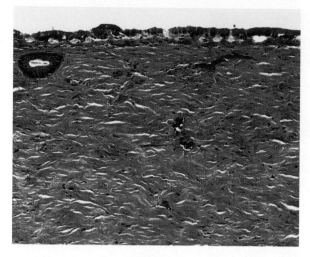

Figure 15-11
CHOLEDOCHAL CYST
The wall consists of dense fibrous tissue and is lined by cuboidal biliary type epithelium.

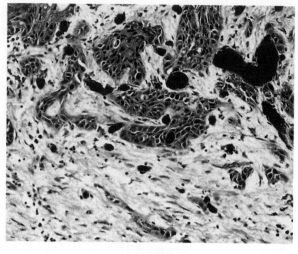

Figure 15-13
CHOLEDOCHAL CYST
Moderately differentiated squamous cell carcinoma infiltrates the wall of a choledochal cyst.

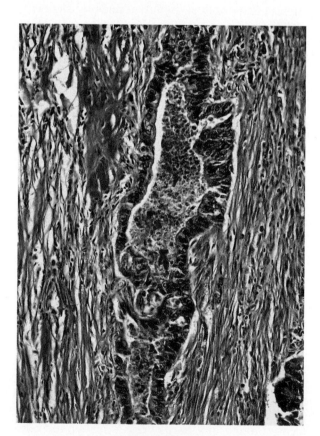

Figure 15-12
CHOLEDOCHAL CYST
Adenocarcinoma arising in the choledochal cyst shown in figure 15-10. A neoplastic gland is seen within the fibrotic wall of the cyst. (Courtesy of Dr. Jesus Aguirre, Mexico City, Mexico.)

extrahepatic ducts. Type V is an intrahepatic ductal cyst, either single or multiple. Type V is also known as *Caroli's disease* when associated with hepatic fibrosis.

An association between choledochal cysts and carcinoma is well established (30). It has been estimated that 2.5 to 15 percent of patients with choledochal cysts develop carcinoma. The frequency of carcinoma, however, varies with age. In patients less than 10 years, the incidence is less than 1 percent; in those between 10 and 20 years, the incidence is 6.8 percent; and in those over 20 years of age, it rises to 15 percent (22,31). Histologically, the cyst wall is composed of dense fibrous connective tissue which usually lacks an epithelial lining, although scattered islands of intact mucosa may be seen (fig. 15-11). There is usually focal or diffuse inflammation in the wall, which tends to be more pronounced in older patients. Adenocarcinoma is the most common malignant tumor complicating biliary cysts, although squamous cell carcinomas, adenosquamous carcinomas, carcinoid tumors, undifferentiated spindle and giant cell carcinomas, and even an embryonal rhabdomyosarcoma have been reported (figs. 15-12, 15-13). The most common site for the tumor is the posterior wall of the cyst. Tumors most commonly arise in cysts classified as types I and IV and are uncommon in types II, III, and V (27). In all excised cysts, the pathologist should carefully evaluate the specimen for carcinoma. Severe or fatal peritonitis can result from rupture of a cyst.

Stones are present in about 25 percent of cysts. They are more likely to be found in older patients. Choledochal cysts can occur in association with congenital hepatic fibrosis (21,24). Because of its location, the choledochocele is usually lined by duodenal mucosa both inside and out, but some may have a biliary type mucosal lining. Treatment is excision.

THE SURGICAL PATHOLOGY REPORT

The surgical pathology report for a biopsy, segmental extrahepatic bile duct resection, or pancreatoduodenectomy specimen from a malignant tumor should contain the following information:

1. Indicate whether the specimen is received fresh or formalin fixed.

2. Identify the excised segment of the extrahepatic bile duct (common hepatic duct, cystic duct, left or right hepatic ducts). Identify common bile duct, pancreas, main pancreatic duct, stomach, duodenum, and ampulla of Vater if a pancreatoduodenectomy specimen is submitted.

3. Characterize the external surface of the bile duct, pancreas, duodenum, ampulla, and stomach, including color, congestion, hemorrhage, adhesions, or masses.

4. Measure the bile duct and thickness of its wall. If present, state number, size, and color of stones. Measure each of the components of a pancreatoduodenectomy specimen.

5. Indicate presence of stricture causing partial or complete obstruction of the bile duct or presence of cyst (choledochal cyst).

6. Describe size, color and consistency of the tumor. Polypoid, nodular, diffusely infiltrating, or combined gross features should be described.

7. Describe appearance of adjacent non-neoplastic mucosa: granular, hemorrhagic, ulcerated, etc.

8. Record intestinal or antral gland metaplasia in adjacent mucosa.

9. Indicate histologic type, grade, and pathologic stage of tumor. Record depth of invasion; extension into muscular wall, periductal connective tissue, pancreas, duodenum, or ampulla of Vater; pyloric and intestinal metaplasia as well as dysplasia or carcinoma in situ in adjacent bile duct mucosa; and perineural and vascular invasion.

10. State status of proximal and distal margins of resection: free or involved by tumor; include common bile duct, and pancreatic, duodenal, and gastric margins in pancreatoduodenectomy specimens.

11. State status of lymph nodes with or without metastasis.

12. State status of gallbladder, pancreas, stomach, and duodenum if submitted.

13. Include results of immunoperoxidase stains, flow cytometry, and electron microscopy.

REFERENCES

Embryonal Rhabdomyosarcoma

1. Akers DR, Needham ME. Sarcoma botryoides (rhabdomyosarcoma) of the bile ducts with survival. J Pediatr Surg 1971;6:474–9.
2. Davis GL, Kissane JM, Ishak KG. Embryonal rhabdomyosarcoma (sarcoma botryoides) of the biliary tree. Report of five cases and review of the literature. Cancer 1969;24:333–42.
3. Horn RC Jr, Yakovac WC, Kaye R, Koop CE. Rhabdomyosarcoma (sarcoma botryoides) of the common bile duct. Cancer 1955;8:468–72.
4. Isaacson C. Embryonal rhabdomyosarcoma of the ampulla of vater. Cancer 1978;41:365–8.
5. Kindblom LG, Dalberg K. Sarcoma botryoides of the extrahepatic bile ducts. Pathol Res Pract 1980;170:258–66.
6. Lack EE, Perez-Atayde AR, Schuster SR. Botryoid rhabdomyosarcoma of the biliary tract. Am J Surg Pathol 1981;5:643–52.
7. Maurer HM, Gehan EA, Beltangady M, et al. The Intergroup Rhabdomyosarcoma Study II. Cancer 1993;71:1904–22.
8. Newton WA, Gehan EA, Webber BL, et al. Classification of rhabdomyosarcomas and related sarcomas. Pathologic aspects and proposal for a new classification—an Intergroup Rhabdomyosarcoma Study. Cancer 1995;76:1073–85.
9. Parham DM, Webber B, Holt H, Williams WK, Maurer H. Immunohistochemical study of childhood rhabdomyosarcoma and related neoplasms, Results of an Intergroup Rhabdomyosarcoma Study Project. Cancer 1991;67:3072–80.
10. Ruymann FB, Raney RB, Crist WM, Lawrence W Jr, Lindberg RD, Soule EH. Rhabdomyosarcoma of the biliary tree in childhood. A report from the Intergroup Rhabdomyosarcoma Study. Cancer 1985;56:575–81.
11. Scrable H, Witte D, Shimada H, et al. Molecular differential pathology of rhabdomyosarcoma. Genes Chrom Cancer 1989;1:23–35.
12. Taira Y, Nakayama I, Moriuchi A, et al. Sarcoma botryoides arising from the biliary tract of children. Acta Pathol Jpn 1976;26:709–18.

Leiomyosarcoma

13. Braasch JW, Warren KW, Kune GA. Malignant neoplasms of the bile ducts. Surg Clin North Am 1967;47:626–38.
14. Nitshe GA Jr, Suckle HM. Leiomyosarcoma of the ampulla of Vater associated with a tumor of the eighth nerve and neurogenic perforation of duodenum. Am J Clin Pathol 1947;17:827–33.

Carcinosarcoma

15. Edmondson HA. Tumors of the gallbladder and extrahepatic bile ducts. Atlas of Tumor Pathology, 1st Series, Fascicle 26. Washington, D.C.: Armed Forces Institute of Pathology, 1967.

Malignant Lymphoma

16. Brouland J, Molimard J, Nemeth J, Valleur P, Galian A. Primary T-cell rich B-cell lymphoma of the common bile duct. Virchows Arch [A] 1993;423:513–7.
17. Chiu KW, Changchien CS, Chen L, et al. Primary malignant lymphoma of common bile duct presenting as acute obstructive jaundice. J Clin Gastroenterol 1995;20:259–61.
18. Kosuge T, Makuuchi M, Ozaki H, Kinoshita T, Takenaka T, Mukai K. Primary lymphoma of the common bile duct. Hepatogastroenterology 1991;38:235–8.
19. Nguyen GK. Primary extranodal non-Hodgkin's lymphoma of the extrahepatic ducts. Report of a case. Cancer 1982;50:2218–22.

Carcinoma in Choledochal Cyst

20. Arthur GW, Stewart JO. Biliary cysts. Br J Surg 1964;51:671–5.
21. Fujiwara Y, Ohizumi I, Kakizaki G, Fujiwara T. Congenital dilatation of intrahepatic and common bile ducts with congenital hepatic fibrosis. J Pediatr Surg 1976;11:273–4.
22. Komi N, Tamura T, Miyoshi Y, Kunitomo K, Udaka H, Takehara H. Nationwide survey of cases of choledochal cyst. Analysis of coexistent anomalies, complications and surgical treatment in 645 cases. Surg Gastroenterol 1984;3:69-72.
23. Konvolinka CW, Pharr WF. Congenital cystic dilatation of the common bile duct. A review. Am Surg 1970;36:575–80.
24. Lake DN, Smith PM, Wheeler MH. Congenital hepatic fibrosis and choledochus cyst. Br Med J 1977;2:1259–60.
25. Longmire WP Jr, Mandiola SA, Gordon HE. Congenital cystic disease of the liver and biliary system. Ann Surg 1971;174:711–26.
26. O'Neill JA Jr. Choledochal cyst, In: Current problems in surgery, St. Louis: Mosby 1992:365–410.
27. Todani T, Tabuchi K, Watanabe Y, Tobayashi T. Carcinoma arising in the wall of congenital bile duct cysts. Cancer 1979;44:1134–41.
28. Todani T, Watanabe Y, Fujii T, Uemura S. Anomalous arrangement of the pancreaticobiliary ductal system in patients with a choledochal cyst. Am J Surg 1984;147:672–6.
29. Todani T, Watanabe Y, Narusue M, Tabuchi K, Okajima K. Congenital bile duct cysts. Am J Surg 1977;134:263–9.
30. Tsuchiya R, Harada N, Ito T, Furukawa M, Yoshihiro M. Malignant tumors in choledochal cysts. Ann Surg 1977;186:22–8.
31. Voyles CR, Smadja C, Shands C, Blumgart LH. Carcinoma in choledochal cysts age related incidence. Arch Surg 1983;118:986–8.

16

SECONDARY TUMORS OF THE EXTRAHEPATIC BILE DUCTS

Metastases in the extrahepatic bile ducts are extremely rare but are of clinical importance because they can produce obstructive jaundice, simulate sclerosing cholangitis, or resemble primary malignant tumors (3,9). Breast carcinomas in females and prostate adenocarcinomas in males are the most frequent sources of blood-borne metastases in the extrahepatic bile ducts (1,4,9,11). In some patients such metastases occur even in the absence of hepatic or lymph node involvement (4). These cases can be confused with primary malignant tumors or sclerosing cholangitis. Most patients, however, have extensive hepatic metastases at the time of diagnosis. The hepatic metastatic deposits can lead to multifocal strictures of the intrahepatic bile ducts (11).

Rare metastases of renal cell carcinoma in the wall of the common bile duct and ampulla have been reported. Clinically, they lead to gastrointestinal bleeding, obstructive jaundice, or both, and may mimic a primary carcinoma of the periampullary region (2,8). The bulk of the metastatic lesion is usually located in the head of the pancreas, but it frequently extends to the common bile duct and ampulla. The majority of the reported patients had a nephrectomy 8 to 12 years prior to the appearance of the pancreatic and common bile duct lesions (10,14).

Carcinomas of the head of the pancreas often extend to the wall of the common bile duct. Because of morphologic similarities between carcinomas in these two regions, identification of the primary site may become problematic in some cases. The presence of carcinoma in situ in the pancreatic ducts favors a primary tumor in the pancreas, while the demonstration of dysplasia or in situ carcinoma in the bile ducts points to a primary in this location.

Although hepatocellular carcinomas sometimes invade the wall of the intrahepatic bile ducts (6,12), they rarely extend downward into the extrahepatic ducts. We recently encountered such a case which presented as a polypoid mass of the common hepatic duct mimicking a primary tumor.

Involvement of extrahepatic bile ducts by Langerhans' cell histiocytosis (histiocytosis X) has been reported in both children and adults (5a). Because of the fibrosis often associated with the histiocytic infiltration, Langerhans' cell histiocytosis has been confused with sclerosing cholangitis (7) or with biliary atresia (figs. 16-1, 16-2) (5). Most patients have disseminated disease as well as involvement of the intrahepatic bile ducts. Some of the adult patients have not had the bone involvement common with Langerhans' cell histiocytosis (13). Microscopically, the walls of the bile ducts are infiltrated by lymphocytes, plasma cells, eosinophils, multinucleated giant cells, and Langerhans cells that are decorated by antibodies to S-100 protein and CD1a.

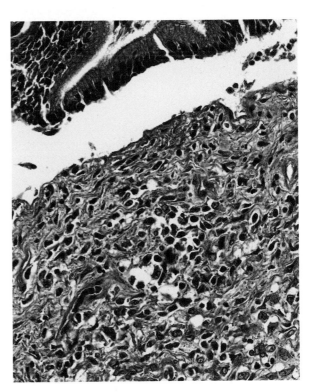

Figure 16-1
LANGERHANS' CELL HISTIOCYTOSIS
The wall of an extrahepatic bile duct at the hilus of the liver contains a mixed cellular infiltrate rich in Langerhans histiocytes and eosinophils. (Courtesy of Dr. Cecilia Ridaura, Mexico City, Mexico.)

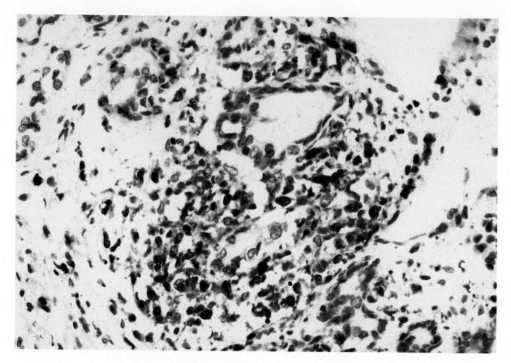

Figure 16-2
LANGERHANS' CELL HISTIOCYTOSIS
Most histiocytes around intramural glands are S-100 protein positive indicating a Langerhans cell phenotype. (Courtesy of Dr. Cecilia Ridaura, Mexico City, Mexico.)

REFERENCES

1. Andry G, Turnbull AD, Botet J, Kurtz RC. Cholesonographic characteristics of cystic duct metastasis causing acute acalculous cholecystitis: case report. J Surg Oncol 1986;31:178–81.
2. Bolkier M, Ginesin Y, Moskovitz B, Munichor M, Levin DR. Obstructive jaundice caused by metastatic renal cell carcinoma. Eur Urol 1991;19:87–8.
3. Chen M, Mullane MR. Metastatic prostatic carcinoma presenting as cholangiocarcinoma (Klatskin tumor). Ann Int Med 1990;112:881–4.
4. Engel JJ, Trujillo Y, Spellberg M. Metastatic carcinoma of the breast: a cause of obstructive jaundice. Gastroenterology 1980;78:132–5.
5. Heitnev R, Morton S, Rabinowitz L, Rosen EU. Type I histiocytosis presenting as biliary atresia. A case report. S Afr Med J 1978;53:768–70.
5a. Kaplan KJ, Goodman ZD, Ishak KG. Liver involvement in Langerhans' cell histiocytosis. Mod Pathol 1999;12:370–8.
6. Kojiro M, Kawabata K, Kawano Y, et al. Hepatocellular carcinoma presenting as intrabile duct tumor growth. A clinicopathologic study of 25 cases. Cancer 1982;49:2144–7.
7. LeBlanc A, Hadchonel M, Jehan P, Odievre M, Alagille D. Obstructive jaundice in children with histiocytosis X. Gastroenterology 1981;80:134–9.
8. Leslie KA, Tsao JI, Rossi RL, Braasch JW. Metastatic renal cell carcinoma to ampulla of Vater. An unusual lesion amenable to surgical resection. Surgery 1996;119:349–51.
9. Popp JW, Schapiro RH, Warshaw AL. Extrahepatic biliary obstruction caused by metastatic breast carcinoma. Ann Int Med 1979;91:568–71.
10. Robertson GS, Gertler SL. Late presentation of metastatic renal cell carcinoma as a bleeding ampullary mass. Gastrointest Endosc 1990;36:304–6.
11. Taylor J, Lindor K. Metastatic prostate cancer simulating sclerosing cholangitis. J Clin Gastroenterol 1993;16:143–5.
12. Terada T, Nakanuma Y, Kawai K. Small hepatocellular carcinoma presenting as intrabiliary pedunculated polyp and obstructive jaundice. J Clin Gastroenterol 1989;11:578–83.
13. Thompson HH, Pitt HA, Lewin KJ, Longmire WP Jr. Sclerosing cholangitis and histiocytosis X. Gut 1984;25:526–30.
14. Venu RP, Rolny P, Geenen JE, et al. Ampullary tumor caused by metastatic renal cell carcinoma. Dig Dis Sci 1991;36:376–8.

17
TUMOR-LIKE LESIONS OF THE EXTRAHEPATIC BILE DUCTS

Tumor-like lesions are occasionally found in the extrahepatic bile ducts. They primarily include heterotopia and amputation neuromas.

PANCREATIC HETEROTOPIA

Heterotopic tissues, including pancreas and gastric mucosa, have been found in the extrahepatic bile ducts. Heterotopic pancreas is exceedingly rare and appears to be less common than in the gallbladder (1). To our knowledge only five cases have been reported. However, ectopic pancreatic tissue in the wall of the extrahepatic bile ducts is often symptomatic. In one patient obstruction of the cystic duct led to hydrops of the gallbladder (2). Obstruction of the common hepatic duct by ectopic pancreas produced jaundice in three patients (4–6). Heterotopic pancreas of the common bile duct mimicked carcinoma of the head of the pancreas in another patient (3). We have seen one example of ectopic pancreas that coexisted with adenocarcinoma of the extrahepatic bile ducts.

AMPUTATION NEUROMA

Amputation neuromas, which can occur many years after cholecystectomy, result from the proliferation of transected nerves (7–9). Clinically, they are responsible for some cases of postcholecystectomy pain. These neuromas may rarely grow into the lumen of the bile ducts, mimicking a true neoplasm and causing obstructive jaundice (10).

Amputation neuromas are most commonly located in the stump of the cystic duct, although other ducts can also be involved following surgery. Grossly, they are nodular and have a gray-white, whorled cut surface. Histologically similar to neuromas in other sites, they show a conglomeration of distorted nerve fibers supported by variable amounts of fibrous tissue (fig. 17-1).

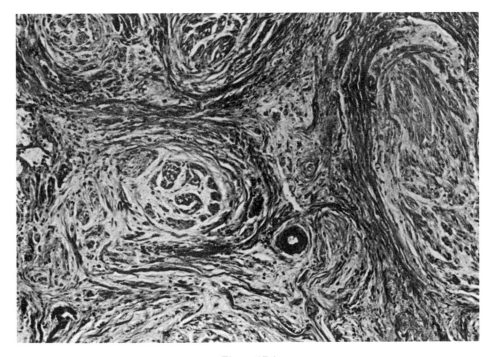

Figure 17-1
AMPUTATION NEUROMA OF THE CYSTIC DUCT
Distorted and hypertrophied nerve trunks are separated by fibrous tissue. (Fig. 161 from Fascicle 22, 2nd Series.)

REFERENCES

Pancreatic Heterotopia

1. Ben-Baruch D, Sandbank Y, Wolloch Y. Heterotopic pancreatic tissue in the gallbladder. Acta Chir Scand 1986;152:557–8.
2. Inceoglu R, Dosluoglu HH, Kullu S, et al. An unusual cause of hydropic gallbladder and biliary colic–heterotopic pancreatic tissue in the cystic duct: report of a case and review of the literature. Jpn J Surg 1993;23:532–4.
3. O'Reilly DJ, Craig RM, Lorenzo G, et al. Heterotopic pancreas mimicking carcinoma of the head of the pancreas: a rare cause of obstructive jaundice. J Clin Gastroenterol 1983;5:165–8.
4. Pang L. Pancreatic heterotopia: a reappraisal and clinicopathologic analysis of 32 cases. Southern Med J 1988;81:1264–75.
5. Schu W, Copeland R, Fromm D, Elbadawi A. Obstruction of the common hepatic bile duct by ectopic pancreas. NY State J Med 1988;4:197–8.
6. Weber CM, Zito PF, Becker SM. Heterotopic pancreas: an unusual cause of obstruction of the common bile duct. Am J Gastroenterol 1968;49:153–9.

Amputation Neuroma

7. Bartlett MK, McDermott WF Jr. Amputation neuroma of the bile ducts with obstructive jaundice. N Engl J Med 1954;251:213–6.
8. Cattell RB, St. Ville J. Amputation neuromas of the biliary tract. Arch Surg 1961;83:242–6.
9. Joske RA, Finlay-Jones LR. Amputation neuroma of the cystic-duct stump. Br J Surg 1966;53:766–8.
10. Larson D, Sorsteen KA. Traumatic neuroma of the bile ducts with intrahepatic extension causing obstructive jaundice. Hum Pathol 1984;15:287–90.

18

PRIMARY SCLEROSING CHOLANGITIS

Recognized since 1924, primary sclerosing cholangitis (PSC) has become an important consideration in the differential diagnosis of extrahepatic bile duct cancer.

Definition. PSC is a progressive cholestatic disease morphologically manifested by chronic inflammation, focal stenosis, and fibrous thickening of the extrahepatic and intrahepatic bile ducts (fig. 18-1). It has an uncertain but generally poor prognosis, no defined etiology, and is usually treated empirically (14,42). Most likely the disease has an autoimmune basis since it is frequently associated with other autoimmune disorders. There is a well-established association with inflammatory bowel disease (27). Death usually results from liver failure or less frequently from septice-

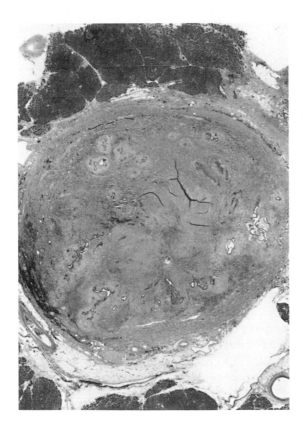

Figure 18-1
PRIMARY SCLEROSING CHOLANGITIS
Cross section through the common bile duct shows obliteration of the lumen and fibrous thickening of the wall. (Fig. 196 from Fascicle 22, 2nd Series.)

mia secondary to biliary obstruction. The disease is uncommon, occurring less often than secondary types of sclerosing cholangitis from which it should be differentiated (21).

Pathologic Findings. Clinically and morphologically the disease resembles cancer. The clinical manifestations, progressive jaundice in the absence of stones, infection, or previous surgery, often suggest a diagnosis of extrahepatic bile duct carcinoma (4). Histologically, the extrahepatic bile ducts show an intact or ulcerated mucosa, periglandular lymphocytic infiltration, glandular distortion, fibrosis, and stenosis (fig. 18-2). The bile ducts may be focally or diffusely thickened. At laparotomy, they are often described as rope-like as a result of fibrosis. In many cases, biopsy of the liver reveals pericholangitis, portal fibrosis, ductopenia, and cholestasis changes which are often difficult to separate from primary biliary cirrhosis. The fibrous obliterative cholangitis that leads to the characteristic onion skin lesion is rarely seen in biopsy specimens. The disease may also involve the pancreatic ducts (20) as well as the gallbladder (15). Liver transplantation is the treatment of choice for patients with end-stage liver disease secondary to PSC.

While biopsies of the bile ducts are helpful in the diagnosis, the histologic changes are nonspecific and often not diagnostic (22). It is often impossible to separate histologically the primary from the secondary types of sclerosing cholangitis. A diagnosis of PSC is usually based on the characteristic beaded and irregular appearance of the bile ducts seen on retrograde or transhepatic cholangiography. A liver biopsy may be more helpful than a biopsy of the extrahepatic ducts. Liver biopsies, however, are rarely definitive although they are useful for evaluating prognosis. Biopsy of the extrahepatic bile ducts is indicated if carcinoma is suspected.

Seventy to 90 percent of patients with PSC have either preexisting or coexisting ulcerative colitis (1). Conversely, less than 10 percent of patients with ulcerative colitis develop some form of hepatobiliary disease (35). The types of secondary cholangitis that should be excluded

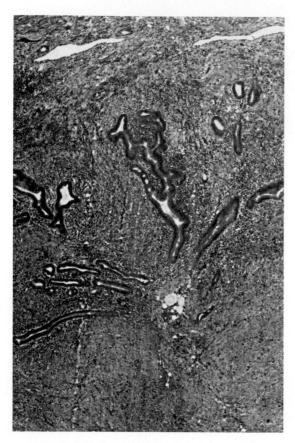

Figure 18-2
PRIMARY SCLEROSING CHOLANGITIS
Higher magnification of figure 18-1 shows distortion and proliferation of intramural glands which lie in dense fibrous tissue that contains some inflammatory cells (X43). (Figure 197 from Fascicle 22, 2nd Series.)

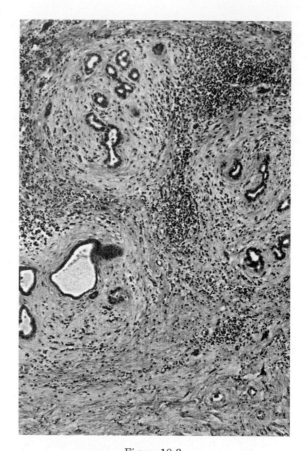

Figure 18-3
PRIMARY SCLEROSING CHOLANGITIS
Higher magnification of figure 18-1. The distorted glands are arranged in lobules, and are surrounded by concentric rings of fibrous tissue. Chronic inflammatory cells are also present (X80). (Fig. 198 from Fascicle 22, 2nd Series.)

are caused by infection, stones, congenital anomalies, trauma such as penetrating wounds, and previous surgery, the most common cause.

As a result of fibrosis and inflammation, the glands are often distorted and displaced, changes which can resemble a well-differentiated adenocarcinoma (fig. 18-3). On the other hand, in well-differentiated carcinomas, the neoplastic glands can grow along the wall of the bile ducts without producing a nodular mass. These glands, along with the attendant desmoplasia and inflammation, can resemble the changes seen in sclerosing cholangitis.

Carcinoma. The development of extrahepatic bile duct carcinoma is a major complication. While often associated with longstanding disease, carcinomas can occur any time after a

diagnosis of PSC has been established. Five to 10 percent of patients develop carcinoma. Most of these tumors are either well- or moderately differentiated adenocarcinomas (44).

Occasionally multifocal in origin (33), carcinomas can arise in any segment of the extrahepatic bile ducts. Small carcinomas are sometimes found at autopsy in patients who have died from PSC without having evidence of cancer clinically. Overall, the prevalence of bile duct carcinoma found at autopsy in patients with PSC is 42 percent (33). Because of its association with carcinoma, PSC should be considered a premalignant condition. Flat or papillary dysplasia as well as in situ carcinoma are seen in a number of patients (23). The presence of dysplasia may affect decisions about liver transplantation.

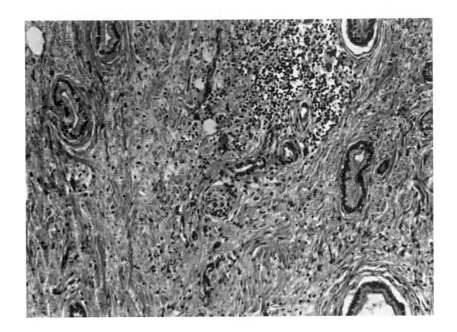

Figure 18-4
LEFT HEPATIC DUCT
ADENOCARCINOMA
A well-differentiated adenocarcinoma of the left hepatic
duct shows scattered glands
separated by dense fibrous
stroma in which are some inflammatory cells. This histologic pattern can be mistaken
for primary sclerosing cholangitis (X125). (Fig. 199 from Fascicle 22, 2nd Series.)

The lesion interpreted as cholangitis glandu- laris proliferans is characterized by a nodular pro- liferation of the intramural glands of the ex- trahepatic bile ducts (12,32). It is not related to PSC since it has been seen in association with secondary cholangitis as well as with carcinoma of the bile ducts. Moreover, it is not typically associated with inflammatory bowel disease.

Differential Diagnosis. Although most bi- opsies of the extrahepatic bile ducts are per- formed to exclude cancer, the differential diag- nosis between sclerosing cholangitis and infiltrating carcinoma can be difficult, especially with a small biopsy, and may not be possible in some cases. The difficulties have been repeat- edly emphasized (2,21,30). In addition to the usual criteria for malignancy, the following should be noted. The presence of normal mucosa in a biopsy does not exclude carcinoma, since tumor may extend along the bile duct for some distance beneath the mucosa. Nuclear hyper- chromatism and epithelial atypia are found in both conditions, but tend to be more pronounced in carcinoma. Cancerous glands, on the other hand, infiltrate the wall in a random and diffuse manner and often extend into the periductal tissues (fig. 18-4). In contrast to glands in sclero-

sing cholangitis that are p53 and carcinoembry- onic antigen (CEA) negative or stain faintly along the apical cytoplasm, neoplastic glands usually are p53 and CEA positive (fig. 18-5). Perineural invasion is a common and important feature of carcinoma.

In contrast, the glands of sclerosing cholang- itis are usually arranged in well-defined lobular patterns. In addition, the fibrosis is usually ar- ranged concentrically around the glands, a fea- ture that is uncommon in carcinoma. Finally, in carcinoma, the number of neoplastic glands may exceed the number of normal glands expected in the section. In general, the pattern of invasion and gland arrangement may be more helpful than the appearance of individual glands. Some cases may require the presence of regional me- tastasis before a diagnosis can be safely made. Bile should be collected for cytology in all cases.

Clinically, it is difficult to determine whether patients with PSC have carcinoma in the bile ducts, especially small carcinomas. Endoscopic cholangiography, ultrasound, and computed tomographic scanning usually do not reveal car- cinoma. In some patients, serum levels of CA19- 9 and CEA are increased (31), but these markers lack specificity.

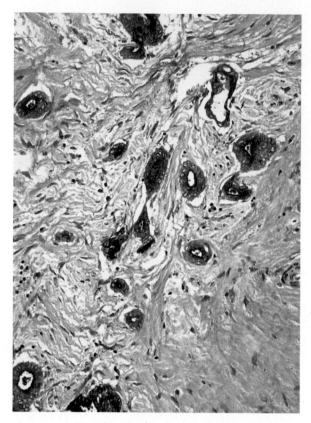

Figure 18-5
WELL-DIFFERENTIATED ADENOCARCINOMA
OF THE LEFT HEPATIC DUCT
The small glands of this well-differentiated adenocarcinoma of the left hepatic duct are CEA positive.

Although an infrequent occurrence, carcinomas metastatic to the extrahepatic bile ducts can simulate sclerosing cholangitis clinically and radiographically (39).

Association with Other Diseases. Sclerosing cholangitis often occurs in association with other immunologic disorders, usually with ulcerative colitis. It has also occurred with retroperitoneal fibrosis, mediastinal fibrosis, Peyronie's disease (43), Riedel's struma, dermatitis herpetiformis (19), Crohn's disease (1,36), Sjogren's syndrome (28,37), pseudotumor of the orbit (6), systemic sclerosis (11), and diabetes mellitus (16). PSC has occurred in a renal transplant recipient (41) and in chil-

dren (9,29,38,45). It has also been associated with angioimmunoblastic lymphadenopathy (3), Hodgkin's disease (24), and Langerhans' histiocytosis X especially in children (9,40). The first symptoms can occur in the neonatal period or in children less than 3 years of age (9). Because of its association with other diseases, PSC is probably one manifestation of a larger disease complex that includes ulcerative colitis, primary biliary cirrhosis, and other progressive inflammatory conditions. Sclerosing cholangitis has also been associated with the acquired immunodeficiency syndrome (AIDS) (34).

Pathogenesis. The pathogenesis of PSC is unknown but genetic and immunologic factors are thought to be involved. The disease is invariably accompanied by abnormalities of immune regulation that in all probability reflect its etiology, although it is uncertain whether these abnormalities are primary or secondary. PSC is often associated with HLA phenotypes B8, DR3, and DR2, and the DRW 52a haplotypes often found in other autoimmune disorders.

A variety of immunologic abnormalities have been reported. They include a deficiency of suppressor T-cell activity (17), autoantibodies reactive against a peptide found in both colon and biliary epithelium (25), and autoantibodies reactive against the perinuclear cytoplasmic components of neutrophils (10,13). These neutrophilic autoantibodies are found in 60 to 80 percent of patients. Similar antibodies are also found in patients with ulcerative colitis. Some believe, on the basis of experimental studies, that cellular immune responses to specific biliary antigens are involved in progressive bile duct destruction (26).

The serum mitochondrial antibody test, which is positive in a large percentage of patients with primary biliary cirrhosis, is usually negative in cases of sclerosing cholangitis (7).

The higher incidence of bile duct carcinoma in patients with ulcerative colitis and the role of PSC are further discussed on page 182. Numerous reviews on the pathogenesis and etiology of sclerosing cholangitis have been published (5,8,18,42,46).

REFERENCES

1. Aadland E, Schrumpf E, Fausa O, et al. Primary sclerosing cholangitis: a long-term follow-up study. Scand J Gastroenterol 1987;22:655–64.
2. Altemeier WA, Gall EA, Culbertson WR, Inge WW. Sclerosing carcinoma of the intrahepatic (hilar) bile ducts. Surgery 1966;60:191–200.
3. Bass NM, Chapman RW, O Reilly A, Sherlock S. Primary sclerosing cholangitis associated with angioimmunoblastic lymphadenopathy. Gastroenterology 1983;85:420–4.
4. Beachley MC, Lankau CA Jr. Sclerosing cholangitis simulating periampullary carcinoma. Milit Med 1976;141:475–6.
5. Boberg KM, Lundin KE, Schrumpf E. Etiology and pathogenesis in primary sclerosing cholangitis. Scand J Gastroenterol 1994;29(Suppl 204):47–58.
6. Caroli J, Rosner D. Cholangitis. In: Bockus HL, ed. Gastroenterology, Vol. III. Philadelphia: WB Saunders, 1976:865–74.
7. Chapman RW, Arborgh BA, Rhodes JM, et al. Primary sclerosing cholangitis: a review of its clinical features, cholangiography, and hepatic histology. Gut 1980;21:870–7.
8. Crippin JS, Lindor KD. Primary sclerosing cholangitis: etiology and immunology. Eur J Gastroenterol Hepatol 1992;4:261–5.
9. Debray D, Pariente D, Urvoas E, Hadchouel M, Bernard O. Sclerosing cholangitis in children. J Pediatr 1994;124:49–56.
10. Duerr RH, Targan SR, Landers CJ, et al. Neutrophil cytoplasmic antibodies: a link between primary sclerosing cholangitis and ulcerative colitis. Gastroenterology 1991;100:1385–91.
11. Fraile G, Rodriguez-Garcia JL, Moreno A. Primary sclerosing cholangitis associated with systemic sclerosis. Postgrad Med J 1991;67:189–92.
12. Graham SM, Barwick K, Cahow CE, Baker CC. Cholangitis glandularis proliferans. A histologic variant of primary sclerosing cholangitis with distinctive clinical and pathological features. J Clin Gastroenterol 1988;10:579–83.
13. Hardarson S, LaBrecque DR, Mitros FA, Neil GA, Goeken JA. Antineutrophil cytoplasmic antibody in inflammatory bowel and hepatobiliary diseases. High prevalence in ulcerative colitis, primary sclerosing cholangitis and autoimmune hepatitis. Am J Clin Pathol 1993;99:277–81.
14. Harnois DM, Lindor KD. Primary sclerosing cholangitis. Evolving concepts in diagnosis and treatment. Dig Dis 1997;15:23–41.
15. Jeffrey GP, Reed WD, Carrello S, Shilkin KB. Histological and immunohistochemical study of the gallbladder lesion in primary sclerosing cholangitis. Gut 1991;32:424–9.
16. Kay M, Wyllie R, Michener W, Caulfield M, Steffen R. Associated ulcerative colitis, sclerosing cholangitis, and insulin-dependent diabetes mellitus. Cleve Clin J Med 1993;60:473–8.
17. Kilby AE, Krawitt EL, Albertini RJ, Chastenay BF, John A. Suppressor T-cell deficiency in primary sclerosing cholangitis. Case and family study. Dig Dis Sci 1991;36:1213–6.
18. Lee YM, Kaplan MM. Primary sclerosing cholangitis. N Eng J Med 1995;332:924–33.
19. Lewis HM, Goldin R, Leonard JN. Dermatitis herpetiformis and primary sclerosing cholangitis. Clin Exp Dermatol 1993;18:363–5.
20. Lindström E, Bodemar G, Rydén BO, Ihse I. Pancreatic ductal morphology and exocrine function in primary sclerosing cholangitis. Acta Chir Scand 1990;156:451–6.
21. Longmire WP Jr. When is cholangitis sclerosing? Am J Surg 1978;135:312–30.
22. Ludwig J. Surgical pathology of the syndrome of primary sclerosing cholangitis. Am J Surg Pathol 1989;13(Suppl 1):43–9.
23. Ludwig J, Wahlstrom HE, Batts KP, Wiesner RH. Papillary bile duct dysplasia in primary sclerosing cholangitis. Gastroenterology 1992;102:2134–8.
24. Man KM, Grejet A, Keeffe EB, Garcia-Kennedy R, Imperial JC, Esquivel CO. Primary sclerosing cholangitis and Hodgkin's disease. Hepatology 1993;18:1127–31.
25. Mandal A, Dasgupta A, Jeffers L, et al. Autoantibodies in sclerosing cholangitis against a shared peptide in biliary and colon epithelium. Gastroenterology 1994;106:185–92.
26. McFarlane IG, Wojcicka BM, Tsantoulas C, Portman BC, Eddleston AL, Williams R. Leukocyte migration inhibition in response to biliary antigens in primary biliary cirrhosis, sclerosing cholangitis, and other chronic liver diseases. Gastroenterology 1979;76:1333–40.
27. Mihas AA, Murad TM, Hirschowitz BI. Sclerosing cholangitis associated with ulcerative colitis. Light and electron microscopy studies. Am J Gastroenterol 1978;70:614–9.
28. Montefusco PP, Geiss AC, Bronzo RL, Randall S, Kahn E, McKinley MJ. Sclerosing cholangitis, chronic pancreatitis, and Sjogren's syndrome: a syndrome complex. Am J Surg 1984;147:822-6.
29. Ong JC, O Loughlin EV, Kamath KR, Dorney SF, de Silva M, Gaskin KJ. Sclerosing cholangitis in children with inflammatory bowel disease. Aust NZ J Med 1994;24:149–53.
30. Peck JJ, Kern WH, Mikkelsen WP. Sclerosis of extrahepatic bile ducts. Arch Surg 1974;108:798–800.
31. Ramage JK, Donaghy A, Farrant JM, Iorns R, Williams R. Serum tumor markers for the diagnosis of cholangiocarcinoma in primary sclerosing cholangitis. Gastroenterology 1995;108:865–9.
32. Richardson AJ, Grierson JM, Tait N, Williams SJ, Little JM. A case of cholangitis glandularis proliferans and cholangiocarcinoma of the common bile duct. HPB Surg 1993;6:205–9.
33. Rosen CB, Nagorney DM, Wiesner RH, Coffey RJ, LaRusso NF. Cholangiocarcinoma complicating primary sclerosing cholangitis. Ann Surg 1991;213:21–5.
34. Schneiderman DJ, Cello JP, Laing FC. Papillary stenosis and sclerosing cholangitis in the acquired immune deficiency syndrome. Ann Intern Med 1987;106:546–9.

35. Schrumpf E, Fausa O, Elgjo K, Kolmannskog F. Hepatobiliary complications of inflammatory bowel disease. Semin Liver Dis 1988;8:201–9.

36. Segal I, Ou Tim L, Rubin A, et al. Rare and unusual manifestations of Crohn's disease with pyoderma gangrenosum and sclerosing cholangitis. S Afr Med J 1979;55:596–9.

37. Sjogren I, Wengle B, Korsgren M. Primary sclerosing cholangitis associated with fibrosis of the submandibular glands and the pancreas. Acta Med Scand 1979;205:139–41.

38. Spivak W, Grand RJ, Eraklis A. A case of primary sclerosing cholangitis in childhood. Gastroenterology 1982;82:129–32.

39. Taylor J, Lindor K. Metastatic prostate cancer simulating sclerosing cholangitis. J Clin Gastroenterol 1993;16:143–5.

40. Thompson HH, Pitt HA, Lewin KJ, Longmire WP Jr. Sclerosing cholangitis and histiocytosis X. Gut 1984; 25:526–30.

41. Thompson HH, Pitt HA, Tompkins RK, Longmire WP Jr. Primary sclerosing cholangitis. Ann Surg 1982; 196:127–36.

42. Ueno Y, LaRusso NF. Primary sclerosing cholangitis. J Gastroenterol 1994;29:531–43.

43. Viteri AL, Hardin WJ, Dyck WP. Peyronie's disease and sclerosing cholangitis in a patient with ulcerative colitis. Dig Dis Sci 1979;24:490–1.

44. Weinbren K, Mutum SS. Pathological aspects of cholangiocarcinoma. J Pathol 1983;139:217–38.

45. Werlin SL, Glicklich M, Jona J, Starshak RJ. Sclerosing cholangitis in childhood. J Pediatr 1980;96:433–5.

46. Wiesner RH. Current concepts in primary sclerosing cholangitis. Mayo Clin Proc 1994;69:969–82.

❖❖❖

19

BENIGN EPITHELIAL TUMORS OF THE AMPULLARY REGION

Within the ampulla there is a transition from the pancreatobiliary type epithelium of the distal common and pancreatic ducts to the intestinal type epithelium of the periampullary duodenum. Therefore, ampullary epithelial neoplasms may resemble tumors of either the duodenum (and the intestines in general) or the pancreatobiliary ducts. Most noninvasive ampullary epithelial neoplasms resemble adenomas of the intestines and are designated using analogous terminology. Some predominantly exophytic ampullary tumors exhibit a greater complexity of architecture and fewer "intestinal features." These papillary tumors resemble some of the exophytic tumors of the pancreatic and biliary ducts which have been designated intraductal papillary-mucinous neoplasms in the pancreas (3,4,6) and papillary adenomas, papillary carcinomas, or papillomatosis in the bile ducts. Although a spectrum of atypia exists within pancreatobiliary type papillary tumors of the ampulla, all of the cases we have observed have exhibited sufficient cyto-architectural atypia to justify the term papillary carcinoma; these tumors are discussed in chapter 20. Although it is possible for a benign counterpart with minimal or no atypia (pancreatobiliary type papillary adenoma) to exist, we have not observed such a tumor. In contrast to the gallbladder, adenomas of the pyloric gland type have not been described in the ampulla.

INTESTINAL TYPE ADENOMA

Intestinal type adenomas are benign epithelial neoplasms exhibiting tubular, papillary, or mixed patterns and resembling adenomas of the small and large intestines. More than 95 percent of benign ampullary neoplasms are adenomas of intestinal type. The frequency of tubular, papillary, and tubulopapillary adenomas is similar in sporadic cases (2), although tubular adenomas are more common among patients with polyposis (1,5). In keeping with the intestinal model, dysplasia is a prerequisite for the diagnosis of adenoma and may be of mild, moderate, or severe degree; most dysplasias are mild or moderate (2). However, the degree of dysplasia may vary in differ-

ent regions of the tumor. In addition, foci of in situ or invasive carcinoma may be present. Therefore, extensive sampling of the lesion should be performed to exclude carcinoma.

Epidemiology. Although adenomas involving the small intestine are uncommon, they tend to occur within the duodenum and specifically near the ampulla (8,11,19,21,30). Fifty-five percent of small intestinal adenomas involve the ampulla and another 25 percent involve the extra-ampullary duodenum (19). The incidence of ampullary adenomas at autopsy ranges from 0.04 to 0.12 percent (9,23,25). As of 1982, only 103 adenomas had been reported, some of which contained invasive carcinoma (18,26). However, increased recognition has resulted in many more cases being reported in the last 15 years.

Ampullary adenomas may occur sporadically or may be associated with familial adenomatous polyposis (FAP) and Gardner's syndrome (7,15, 24,27). The prevalence of ampullary or peri-ampullary duodenal adenomas in patients with FAP ranges from 50 to 95 percent (7,13,16,17, 31). Ampullary adenomas are more frequent than duodenal adenomas and tend to exhibit higher grades of dysplasia (24). There does not appear to be any association with the other extracolonic manifestations of FAP (15). Ampullary adenomas usually become symptomatic later than colorectal adenomas, generally 10 to 15 years after colectomy (17); however, screening of asymptomatic patients has shown adenomas to occur within 3 years after colectomy (24). In some cases the ampullary adenoma may be detected before the colon polyps (or carcinoma) (22). Thus, the colon should be examined in patients with ampullary adenoma, especially if the adenomas are multiple. In more than 60 percent of cases, patients with FAP have more than five adenomas in the duodenum and ampulla (17). In the absence of adenomas, ampullary biopsies from FAP patients may show hyperplasia of the villous and crypt epithelium, a change which may represent a precursor to adenoma (13). Ampullary adenomas in nonpolyposis patients are rare (20), however, increasing recognition of the high incidence in polyposis has resulted in many cases of ampullary adenoma being reported (7,15,17,24). In addition, patients with FAP are currently being detected at younger ages, allowing curative colectomy before the development of colorectal carcinoma; thus, polyposis patients are now living long enough for ampullary and duodenal adenomas to become manifest.

Ampullary adenomas are considered premalignant lesions (10,12,14,18,29,30), with papillary adenomas having a greater risk for malignant transformation than tubular adenomas (9,28). The morphologic sequence in the transformation of adenoma to carcinoma in the ampulla is similar to that of the large intestine. The likelihood of finding carcinoma in an ampullary adenoma is greater than for adenomas of similar size in the large intestine or even in the extra-ampullary duodenum (19,22). About 25 to 50 percent of ampullary tumors showing adenoma on biopsy contain carcinoma in the resected specimen (21,22). The lack of severe dysplasia or invasive carcinoma in an endoscopically biopsied adenoma must therefore be interpreted with caution (11). Surgical excision may be indicated if the lesion is too large to permit complete endoscopic removal (30).

Clinical Features. Patients with sporadic ampullary adenomas range from 33 to 81 years of age, with a mean age of 61 years; females outnumber males by 2.6 to 1 (33,38,40,42,45). Polyposis patients with ampullary adenomas are younger (mean, 41 years), probably because of both earlier onset as well as earlier detection due to screening endoscopy (32,37). In patients with polyposis the female to male ratio is 1 to 1 (32,35,37,44).

Because of the anatomy of the ampulla, patients with ampullary adenomas generally present with biliary obstruction. Patients with sporadic adenomas often present with jaundice; but abdominal pain, weight loss, and occasionally, pancreatitis can also occur (39,41–43,46,47). Although massive upper gastrointestinal hemorrhage is unusual, occult blood may be found in the stool. A distended, palpable gallbladder is an unusual finding (38). Elevations of serum bilirubin, serum glutamic-oxaloacetic transaminase (SGOT), serum glutamic-pyruvic transaminase (SGPT), and alkaline phosphatase may be present, occasionally in the absence of clinical symptoms (36,41,42). Patients with pancreatitis may have elevations in

serum amylase. Some patients have had coincident cholelithiasis or choledocholithiasis (42,45). Patients with polyposis are generally asymptomatic and ampullary adenomas are detected during screening endoscopy.

The diagnosis of ampullary adenoma can be made by endoscopic biopsies. Exophytic nodular or papillary growths are seen endoscopically. Intra-ampullary adenomas may appear only as a prominent bulge underlying intact periampullary duodenal mucosa. Ulceration is a worrisome feature for malignancy. In patients with FAP, the entire periampullary duodenum may contain polyps, although those involving the ampulla are generally the most prominent. Multiple biopsies taken after a papillotomy will increase the diagnostic yield, especially for intra-ampullary tumors.

Ampullary adenomas are cured by complete excision, although pancreatoduodenectomy may be necessary for large lesions. In patients who have had local excision, there may be recurrence (34,43), either because of incomplete removal or development of a new tumor in the adjacent mucosa. The latter event is common in patients with FAP.

Gross Findings. Gross examination of ampullary adenomas generally reveals pale soft polyps or plaques projecting into the duodenal lumen (fig. 19-1) when the tumors are exophytic (49). Less commonly, the tumor may be confined within the ampulla (intra-ampullary), resulting in a prominent bulging papilla covered with intact mucosa (53). Papillary adenomas often have a characteristic villiform appearance. In patients presenting with symptoms, most ampullary adenomas are between 1 and 3 cm (53). Patients with FAP may also have numerous duodenal adenomas (fig. 19-2). Endoscopy for screening purposes may biopsy adenomatous mucosa in a minimally granular or even normal-appearing ampulla (48,50,51). Intraoperatively, ampullary adenomas may be overlooked since they may not be palpable through the duodenal wall due to their soft consistency (52).

Microscopic Findings. Histologically, ampullary adenomas may be either exophytic into the duodenum (fig. 19-3) or, less often, contained within the ampulla (fig. 19-4). In many cases the adenomatous epithelium involves more than one anatomic location in the periampullary region (58). Most commonly, there is

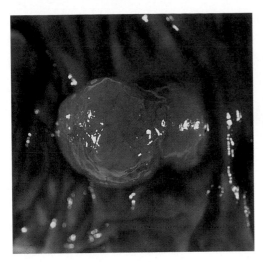
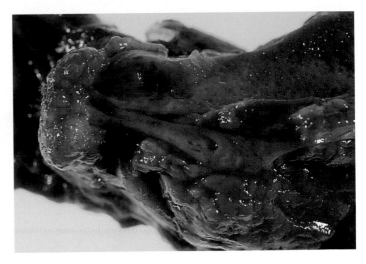

Figure 19-1
GROSS APPEARANCE OF SPORADIC AMPULLARY ADENOMA

Left: A single circumscribed, exophytic tumor projects from the surface of the papillae. The surface is smooth without areas of ulceration.

Right: On cut section the tumor involves the distal aspect of both pancreatic and biliary ducts, although the predominant component extends into the duodenal lumen.

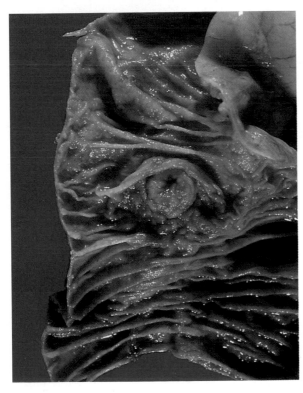
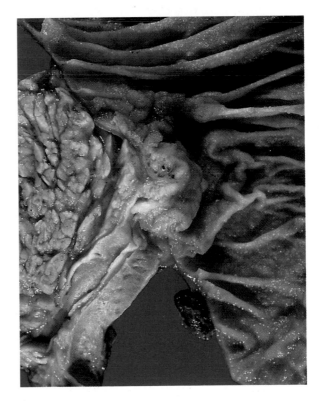

Figure 19-2
GROSS APPEARANCE OF AMPULLARY AND PERIAMPULLARY DUODENAL ADENOMAS IN A PATIENT
WITH FAMILIAL ADENOMATOUS POLYPOSIS

Left: Viewed from the duodenal lumen, the largest adenoma involves the ampulla itself (center), with numerous smaller polyps scattered around the ampulla and in lesser numbers elsewhere within the duodenum.

Right: Cut section through the ampulla reveals nodular thickening of the ampullary and periampullary duodenal mucosae. Portions of the adenoma extend into the distal pancreatic and biliary ducts.

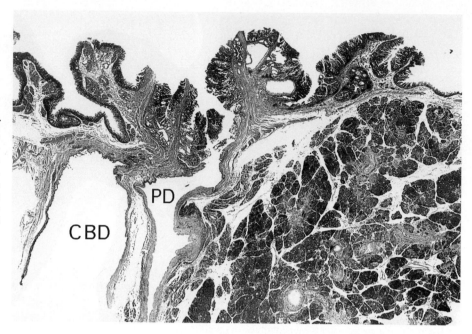

Figure 19-3
PAPILLARY ADENOMA
Low-power appearance of ampullary intestinal type adenoma. The mucosa of the ampulla and periampullary duodenum is thickened and villiform. There was biliary obstruction due to the lesion, with resulting dilatation of the common bile duct (CBD). The pancreatic duct (PD) is of normal caliber.

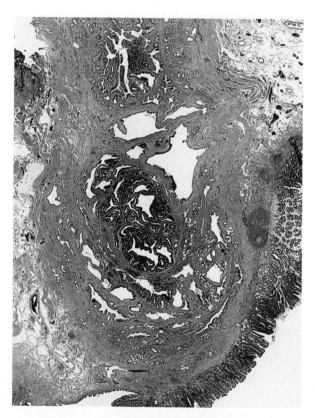

Figure 19-4
SMALL TUBULAR ADENOMA
In this patient with familial adenomatous polyposis, an early adenoma is entirely confined within the ampulla. Dilated periampullary ductules surround the tumor.

involvement of the periampullary duodenal mucosa (including the mucosa of the papilla) along with the ampullary channel, and extension into the distal bile duct or pancreatic duct is frequent (fig. 19-5). At the periphery of the lesion, adenomatous changes may extend in a flat configuration for a variable distance into the pancreatic or biliary ducts (fig. 19-6).

Tubular adenomas are usually smaller than the papillary or tubulopapillary variety and exhibit a polypoid configuration (57). They consist of tubular glands resembling the basal portions of the intestinal crypts (fig. 19-7). The nuclei are oval, hyperchromatic, and pseudostratified. Because of the normal villous architecture of the duodenum and valves of Wirsung within the ampulla, a small degree of villiform growth is acceptable in tubular adenomas. Papillary intestinal type adenomas (also known as villous adenomas) are usually sessile. The proliferating cells line simple papillae, which vary in length and may branch (fig. 19-8). Perhaps because they are usually larger than tubular adenomas (up to 5 cm), papillary adenomas have a greater incidence of coexistent severe dysplasia or intramucosal carcinoma. Tubulopapillary (or tubulovillous) adenomas contain more than 25 percent of both tubular and papillary elements (fig. 19-9).

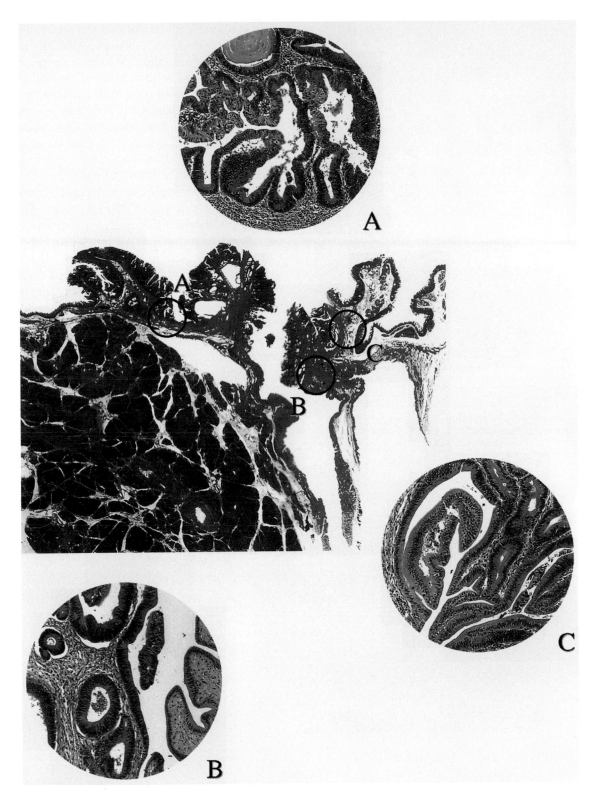

Figure 19-5
FAMILIAL ADENOMATOUS POLYPOSIS
In this case, adenomatous changes involve the duodenum, distal common bile duct, and distal pancreatic duct (as shown in the insets) in addition to the ampulla itself.

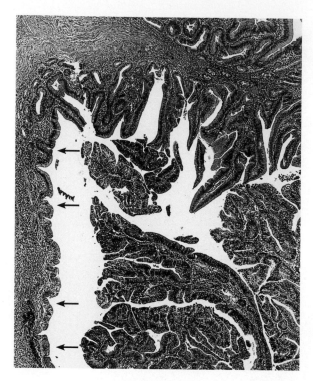

Figure 19-6
AMPULLARY PAPILLARY ADENOMA
At the periphery of this ampullary papillary adenoma, there is extension of adenomatous epithelium with a flat configuration along the common bile duct proximal to the tumor (arrows).

In cases with mild dysplasia, the relatively uniform nuclei are basally situated and the apical cytoplasm is amphophilic. Moderate dysplasia results in increased stratification of the nuclei, including frequent extension to the luminal border, and moderate variability in their size and shape. Mitotic figures are frequent and often nonbasal. Mild architectural complexity may be present, with branching glands; however, cribriforming is absent. In severe dysplasia, the glandular architecture is more complex, cribriformed glands are present, and the nuclei display more marked cytologic abnormalities and a relative lack of polarity with mitoses at all levels (fig. 19-10A). Carcinoma in situ is present when the cyto-architectural atypia is so pronounced that the individual cells and glands have features indistinguishable from those of invasive carcinoma (fig. 19-10B,C). Small amounts of necrotic debris may be found in the glandular lumens. In carcinoma in situ, the atypical cellular proliferation is limited to the basement membrane of the glands; there is no stromal reaction and no infiltrative or expansile growth (fig. 19-11).

Cytologically, adenomas are characterized by small clusters and sheets of elongated columnar cells. The basally located nuclei are also elongated

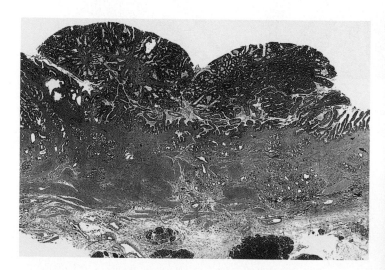

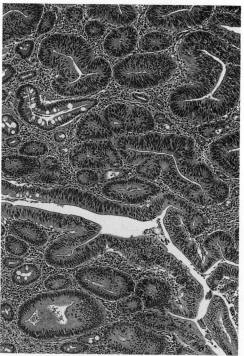

Figure 19-7
TUBULAR ADENOMA INVOLVING THE AMPULLARY PORTION OF THE DISTAL COMMON BILE DUCT
Above: At low power, the tumor consists largely of simple, tubular glands.
Right: At higher power, the involved glands are lined by pseudostratified cells with elongated, atypical nuclei. There is no significant papillae formation.

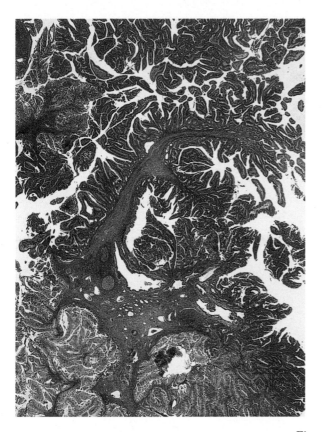 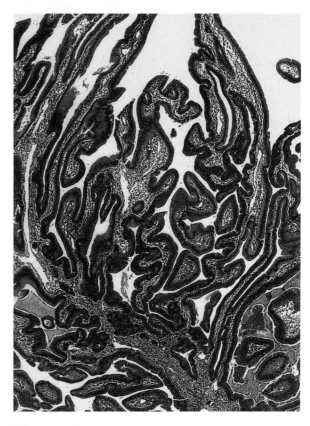

Figure 19-8
PAPILLARY INTESTINAL TYPE ADENOMA
Left: This papillary intestinal type adenoma exhibits a marked villiform architecture, with large papillary fronds containing numerous secondary papillae at low power.
Right: In this example, areas of complexity reflect foci of high-grade dysplasia. In more simple areas, the papillae are lined by a single layer of pseudostratified cells resembling those of tubular adenomas.

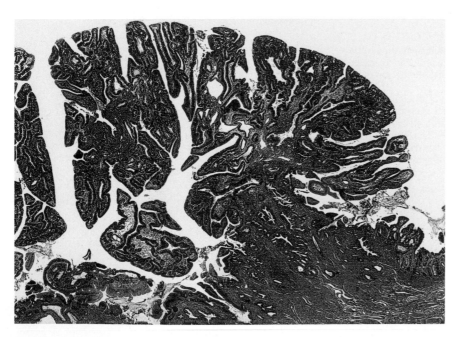

Figure 19-9
TUBULOPAPILLARY
ADENOMA
This tubulopapillary adenoma contains a mixture of tubular and papillary architectural patterns.

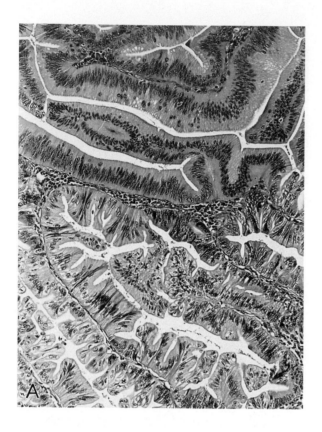

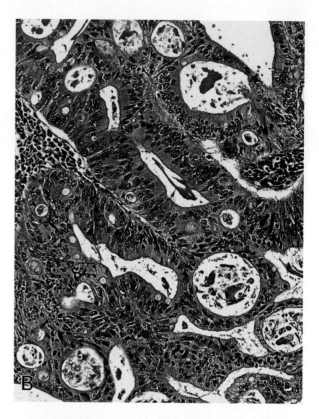

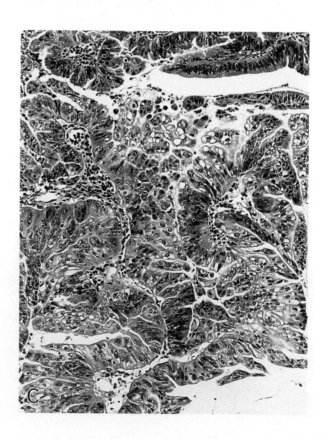

Figure 19-10
SEVERE DYSPLASIA/CARCINOMA IN SITU

A: There is architectural atypia including micropapillary formation and early cribriforming in addition to nuclear atypia. Note the residual foci of mild dysplasia (top) in this carcinoma in situ.

B,C: The cytoarchitectural atypia is sufficiently marked that the features are indistinguishable from those of invasive carcinoma. Extensive cribriforming, with luminal necrotic debris, is shown in B. Exuberant micropapillary formations with marked nuclear atypia are depicted in C. In both instances, however, there is no invasion and the basement membrane appears intact.

and are uniform, with inconspicuous nucleoli and a fine chromatin pattern (59,60). The presence of significant nuclear atypia or an increased nuclear:cytoplasmic ratio suggests that severe dysplasia or carcinoma is also present.

As in intestinal adenomas, there may be "pseudoinvasion" characterized by extravasation of mucin from the glands at the base of the lesion into the subjacent stroma. The mucin often elicits an inflammatory reaction which may be accompanied by recent or old hemorrhage. However, no malignant cells are found within the mucin or in the stroma. Extension of the adenomatous epithelium into submucosal glands (such as Brunner's glands) or into the periductal ductules surrounding the distal pancreatic and bile ducts may simulate invasive carcinoma (fig. 19-12). Cystic changes may be superimposed upon the adenomatous glands.

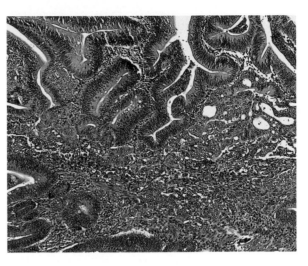

Figure 19-11
INTRAMUCOSAL INVASIVE CARCINOMA
INVOLVING AN ADENOMA
In this example, residual adenomatous glands are surrounded by small clusters of cells and cribriformed nests which are no longer surrounded by the native basement membrane.

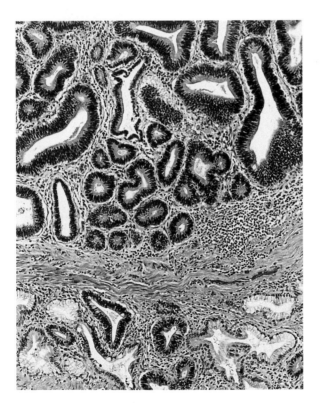 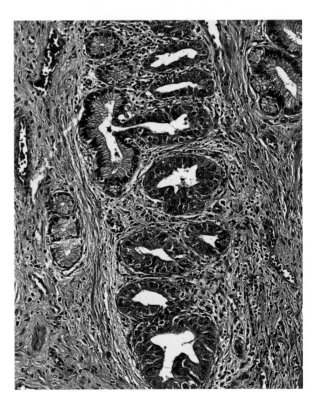

Figure 19-12
TUBULAR ADENOMA
Left: Adenomatous changes may extend into periampullary glands and ductules. At the base of this adenoma some of the periampullary ductules exhibit pseudostratified nuclei whereas adjacent ductules remain uninvolved.
Right: The adenomatous foci involving ductules exhibit severe dysplasia while the individual glands resemble invasive carcinoma since they are situated deep within the stroma.

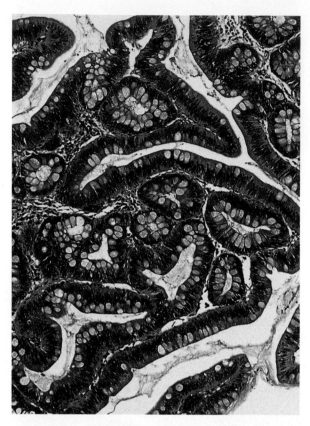

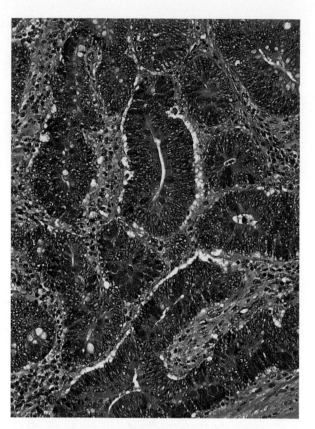

Figure 19-13
GOBLET CELLS IN TUBULAR ADENOMA
Goblet cells may be focally abundant in ampullary adenomas. They usually occur in regions with low-grade dysplasia.

Figure 19-14
PANETH CELLS IN TUBULAR ADENOMA
Numerous Paneth cells in an ampullary adenoma.

Most of the tall columnar cells making up adenomas contain modest amounts of mucin within the apical cytoplasm. Interspersed goblet cells are common in both tubular and papillary adenomas, generally occurring in areas of mild or moderate dysplasia (fig. 19-13). Goblet cells stain with Alcian blue and periodic acid–Schiff. Neutral mucins, sialomucins, and sulphomucin can be detected histochemically in ampullary adenomas, and the sulphomucins are more frequently and intensely positive in areas of severe dysplasia or carcinoma in situ (56).

Immunohistochemical Findings. Particularly numerous in ampullary adenomas relative to their intestinal counterparts are Paneth cells (54–56), which may be detected immunohistochemically with stains for lysozyme (fig. 19-14). These cells are scattered throughout the adenoma, often concentrated in the basal portions of the glands. Endocrine cells are also found in intestinal type adenomas and may be numerous (56). They may be revealed in abundance after immunohistochemical staining for chromogranin or serotonin (fig. 19-15). Paneth cells and endocrine cells are less numerous in adenomas with greater degrees of dysplasia or a more papillary architecture (56).

Immunohistochemical staining for carcinoembryonic antigen (CEA) and CA19-9 reveal predominantly surface membrane positivity in adenomas with mild or moderate dysplasia, with only focal weak cytoplasmic staining. In areas of severe dysplasia or carcinoma in situ, however, there may be intense cytoplasmic staining for these markers (61).

Differential Diagnosis. The differential diagnosis of intestinal type adenomas on biopsy includes reactive atypia associated with other benign lesions or inflammatory conditions. The epithelial component of adenomyoma (or adenomyomatous hyperplasia) may display oval,

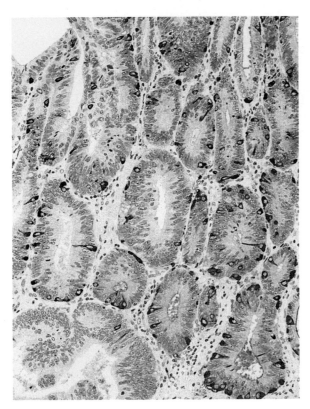 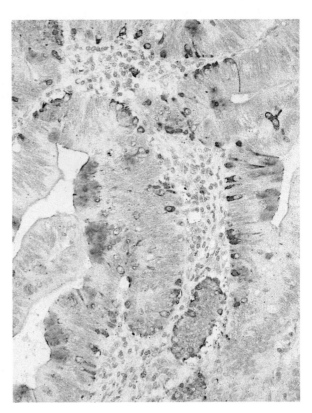

Figure 19-15

ENDOCRINE AND PANETH CELLS IN AMPULLARY ADENOMAS

Left: Endocrine cells are often numerous. Although generally difficult to detect by routine microscopy, they are highlighted by immunohistochemical staining for chromogranin.

Right: Double immunohistochemical staining for chromogranin (brown reaction product) and muramidase (blue reaction product) shows the distribution of Paneth and endocrine cells. Note the basal localization of most endocrine cells and the apical distribution of Paneth cell granules.

slightly pseudostratified nuclei simulating adenomatous changes; however, the glands are intimately mixed with fascicles of smooth muscle. Reactive epithelial atypia associated with inflammatory conditions commonly exhibits large nuclei with an open chromatin pattern, thick nuclear membranes, and prominent nucleoli (fig. 19-16). There is generally no pseudostratification. Paradoxically, reactive atypia more commonly resembles a carcinoma than an adenoma.

FLAT CARCINOMA IN SITU

Although most preneoplastic tumors of the ampulla exhibit a polypoid configuration (adenomas), occasionally there are foci of flat or micropapillary carcinoma in situ associated with invasive carcinoma. Rarely, these lesions are encountered in the absence of an invasive component.

We have observed two clinically symptomatic patients with flat carcinoma in situ involving the ampulla. The neoplastic population was present on the surface as well as within the submucosal ductules (fig. 19-17), and involved the distal bile duct and pancreatic duct in addition to the ampulla. No invasive carcinoma was present. Thus, these lesions resembled the flat in situ carcinomas of the gallbladder and bile ducts. Although similar changes may be seen focally at the periphery of adenomas, pure nonpolypoid in situ carcinoma appears to be rare in the ampulla. Cytologically, there was marked atypia with a high nuclear: cytoplasmic ratio. One case exhibited abundant micropapillae which lacked fibrovascular cores. The typical pseudostratified cells of adenomas were absent, further distinguishing these lesions. Presumably, flat or micropapillary carcinoma in situ also represents a precursor to invasive carcinoma.

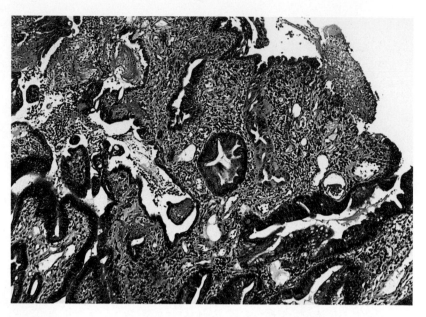

Figure 19-16
REACTIVE EPITHELIAL ATYPIA
An ampullary biopsy shows marked inflammation with reactive changes, simulating adenomatous epithelium. In some areas there is nuclear stratification but elsewhere the glands show enlarged, atypical nuclei with single prominent nucleoli, reparative atypia which may be mistaken for carcinoma.

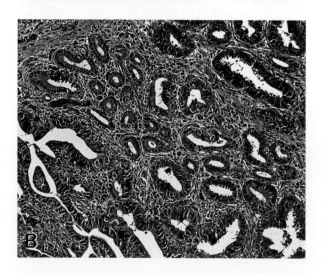

Figure 19-17
FLAT CARCINOMA IN SITU INVOLVING THE AMPULLA
Although preneoplastic changes in this location are generally present in the context of a polypoid lesion, a rare case exhibits flat or micropapillary carcinoma in situ without a significant polyploid component.

A: At low power, micropapillary structures can be seen involving the periampullary ductules surrounding the distal biliary and pancreatic ducts, longitudinal sections of which are present at the right.

B: At higher power, the markedly atypical flat proliferation replaces the epithelium of the periampullary ductules, some of which are uninvolved.

C: In another case, the proliferation exhibits micropapillary formations which lack fibrovascular cores.

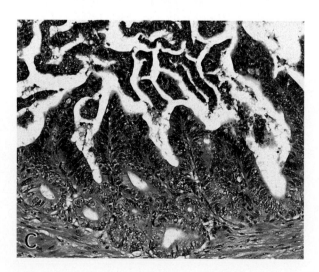

REFERENCES

General

1. Domizio P, Talbot IC, Spigelman AD, Williams CB, Phillips RK. Upper gastrointestinal pathology in familial adenomatous polyposis: results from a prospective study of 102 patients. J Clin Pathol 1990;43:738–43.
2. Komorowski RA, Beggs BK, Geenan JE, Venu RP. Assessment of ampulla of Vater pathology. An endoscopic approach. Am J Surg Pathol 1991;15:1188–96.
3. Nagai E, Ueki T, Chijiwa K, Tanaka M, Tsuneyoshi M. Intraductal papillary mucinous neoplasms of the pancreas associated with so-called mucinous ductal ectasia. Histochemical and immunohistochemical analysis of 29 cases. Am J Surg Pathol 1995;19:576–89.
4. Nishihara K, Fukuda T, Tsuneyoshi M, Komirami T, Maeda S, Saku M. Intraductal papillary neoplasm of the pancreas. Cancer 1993;72:689–96.
5. Odze R, Gallinger S, So K, Antonioli D. Duodenal adenomas in familial adenomatous polyposis: relation of cell differentiation and mucin histochemical features to growth pattern. Mod Pathol 1994;7:376–84.
6. Sessa F, Solcia E, Capella C, et al. Intraductal papillary mucinous tumors represent a distinct group of pancreatic neoplasms: an investigation of tumor cell differentiation and K-ras, p53 and c-erbB-2 abnormalities in 26 patients. Virchows Arch 1994;425:357–67.

Epidemiology

7. Alexander JR, Andrews JM, Buchi KN, Lee RG, Becker JM, Burt RW. High prevalence of adenomatous polyps of the duodenal papilla in familial adenomatous polyposis. Dig Dis Sci 1989;34:167–70.
8. Attanoos R, Williams GT. Epithelial and neuroendocrine tumors of the duodenum. Semin Diag Pathol 1991;8:149–62.
9. Baggenstoss AH. Major duodenal papilla. Variations of pathologic interest and lesions of the mucosa. Arch Pathol 1938;26:853–68.
10. Benediktsdottir K, Lundell L, Thulin A. Premalignant lesions of the periampullary region. Report of two cases. Ann Chir Gynaecol 1981;70:86–9.
11. Bugra D, Alper A, Goksen Y, Emre A. Villous tumors of the duodenum. Hepatogastroenterology 1991;38:84–5.
12. Cattell RB, Pyrtek LJ. Premalignant lesions of the ampulla of Vater. Surg Gyn Obstet 1949;90:21–30.
13. Domizio P, Talbot IC, Spigelman AD, Williams CB, Phillips RK. Upper gastrointestinal pathology in familial adenomatous polyposis: results from a prospective study of 102 patients. J Clin Pathol 1990;43:738–43.
14. Kozuka S, Tsubone M, Yamaguchi A, Hachisuka K. Adenomatous residue in cancerous papilla of Vater. Gut 1981;22:1031–4.
15. Kurtz RC, Sternberg SS, Miller HH, Decosse JJ. Upper gastrointestinal neoplasia in familial polyposis. Dig Dis Sci 1987;32:459–65.
16. Noda Y, Watanabe H, Iida M, et al. Histologic follow-up of ampullary adenomas in patients with familial adenomatosis coli. Cancer 1992;70:1847–56.
17. Odze R, Gallinger S, So K, Antonioli D. Duodenal adenomas in familial adenomatous polyposis: relation of cell differentiation and mucin histochemical features to growth pattern. Mod Pathol 1994;7:376–84.
18. Oh C, Jemerin EE. Benign adenomatous polyps of the papilla of Vater. Surgery 1965;57:495–503.
19. Perzin KH, Bridge MF. Adenomas of the small intestine: a clinicopathologic review of 51 cases and a study of their relationship to carcinoma. Cancer 1981;48:799–819.
20. Rosenberg J, Welch JP, Pyrtek LJ, Walker M, Trowbridge P. Benign villous adenomas of the ampulla of Vater. Cancer 1986;58:1563–8.
21. Ryan DP, Schapiro RH, Warshaw AL. Villous tumors of the duodenum. Ann Surg 1986;203:301–6.
22. Seifert E, Schulte F, Stolte M. Adenoma and carcinoma of the duodenum and papilla of Vater: a clinicopathologic study. Am J Gastroenterol 1992;87:37–42.
23. Shapiro P, Lifvendahl RA. Tumors of the extrahepatic bile ducts. Arch Pathol 1931;95:61–79.
24. Shemesh E, Bat L. A prospective evaluation of the upper gastrointestinal tract and periampullary region in patients with Gardner syndrome. Am J Gastroenterol 1985;80:825–7.
25. Sobol S, Cooperman AM. Villous adenoma of the ampulla of Vater. An unusual cause of biliary colic and obstructive jaundice. Gastroenterology 1978;75:107–9.
26. Starling JR, Turner JH. Villous adenoma involving the ampulla of Vater: treatment by submucosal resection and double sphincteroplasty. Am Surg 1982;48:188–90.
27. Stevenson JK, Reid BJ. Unfamiliar aspects of familial polyposis coli. Am J Surg 1986;152:81–6.
28. Stolte M, Pscherer C. Adenoma-carcinoma sequence in the papilla of Vater. Scand J Gastroenterol 1996;31:376–82.
29. Uchida Y, Tomonaki K, Shibata O, et al. Carcinoma in adenoma of the papilla of Vater. Jpn J Surg 1986;16:371–6.
30. Witteman BJ, Janssens AR, Terpstra JL, Eulderink F, Welvaart K, Lamers CB. Villous tumors of the duodenum. Presentation of five cases. Hepatogastroenterology 1991;38:550–3.
31. Yao T, Iida M, Ohsato K, Watanabe H, Omae T. Duodenal lesions in familial polyposis of the colon. Gastroenterology 1977;73:1086–92.

Clinical Features

32. Alexander JR, Andrews JM, Buchi KN, Lee RG, Becker JM, Burt RW. High prevalence of adenomatous polyps of the duodenal papilla in familial adenomatous polyposis. Dig Dis Sci 1989;34:167–70.
33. Cattell RB, Pyrtek LJ. Premalignant lesions of the ampulla of Vater. Surg Gyn Obstet 1949;90:21–30.

34. Celik C, Venditti JA Jr, Satchidanand S, Freier DT. Villous tumors of the duodenum and ampulla of Vater. J Surg Oncol 1986;33:268–72.
35. Domizio P, Talbot IC, Spigelman AD, Williams CB, Phillips RK. Upper gastrointestinal pathology in familial adenomatous polyposis: results from a prospective study of 102 patients. J Clin Pathol 1990;43:738–43.
36. Lewis JH, Shorb PE, Nochomovitz LE. Benign duodenal villous adenoma obstructing the ampulla of Vater: a surgical dilemma. South Med J 1985;78:1507–11.
37. Odze R, Gallinger S, So K, Antonioli D. Duodenal adenomas in familial adenomatous polyposis: relation of cell differentiation and mucin histochemical features to growth pattern. Mod Pathol 1994;7:376–84.
38. Oh C, Jemerin EE. Benign adenomatous polyps of the papilla of Vater. Surgery 1965;57:495–503.
39. Ohmori K, Kinoshita H, Shiraha Y, Satake K. Pancreatic duct obstruction by a benign polypoid adenoma of the ampulla of Vater. Am J Surg 1976;132:662–3.
40. Perzin KH, Bridge MF. Adenomas of the small intestine: a clinicopathologic review of 51 cases and a study of their relationship to carcinoma. Cancer 1981;48:799–819.
41. Ponchon T, Berger F, Chavaillon A, Bory R, Lambert R. Contribution of endoscopy to diagnosis and treatment of tumors of the ampulla of Vater. Cancer 1989;64:161–7.
42. Rosenberg J, Welch JP, Pyrtek LJ, Walker M, Trowbridge P. Benign villous adenomas of the ampulla of Vater. Cancer 1986;58:1563–8.
43. Ryan DP, Schapiro RH, Warshaw AL. Villous tumors of the duodenum. Ann Surg 1986;203:301–6.
44. Shemesh E, Bat L. A prospective evaluation of the upper gastrointestinal tract and periampullary region in patients with Gardner syndrome. Am J Gastroenterol 1985;80:825–7.
45. Sobol S, Cooperman AM. Villous adenoma of the ampulla of Vater. An unusual cause of biliary colic and obstructive jaundice. Gastroenterology 1978;75:107–9.
46. White SH, Nazarian NA, Smith AM, et al. Periampullary adenoma causing pancreatitis. Br Med J 1981;283:527.
47. Yamaguchi K, Enjoji M. Adenoma of the ampulla of Vater: putative precancerous lesion. Gut 1991;32:1558–61.

Gross Features

48. Alexander JR, Andrews JM, Buchi KN, Lee RG, Becker JM, Burt RW. High prevalence of adenomatous polyps of the duodenal papilla in familial adenomatous polyposis. Dig Dis Sci 1989;34:167–70.
49. Blackman E, Nash SV. Diagnosis of duodenal and ampullary epithelial neoplasms by endoscopic biopsy: a clinicopathologic and immunohistochemical study. Hum Pathol 1985;16:901–10.
50. Domizio P, Talbot IC, Spigelman AD, Williams CB, Phillips RK. Upper gastrointestinal pathology in familial adenomatous polyposis: results from a prospective study of 102 patients. J Clin Pathol 1990;43:738–43.
51. Iida M, Yao T, Itoh H, Ohsato K, Watanabe H. Endoscopic features of adenoma of the duodenal papilla in familial polyposis of the colon. Gastrointest Endosc 1981;27:6–8.
52. Sobol S, Cooperman AM. Villous adenoma of the ampulla of Vater. An unusual cause of biliary colic and obstructive jaundice. Gastroenterology 1978;75:107–9.
53. Yamaguchi K, Enjoji M. Adenoma of the ampulla of Vater: putative precancerous lesion. Gut 1991;32:1558–61.

Microscopic Features

54. Ferrell LD, Beckstead JH. Paneth-like cells in an adenoma and adenocarcinoma in the ampulla of Vater. Arch Pathol Lab Med 1991;115:956–8.
55. Komorowski RA, Cohen EB. Villous tumors of the duodenum: a clinicopathologic study. Cancer 1981;47:1377–86.
56. Odze R, Gallinger S, So K, Antonioli D. Duodenal adenomas in familial adenomatous polyposis: relation of cell differentiation and mucin histochemical features to growth pattern. Mod Pathol 1994;7:376–84.
57. Perzin KH, Bridge MF. Adenomas of the small intestine: a clinicopathologic review of 51 cases and a study of their relationship to carcinoma. Cancer 1981;48:799–819.
58. Starling JR, Turner JH. Villous adenoma involving the ampulla of Vater: treatment by submucosal resection and double sphincteroplasty. Am Surg 1982;48:188–90.
59. Veronezi-Gurwell A, Wittchow RJ, Bottles K, Cohen MB. Cytologic features of villous adenoma of the ampullary region. Diagn Cytopathol 1996;14:145–9.
60. Witte S. Brush cytology of the papilla of Vater. Scand J Gastroenterol 1979;54:55–8.
61. Yamaguchi K, Enjoji M. Adenoma of the ampulla of Vater: putative precancerous lesion. Gut 1991;32:1558–61.

✧✧✧

20

MALIGNANT EPITHELIAL TUMORS OF THE AMPULLA

Carcinoma is the most common tumor that involves the ampulla. More than 90 percent of ampullary epithelial neoplasms are malignant (1, 2). Because of their often dramatic clinical presentation and potentially curable nature, tumors in this location have received considerable attention in the literature, even though they are not common.

Because the vaterian system is complex, with various anatomic components, the origin of a carcinoma involving the ampulla may be difficult to determine. The ampulla may be completely overgrown even by small carcinomas, making it impossible to determine whether the tumor originated in the periampullary duodenum, the distal common bile duct, the head of the pancreas, or in the ampulla. In the literature the term, "periampullary" is often used to refer to tumors anywhere in the region of the head of the pancreas, including any of these four sites (3–5,7). The similarity in histologic appearance among tumors arising in these locations further complicates the identification of the primary site. Moreover, preneoplastic lesions accompanying invasive carcinomas may involve more than one site. Fortunately, most pancreatic ductal carcinomas do not arise from the main ducts, and ampullary involvement by pancreatic carcinoma usually consists of peripheral extension, which is readily apparent. Distal bile duct carcinomas may also be distinguished by their fusiform growth along the bile duct. However, distinguishing periampullary duodenal carcinomas from true ampullary carcinomas may be impossible. Some authors consider ampullary and duodenal neoplasms together when discussing endoscopic appearance, biopsy diagnosis, etcetera (2). Because ampullary carcinomas and periampullary duodenal carcinomas often cannot be distinguished and because they share many clinical, histologic, and molecular features, it is appropriate to consider them collectively as "ampullary" carcinomas (6,8).

EPIDEMIOLOGY

Carcinomas of the ampullary region are uncommon; however, they occur more frequently in the ampullary region than elsewhere in the small intestine (10). They represent 1 percent of all carcinomas and 5 percent of all gastrointestinal carcinomas (9). The estimated lifetime incidence in the general population is 0.01 to 0.04 percent (12). The incidence of ampullary carcinoma in autopsy series has varied from 0.06 to 0.21 percent (11). In addition to carcinomas of the distal bile duct, duodenum, and head of pancreas, carcinoma of the ampulla is one of the tumors manifested by a mass in the region of the head of the pancreas, where it comprises 5 to 10 percent of carcinomas. Among 1,545 patients with carcinomas in the region of the head of the pancreas admitted to the surgical service at Memorial Sloan-Kettering Cancer Center, 129 (8.3 percent) were found to have ampullary tumors (Table 20-1). This percentage may be inflated, since the patient population is biased towards those with potentially resectable tumors, and ampullary carcinomas are more frequently resectable than carcinomas originating in the distal bile duct or head of the pancreas.

Ampullary carcinoma is more common in older adults, with a peak age incidence in the eighth decade (fig. 20-1). The age range of 880 patients from 20 reported series was 20 to 91 years, with a mean of 61.9 years. Males are affected somewhat more commonly than females: the male to female ratio based on 931 cases from the literature is 1.48 to 1.

Table 20-1

LOCATION OF CARCINOMAS IN THE REGION OF THE HEAD OF THE PANCREAS IN PATIENTS EVALUATED BY THE DEPARTMENT OF SURGERY AT MSKCC*, 1983–1995

Site	No. Patients (% of total)	No. Resected (%)
Ampulla	129 (8.3)	100 (78)
Duodenum	98 (6.3)	59 (60)
Pancreas (head)	1180 (76.4)	296 (25)

*MSKCC - Memorial Sloan-Kettering Cancer Center

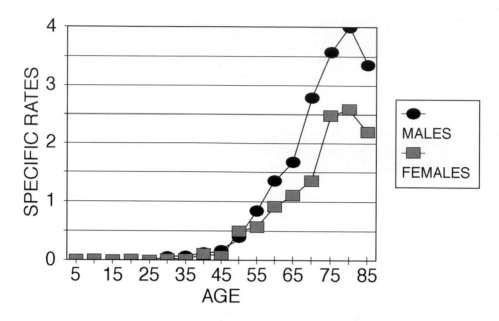

Figure 20-1
AGE-SPECIFIC RATES FOR CANCERS OF THE AMPULLA OF VATER
The data are taken from the Surveillance, Epidemiology, and End Results Program, National Cancer Institute for the years 1981–1990. The rates reflect histologically proven invasive cancers only and include all histologic types.

ASSOCIATED CONDITIONS

A number of predisposing and associated conditions are known for ampullary carcinoma, and some perhaps contribute to the relatively high incidence of carcinomas at this location. Another potential factor is that the ampullary region contains a transition from pancreatobiliary to intestinal epithelium, and such areas of transition are inherently unstable. As early as 1949, Cattell and Pyrtek (18) made the following observation: "Since several types of epithelium meet at the papilla, and this region is stimulated by a variety of digestive enzymes and chemical substances, it becomes an ideal situation for neoplasms to develop, that is, an area of epithelial transition which is constantly being irritated chemically and mechanically."

Adenoma

As is true for carcinomas of both the small and large intestines, many ampullary carcinomas arise from preexisting adenomas. Areas of residual adenoma have been observed in 35 to 90 percent of ampullary carcinomas (14,32,35,46, 47,52,54). The frequency is greater in lesions having a small invasive component (48 percent for carcinomas less than 3 cm [26]) or well-differ-

entiated carcinomas (43) and declines with increasing stage of carcinoma (46,54). In addition, patients whose ampullary adenomas have been locally excised have subsequently developed carcinoma at the same location (23). Noninvasive papillary carcinomas of the ampulla are also precursors to invasive carcinoma, with which they are frequently associated. In addition to areas of residual adenoma, papillary hyperplasia of the surrounding epithelium may accompany ampullary carcinomas (14).

The time required for an ampullary adenoma to progress to carcinoma is not known. Serial follow-up biopsies of patients with familial adenomatous polyposis (FAP) allows the observation of this progression in this selected group at high risk for ampullary carcinoma. In FAP patients, the severity of dysplasia in adenomas followed by serial endoscopy does not significantly progress over 5 to 7 years (37). Since microscopic adenomas can generally be detected within 2 to 3 years of colectomy (44) but carcinomas do not present until 15 to 20 years later (27), it appears that progression from the earliest adenomatous change to invasive carcinoma must occur over many years.

Although the evidence indicates that most ampullary carcinomas arise from adenomas, it is probable that some also arise de novo or from nonpolypoid precursors (flat or micropapillary carcinoma in situ). Extremely small invasive carcinomas have been found with no evidence of a preexisting adenoma. Furthermore, at autopsy, epithelial atypia bordering on severe dysplasia has been observed in the ampullary epithelium in the absence of the architectural features of adenoma (29). More severe atypia is generally found in the distal pancreatobiliary ducts and common channel and may be seen in up to 4 percent of cases (29).

Polyposis

Since ampullary adenomas are common in patients with FAP (or Gardner's syndrome) and are also recognized precursors to invasive adenocarcinoma, it is not surprising that ampullary carcinomas are more frequent in patients with polyposis (16,24,28,37,39). The increase in risk has been estimated to be 100 to 200 fold (27,38, 39), with an estimated lifetime incidence as high as 12 percent (13). Since prophylactic colectomy has reduced the mortality from colonic carcinoma, patients with FAP are at increasingly greater risk for death from ampullary carcinoma (27). Although asymptomatic ampullary adenomas may be detected shortly after the diagnosis of FAP has been established, carcinomas generally are not detected until 15 to 20 years after colectomy, with shorter intervals seen in those patients whose colectomies were performed for carcinoma, as opposed to prophylactically (27). The ampullary carcinomas arising in FAP patients generally occur at a younger age (mean, 45 to 50 years) than in nonpolyposis patients (27,28,39). It is unlikely that all ampullary adenomas in FAP patients progress to carcinoma, as the incidence of ampullary carcinoma in such patients, although much higher than that seen in the general population, is only a fraction of the incidence of adenomas (37). The ampullary carcinomas arising in these patients commonly exhibit areas of residual adenoma; in addition, widespread areas of adenomatous change may be present in the surrounding duodenal mucosa. In one case, adenomas were also found in the common bile duct, duodenum, gallbladder, and pancreatic ducts (31). In some instances mesenteric fibromatoses accompany ampullary carcinomas, also as a manifestation of Gardner's syndrome (34).

Other Neoplasms

Ampullary adenocarcinomas are commonly associated with other malignant tumors: between 10 and 32 percent of patients with ampullary carcinomas have had other primary cancers (19,40,42, 45,50). Based on the data from the Surveillance, Epidemiology, and End Results (SEER) Program, 19.6 percent (167 of 852) of patients with ampullary carcinoma have had second primary neoplasms. In 5 percent, the ampullary carcinoma was diagnosed first; in 14.6 percent the ampullary carcinoma followed another malignant neoplasm. The most frequent association is with colorectal adenocarcinoma. Most commonly, patients with both tumors have FAP, although sporadic associations have also been reported (55). Ampullary carcinomas have also been associated with colorectal carcinomas in patients with the hereditary flat adenoma syndrome (33). Shirai et al. (45) found concurrent superficial gastric adenocarcinomas in 3 of 40 patients undergoing pancreatoduodenectomy for ampullary carcinoma, a potential association which may be specific to Asian patients (53). An increase in ovarian and endometrial carcinomas has also been found (25). Other carcinomas associated with ampullary carcinoma include those of prostate, breast, urinary bladder, lung, endometrium, rectum, lip, and larynx as well as gastrointestinal carcinoid tumors (40,42). Ampullary neoplasms may also be associated with one or more separate papillary tumors of the bile duct (22), intraductal tumors of the pancreatic ducts, or both (36).

Neurofibromatosis

Patients with von Recklinghausen's disease are at risk for a variety of ampullary neoplasms including neurofibromas, carcinoid tumors, and gangliocytic paragangliomas. Ampullary adenocarcinomas have also been reported in these patients (20,30,51).

Miscellaneous Associations

Ampullary carcinoma has been associated with exposure to polycyclic aromatic hydrocarbons and aromatic amino compounds (15). The single case of ampullary carcinoma associated with dermatomyositis/polymyositis may represent a coincidental occurrence, although other malignant tumors have been associated with this condition (49). Cases associated with hemophilia (17), biliary ascariasis (41), and annular pancreas (48) have also been reported. There may be a small increase in the risk of ampullary carcinoma following cholecystectomy (21).

CLINICAL FEATURES

The presenting symptoms of ampullary carcinomas are similar to those of adenomas, although they are generally more pronounced. Biliary obstruction with resultant jaundice is present in 85 percent of patients (56,58,59,61,63, 65), more frequent than in patients with adenomas. The jaundice is usually persistent rather than intermittent (60,64). In contrast to biliary obstruction due to passage of calculi, the biliary obstruction from ampullary neoplasms may be accompanied by a distended, palpable gallbladder (Courvoisier's sign). Although classically described, a palpable gallbladder is an uncommon finding in patients with ampullary carcinoma, being present in only 15 percent of cases (60,64). Gallstones are present in one third of patients (57). Other common symptoms include weight loss and abdominal pain, present in more than half of patients (56,59,62,63,67). Acute pancreatitis is less frequent. Some presenting symptoms are vague, such as indigestion, nausea, or anorexia (60,65,66). Gastrointestinal hemorrhage is generally occult if present.

LABORATORY FINDINGS

The most common laboratory abnormalities encountered in patients with ampullary carcinomas reflect the biliary obstruction. Serum levels of bilirubin, serum glutamic-oxaloacetic transaminase (SGOT), serum glutamic-pyruvic transaminase (SGPT), and alkaline phosphatase are elevated in more than 60 percent of patients (68–70,72), as are lactate dehydrogenase (LDH) levels. Less commonly, the serum albumin is low or the prothrombin time is prolonged, reflecting impaired liver function (73). Nearly half of patients are anemic, a finding often accompanied by guaiac positive stools (73). One case of an ampullary carcinoma with elevated serum alpha-fetoprotein has been reported (71).

DIAGNOSTIC CONSIDERATIONS

Radiographic and Endoscopic Findings

Preoperative evaluation of putative ampullary carcinomas seeks to confirm the presence of a neoplastic process, and to distinguish ampullary or duodenal tumors from carcinomas of the head of the pancreas or common bile duct because the resectability rate varies between these different tumors (from 85 percent for ampullary carcinoma to 22 percent for pancreatic carcinoma [83,90]). In patients with symptoms suggesting a tumor in the region of the head of the pancreas or periampullary area, endoscopy is particularly helpful in establishing a diagnosis. In roughly two thirds of cases, ampullary and duodenal neoplasms are visible endoscopically as exophytic or ulcerated masses (91). Tumors contained within the ampulla appear as a prominent submucosal bulge (84). In patients with FAP there are usually numerous additional small polyps throughout the duodenum (see fig. 19-2). Features of ampullary tumors which should suggest the presence of carcinoma include ulceration or erosion, hemorrhage, necrosis, and a firm or friable consistency (74).

Endoscopic retrograde cholangiopancreatography (ERCP) is also useful for the study of ampullary lesions and their separation from pancreatic and bile duct tumors (90). An accuracy rate of greater than 90 percent for the diagnosis and origin of tumors in this region has been reported (82,90). However, technical factors limit the ability to perform a satisfactory ERCP in 22 percent of patients with suspected periampullary carcinoma (82). Most ampullary neoplasms can be visualized endoscopically, obviating the need for ERCP unless the tumor is covered by intact duodenal mucosa.

Endoscopic ultrasonography (EUS) is effective in the preoperative staging and assessment of resectability of ampullary carcinomas (80,89,92). Tumor size and presence of extramural invasion was correctly assessed significantly more frequently with EUS (78 percent of cases [89]) than with computed tomography (CT) or abdominal ultrasonography (92). Abdominal ultrasound often reveals dilated bile ducts and a distended gallbladder (88); however, the ampullary tumor may not be visualized (76,91). Pancreatic ductal dilatation may also be observed. CT scanning is relatively insensitive for detecting ampullary neoplasms (85,86), which are visualized in only 44 percent of cases (87). Like abdominal ultrasound, secondary dilatation of the pancreatic and biliary ducts may be the only finding (76).

Recently, preoperative laparoscopy has been used to search for signs of unresectability such as metastatic disease or invasion of major vessels (78).

Cytology

Endoscopically obtained cytologic brushings help establish a diagnosis of ampullary carcinoma. The cytologic appearance of normal ampullary lining cells differs from that of the overlying intestinal epithelium. Goblet cells are not generally present, although the apical cytoplasm may show some vacuolation, and there is no obvious brush border (94). The cells appear cylindrical with large oval nuclei; clusters form monolayers with evenly positioned nuclei. Variable degrees of cytologic atypia may be present, including variation in shape and size of nuclei and prominent nucleoli, which often represent reactive atypia on biopsy.

In cytologic brushings of ampullary adenocarcinomas, the cells form three-dimensional clusters or small tubules and exhibit marked cell to cell variation in nuclear size and shape. Multiple prominent nucleoli may be present. Although inadequate sampling may limit the accuracy of cytologic brushings, the problem is less common than with endoscopic biopsy. Fine needle aspiration has also been used to confirm the malignant nature of ampullary tumors; it may be employed either percutaneously or intraoperatively and is associated with fewer complications than core needle or wedge biopsies (79,81).

Biopsy

Largely because of sampling error, endoscopic biopsy has an accuracy rate of only 85 percent in diagnosing ampullary carcinoma (74,95), although multiple biopsies and serial sectioning increases the yield to greater than 90 percent (87). Intra-ampullary carcinomas are covered by intact duodenal mucosa, which makes it difficult to reach the tumor. Also, in 25 to 50 percent of cases biopsy material discloses only adenoma

when deeper portions of the lesion contain invasive carcinoma (74,93,95). For intra-ampullary tumors an endoscopic papillotomy may help access the tumor (84,87,91,95). It is important for the pathologist to note the time interval between papillotomy and biopsy since biopsies of non-neoplastic ampullae taken 2 days after papillotomy have shown significant cytologic atypia, mimicking carcinoma (75). Snare biopsies yield more tissue than forceps biopsies and may therefore be more sensitive in detecting adenocarcinoma within an adenoma (91).

Cytoarchitecturally, malignant glandular epithelium may be seen as detached fragments in endoscopic biopsies. It may be difficult to determine whether these are from portions of an adenoma with severe dysplasia or represent fragments of an invasive carcinoma. The endoscopic appearance of the lesion in such cases may suggest the correct interpretation (74).

Intraoperative biopsy may provide a diagnosis if preoperative biopsies are nondiagnostic. Although core needle biopsy is not indicated for ampullary tumors, open wedge biopsy through a duodenotomy has an accuracy rate approaching 90 percent (77).

PATHOLOGIC FEATURES

Ampullary carcinomas are often small because their location tends to result in early symptoms and detection: 17 percent are less than 1 cm (96) and more than 75 percent are less than 4 cm (99) at presentation. The common bile duct is almost always dilated (96). In half the cases the pancreatic duct is also dilated.

The gross appearance of ampullary carcinoma often depends on the site of origin of the tumor. Most exhibit an exophytic component, often representing a residual adenoma. With larger tumors, it may be difficult to determine the origin (i.e., ampulla versus periampullary duodenum versus distal common bile duct, etc.).

Several gross classification schemes have been proposed. Cubilla and Fitzgerald (97) divided tumors by site of origin into intra-ampullary, periampullary, and mixed (fig. 20-2). Intra-ampullary tumors are largely confined within the ampulla, with minimal surface involvement. As such, they are generally smaller than the other types. Periampullary tumors involve largely the mucosa of

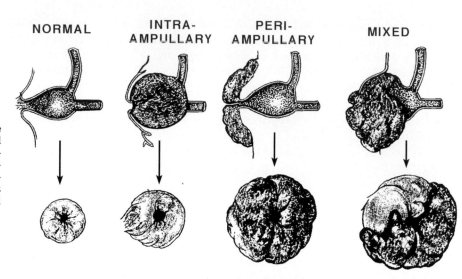

Figure 20-2
GROSS CLASSIFICATION
SYSTEM FOR AMPULLARY
CARCINOMAS DEVISED BY
CUBILLA AND FITZGERALD
Intra-ampullary tumors are
confined within the ampulla and
do not involve the overlying duodenal mucosa of the papilla. Periampullary tumors involve the papillary duodenal mucosa but do not
extend into the ampulla. Mixed
tumors exhibit features of both.

the periampullary duodenum and the luminal
surface of the papilla, whereas mixed tumors com-
bine features of both types. Presumably, once an
intra-ampullary or periampullary tumor enlarges to
involve the respective adjacent structure, it becomes
a mixed type. In the series of Cubilla and Fitzgerald,
61 percent of 33 tumors were intra-ampullary, 24
percent were periampullary, and 15 percent were
mixed. Although this system does allow classification of most gross tumor types encountered in this
region, and there appears to be some relationship
with outcome (see below), the term "periampullary"
is somewhat confusing because it has been applied
to all tumors of the ampullary region. Perhaps
"periampullary duodenal" would be a more specific
designation for this gross configuration.

An alternative classification has been proposed by Tasaka (98) and utilized by Yamaguchi
and Enjoji (100). This classification is based on
the appearance from the duodenal aspect. Tumors with no duodenal luminal component are
intramural protruding; those with a polypoid
configuration, with tumor exposed to the duodenal
lumen, are exposed protruding; those with a central crater-like ulcer are ulcerating. Among 104
cases, 23 percent were intramural protruding, 38.5
percent were exposed protruding, and 38.5 percent
were ulcerated (100). It is not specified in an
exposed protruding tumor whether the involvement is limited to the periampullary duodenum
and papilla or whether there is growth into the
ampulla as well. In comparing this scheme with

that of Cubilla and Fitzgerald (97), it appears
that the intra-ampullary and intramural protruding types are similar; once again, the intramural protruding tumors are the smallest. Most
of the ulcerating and some of the exposed protruding types of Tasaka would be included under
mixed type of Cubilla and Fitzgerald, whereas
most of the periampullary tumors of Cubilla and
Fitzgerald would be included with the exposed
protruding tumors of Tasaka. It is unclear why
the series of cases studied by Cubilla and Fitzgerald contained more intra-ampullary (intramural protruding) tumors (61 percent) than did
that of Yamaguchi and Enjoji (23 percent).

We believe that a combination of the two
schemes outlined above best describes the gross
features that are encountered in tumors of the
periampullary region. We propose four descriptive types: intra-ampullary, periampullary duodenal, mixed exophytic, and mixed ulcerated (fig.
20-3). This classification combines both the appearance from the duodenal lumen as well as the
extent of involvement of the ampulla and periampullary duodenum as determined by cross
sections. A comparison of this classification with
those of Tasaka and of Cubilla and Fitzgerald is
shown in Table 20-2. In our cases, 24 percent of 116
ampullary carcinomas were intra-ampullary, 6
percent were periampullary duodenal, 31 percent
were mixed exophytic, and 39 percent were mixed
ulcerated. Representative gross examples of
each type are shown in figures 20-4–20-9.

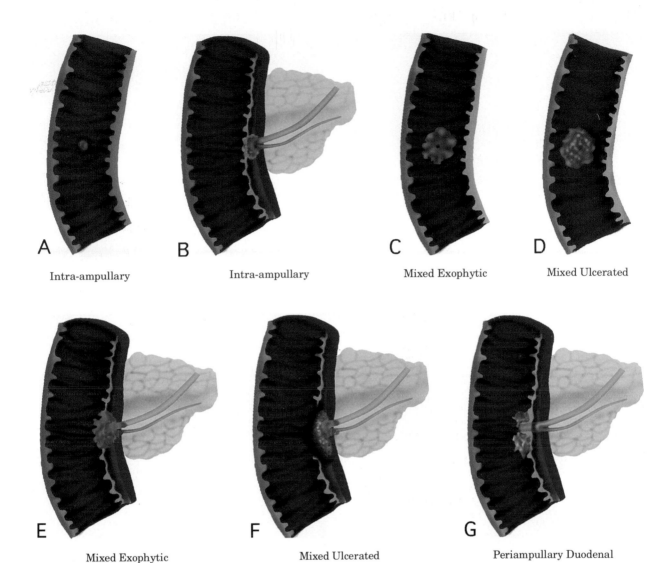

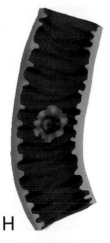

Periampullary
Duodenal

Figure 20-3
SCHEMATIC ILLUSTRATION OF GROSS CLASSIFICATION
OF TUMORS IN THE PERIAMPULLARY REGION

A: From the luminal aspect, intra-ampullary tumors appear as a prominent submucosal bulge underlying the ampullary orifice, which is covered by intact duodenal mucosa.

B: On cut section, intra-ampullary tumors fill the ampulla and may extend into the distal pancreatic and biliary ducts.

C: Mixed exophytic tumors are polyploid lesions projecting into the duodenal lumen.

D: From the luminal aspect, mixed ulcerated tumors exhibit a more flattened configuration than mixed exophytic tumors, with central ulceration and raised edges.

E: On cut section, mixed exophytic tumors also involve the ampulla and may extend into the distal ducts.

F: Often the ampullary orifice is visible within the bed of the ulcer. Mixed ulcerated tumors replace the ampulla on cut section and tend to be larger and more infiltrative than intra-ampullary or mixed exophytic types.

G: On cut section, the tumor surrounds the ampulla and distal ducts but does not involve their lumens.

H: Periampullary duodenal tumors surround the ampulla but do not involve it. From the luminal aspect they may be either exophytic or ulcerated, and the lack of ampullary involvement may be difficult to discern.

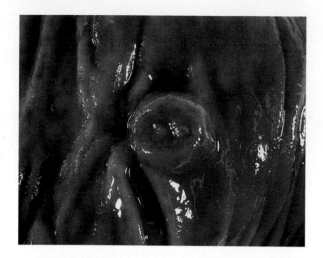
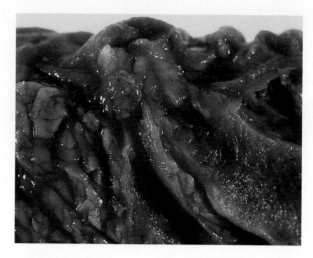

Figure 20-4
INTRA-AMPULLARY CARCINOMA
Left: This intra-ampullary carcinoma is small, producing only slight prominence to the ampulla from the luminal aspect. Minimal tumor is visible through the ampullary orifice.
Right: On cut section, the intact duodenal mucosa overlies the tumor, which appears confined within the ampulla.

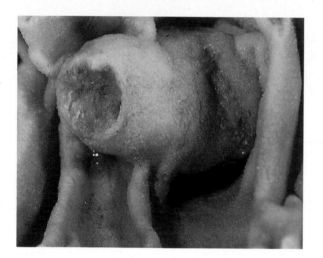
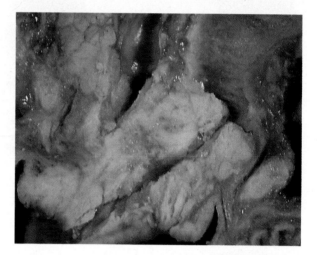

Figure 20-5
INTRA-AMPULLARY CARCINOMA
Left: This larger carcinoma has remained intra-ampullary, with extensive expansion resulting in a finger-like projection into the duodenum.
Right: Cut section demonstrates that most of the tumor is confined within the ampulla and distal common bile duct. (Courtesy of Prof. Gunter Klöppel, Kiel, Germany.)

Microscopic whole mount preparations, which include longitudinal sections of the biliary and pancreatic ducts as well as the ampulla, duodenal wall, and head of pancreas, may also help to illustrate the relationship of ampullary tumors to surrounding structures; some examples are shown in figures 20-10–20-13. It is important to separate primary duodenal carcinomas from periampullary carcinomas, although in some cases it may be very difficult. All of the tumors classified as periampullary duodenal, mixed exophytic, and mixed ulcerated involve the duodenal mucosa and wall to some extent. However, these tumors are generally centered on the ampulla or extensively involve it. When the tumor involves predominantly the duodenum with only

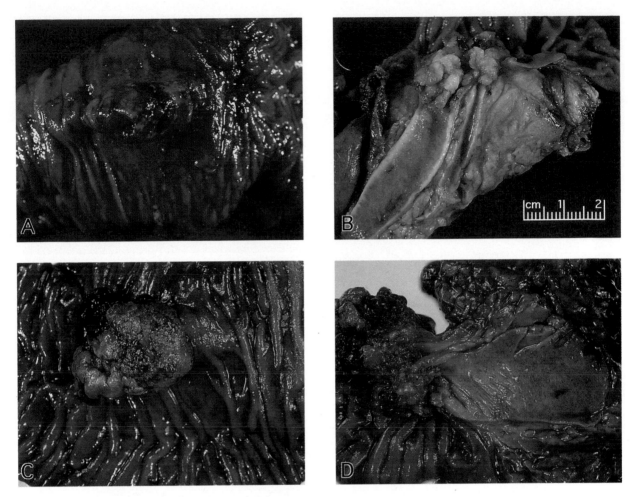

Figure 20-6
MIXED EXOPHYTIC TUMOR

A: From the luminal aspect, the ampulla is replaced by a polyploid tumor grossly involving the duodenal mucosa of the papilla; there is no gross ulceration.

B: Cut section shows the extension of this exophytic tumor into the ampulla and distal ducts.

C: A mixed exophytic tumor with a prominent component of papillary adenoma imparts a granular, bosselated appearance.

D: The papillary nature of this tumor is evident on cut section. The tumor fills the ampulla and dilates the common bile duct.

Table 20-2

COMPARISON OF GROSS CLASSIFICATION SCHEMES FOR AMPULLARY CARCINOMA

Cubilla and Fitzgerald (97)	Tasaka (98)	Proposed
Intra-ampullary	Intramural protruding	Intra-ampullary Intra-ampullary
Periampullary	Exposed protruding	Periampullary duodenal
Mixed		Mixed exophytic
	Ulcerating	Mixed ulcerated

focal peripheral extension into the ampulla, it is best regarded as a duodenal primary. Less commonly, a tumor of the very distal common bile duct may extend into the ampulla; again, the center of the tumor as determined by evaluation of gross or microscopic whole mount preparations can be used as the presumptive site of origin. In some cases, however, microscopic examination may provide conflicting evidence, since in a single case residual adenomatous epithelium may be found in several different locations (e.g., in the duodenum, ampulla, and distal common bile duct) (fig. 20-14). Truly multifocal involvement of the pancreatobiliary tree and ampulla by either papillary

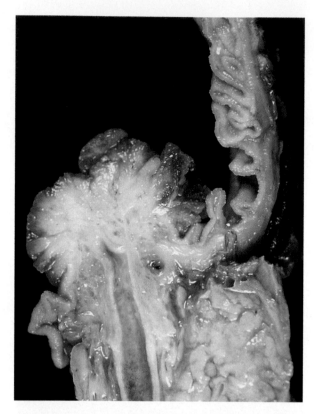

Figure 20-7
EXOPHYTIC MUCINOUS CARCINOMA

This exophytic mucinous carcinoma involves the ampulla and duodenal mucosa but also extends into the common bile duct.

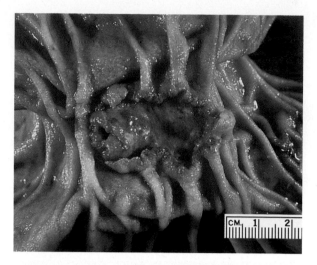

Figure 20-8
PERIAMPULLARY ULCERATED TUMOR

A periampullary ulcerated tumor is seen with the ampullary orifice to the left of the lesion.

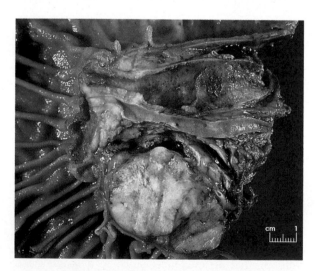

Figure 20-9
EXOPHYTIC MUCINOUS CARCINOMA

Cut section of the tumor in figure 20-8 shows patent pancreatic and biliary ducts which are compressed by the tumor, resulting in marked dilatation of the common bile duct. A large peripancreatic lymph node metastasis is present.

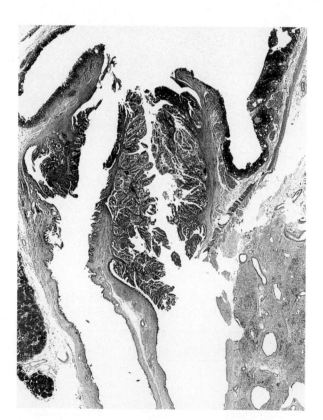

Figure 20-10
MICROSCOPIC WHOLE MOUNT PREPARATION
OF AN INTRA-AMPULLARY CARCINOMA

The tumor is predominantly within the ampulla and distal ducts and has an exophytic, papillary configuration.

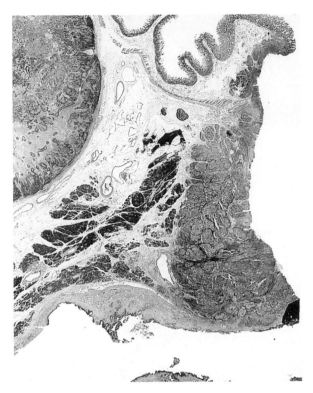

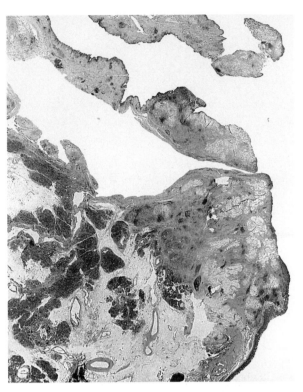

Figure 20-11
PERIAMPULLARY DUODENAL CARCINOMA
This periampullary duodenal carcinoma forms a large ulcerated mass compressing but not obliterating the pancreatic duct, not entirely visualized in this plane of section, and the common bile duct. A residual tubular adenoma is present at the orifice of the common bile duct.

Figure 20-12
PERIAMPULLARY DUODENAL CARCINOMA
In this periampullary duodenal carcinoma, the patency of the ducts is obvious. The tumor invades through the wall of the duodenum into the underlying pancreatic parenchyma.

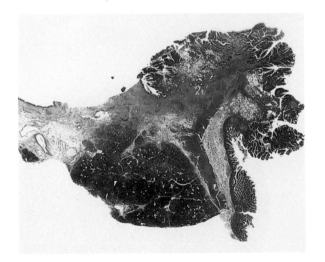

Figure 20-13
MIXED EXOPHYTIC TUMOR
This cross section through a mixed exophytic tumor demonstrates papillary tumor extending into the duodenum (right) as well as into the ampulla on the opposite side of the duodenal muscularis propria (top). A longitudinal section of the distal common bile duct is seen at right.

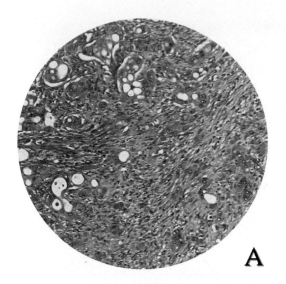

A

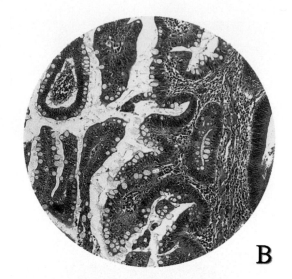

B

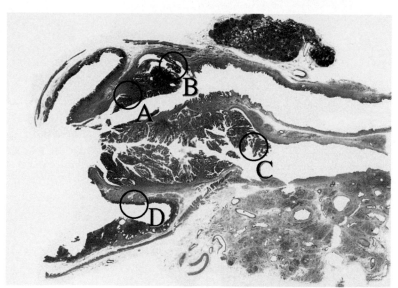

Figure 20-14
INTRA-AMPULLARY CARCINOMA
Multiple foci of adenomatous epithelium surround this intra-ampullary carcinoma and involve the duodenum, bile duct, and pancreatic duct (insets A-D). However, the tumor is centered within the ampulla, where the only invasive carcinoma is present.

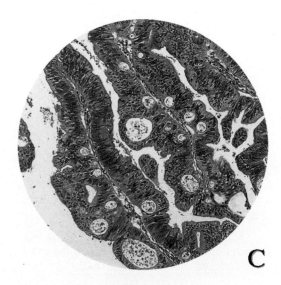

C

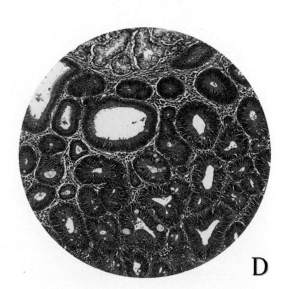

D

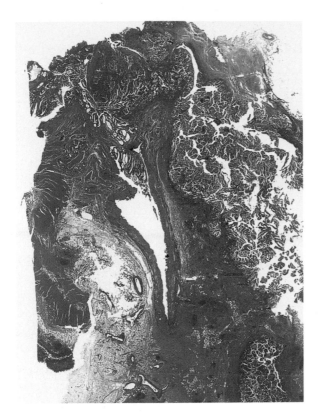

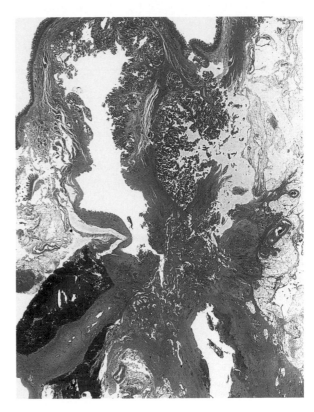

Figure 20-15
MULTICENTRIC TUMOROUS INVOLVEMENT OF THE PANCREATOBILIARY TREE AND AMPULLA
Left: In this example, an invasive carcinoma has developed within the ampulla (top) whereas the pancreatic duct (left) and common bile duct (center) contain only noninvasive papillary tumor.
Right: Conversely, in this example, an invasive carcinoma has developed surrounding the pancreatic duct while the ampulla and bile duct exhibit only papillary tumors.

neoplasms, invasive carcinomas, or both, may also occur (figs. 20-15, 20-16).

MICROSCOPIC FEATURES

Distribution of Histologic Types

Many different histologic types of carcinoma arise in the ampulla, most of which share a gross appearance, clinical features, and natural history. The most common tumor type is adenocarcinoma, which constitutes more than 90 percent of ampullary carcinomas. Table 20-3 shows the distribution of histologic types based on data obtained from the SEER Program of the National Cancer Institute. Table 20-4 shows the different types from our material. Although not all of the terms used for the various entities are identical, there are similar frequencies for most of the histologic types.

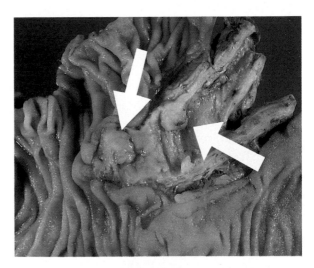

Figure 20-16
CARCINOMAS OF THE
AMPULLA AND COMMON BILE DUCT
Two grossly separate invasive carcinomas involve the ampulla and common bile duct.

Table 20-3

HISTOLOGIC DISTRIBUTION FOR CANCERS OF THE AMPULLA OF VATER, 1982–1991*

Histologic Types	Number of Patients	Percent of Total	Males	Percent of Total	Females	Percent of Total
Carcinoma in situ	22	2.58	12	2.68	10	2.48
Adenocarcinoma, NOS	625	73.36	324	72.32	301	74.5
Papillary adenocarcinoma	83	9.74	41	9.15	42	10.4
Adenocarcinoma, intestinal type	0	0	0	0	0	0
Mucinous adenocarcinoma	33	3.87	16	3.57	17	4.21
Clear cell carcinoma	0	0	0	0	0	0
Signet ring cell carcinoma	4	0.47	2	0.45	2	0.5
Adenosquamous carcinoma	3	0.35	3	0.67	0	0
Squamous cell carcinoma	1	0.12	0	0	1	0.25
Small cell carcinoma	2	0.23	2	0.45	0	0
Adenocarcinoma in villous adenoma	51	5.99	31	6.92	20	4.95
Cholangiocarcinoma	2	0.23	1	0.22	1	0.25
Infiltrating duct carcinoma	7	0.82	3	0.67	4	0.99
Undifferentiated carcinoma	3	0.35	3	0.67	0	0
Total	**836**	**98.12**	**438**	**97.77**	**398**	**98.51**
Carcinoid tumors	3	0.35	1	0.22	2	0.5
Mixed carcinoid-adenocarcinoma	1	0.12	0	0	1	0.25
Total	**4**	**0.47**	**1**	**0.22**	**3**	**0.74**
Sarcoma, NOS	1	0.12	1	0.22	0	0
Rhabdomyosarcoma	0	0	0	0	0	0
Kaposi's sarcoma	0	0	0	0	0	0
Leiomyosarcoma	0	0	0	0	0	0
Malignant fibrous histiocytoma	0	0	0	0	0	0
Angiosarcoma	0	0	0	0	0	0
Total	**1**	**0.12**	**1**	**0.22**	**0**	**0**
Carcinosarcoma	0	0	0	0	0	0
Malignant melanoma	0	0	0	0	0	0
Malignant lymphoma	3	0.35	2	0.45	1	0.25
Others, NOS	8	0.94	6	1.34	2	0.5
Total Invasive	**830**	**97.42**	**436**	**97.32**	**394**	**97.52**
Total Invasive and In Situ	**852**	**100**	**448**	**100**	**404**	**100**

*Data from the Surveillance, Epidemiology, and End Results Program, National Cancer Institute.

Adenocarcinoma. The majority of adenocarcinomas arising in the ampulla are predominantly gland forming (tubular). Within this group, some tumors resemble those of the intestines, while others resemble adenocarcinomas of the pancreas and bile ducts (105,108,110). These variations of histologic appearance presumably reflect the fact that the ampullary region contains several types of epithelium which may give rise to different tumor types. Unfortunately, by the time most of these tumors are detected, they are already too large to determine precisely the epithelium of origin for correlation with the histologic appearance.

Intestinal Type Adenocarcinoma. Most ampullary carcinomas resemble the intestinal type adenocarcinoma of the small and large intestines; more than 85 percent of ampullary carcinomas are classified as intestinal type (102, 109,113). Recognition that some ampullary adenocarcinomas resemble tumors of the pancreas and bile ducts has lead to a reclassification of some tubular adenocarcinomas as pancreatobiliary type (105). When these and other subtypes are considered, approximately half of ampullary adenocarcinomas specifically resemble intestinal adenocarcinomas (Table 20-4).

The histologic appearance of intestinal type adenocarcinoma is essentially indistinguishable from that of tumors of the colorectum (fig. 20-17). In well-differentiated examples, well-formed tubular to elongate glands infiltrate a desmoplastic stroma. Complex cribriformed areas and solid nests may be present. Solid areas predominate in poorly differentiated examples. The glands and cribriform nests characteristically exhibit central necrosis and aggregates of inflammatory cells. The individual cells are columnar and the nuclei are oval and arranged in a pseudostratified configuration in the more basal aspects of the cytoplasm. Although there may be considerable nuclear atypia, the nuclei of adjacent cells generally resemble one another. Variable numbers of mitoses are present. A well-defined brush border often lines the lumina, and interspersed goblet cells may be seen. The amount of desmoplastic stroma varies and is occasionally abundant. Perineural or vascular invasion may be present. Intestinal type adenocarcinomas may produce neutral mucins as well as sialomucins and, less commonly, sulphomucins (106,111).

Areas of residual adenoma may be found within the ampulla, in the surrounding duodenal mucosa, or in both locations. Flat adenomatous changes may also be present in the distal bile duct or pancreatic duct (113). In cases having an adenomatous component with severe dysplasia it may be difficult to determine at what point the tumor is invasive (figs. 20-18–20-20). Involvement of the periampullary ductules by the adenomatous epithelium results in a complex pseudoinfiltrative pattern at the basal aspect of the adenoma obscuring the transition from the adenoma to invasive carcinoma.

Table 20-4

DISTRIBUTION OF HISTOLOGIC TYPES OF AMPULLARY CARCINOMA AT MSKCC*

	No.	(%)
Adenocarcinoma	129	(92)
Intestinal type	69	(49)
Pancreatobiliary type	29	(21)
Poorly differentiated adenocarcinoma	4	(3)
Invasive papillary carcinoma	9	(6)
Mucinous (colloid) carcinoma	15	(11)
Signet ring cell carcinoma	3	(2)
Clear cell carcinoma	0	
Adenosquamous carcinoma	3	(2)
Neuroendocrine carcinoma	3	(2)
Small cell carcinoma	1	(1)
Large cell neuroendocrine carcinoma	2	(2)
Undifferentiated carcinoma	5	(4)
(Not otherwise specified)	3	(2)
With neuroendocrine features	2	(1)
Spindle cell type	0	
Osteoclastic giant cell type	0	
Total cases	**140**	**(100)**

*MSKCC - Memorial Sloan-Kettering Cancer Center.

Pancreatobiliary Type Adenocarcinoma. Pancreatobiliary type adenocarcinomas closely resemble primary tumors of the pancreas or extrahepatic bile ducts. Tumors with this pattern comprise 22 percent of ampullary adenocarcinomas (105). Pancreatobiliary type adenocarcinomas have simple or branching glands and small solid nests of cells surrounded by a strikingly desmoplastic stroma (figs. 20-21, 20-22). Focal papillary and micropapillary formations may be present (110). Necrotic luminal debris is not commonly present. The cuboidal to low columnar cells are generally arranged in a single layer, without nuclear pseudostratification. The nuclei are more rounded than those of intestinal type tumors and often show marked variation in size and shape from one cell to the next. A high degree of nuclear pleomorphism in the presence of architecturally well-formed glands is a characteristic feature (fig. 20-22C). In more poorly differentiated examples, single and small clusters of

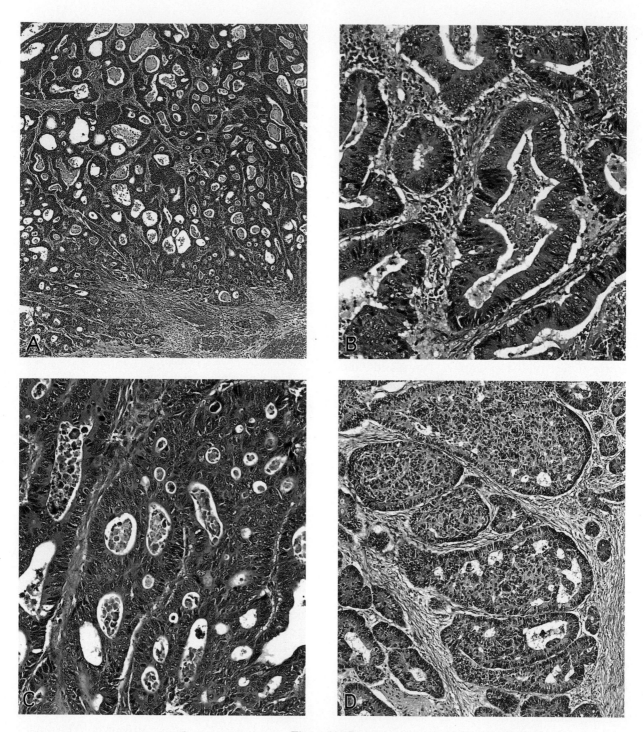

Figure 20-17

HISTOLOGIC APPEARANCE OF INTESTINAL TYPE ADENOCARCINOMA

A: At low power, the tumor has a cribriformed appearance and contains modest amounts of stroma. Nests of carcinoma invade between fascicles of smooth muscle comprising the sphincter of Oddi (bottom). The histologic appearance is indistinguishable from primary adenocarcinoma of the large bowel.

B: In well-differentiated examples, tubular glands are lined by pseudostratified cells containing elongated nuclei. Necrotic debris is present in the gland lumens.

C: Large cribriformed nests of cells are present.

D: In moderately differentiated examples, there are more solid nests but luminal spaces are readily apparent; the nests are relatively large and circumscribed.

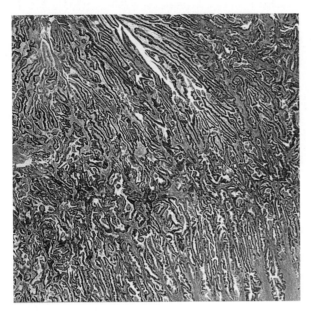

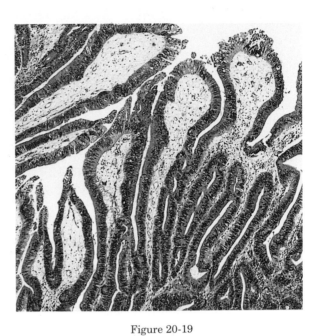

Figure 20-18
GRADUAL EVOLUTION OF INVASIVE
CARCINOMA WITHIN AN AMPULLARY ADENOMA
At low power this tumor is a carcinoma that invades into
duodenal muscularis propria.

Figure 20-19
INVASIVE CARCINOMA
The superficial portions of the lesion consist of papillary
adenoma, with simple papillae lined by mildly to moderately
dysplastic epithelium.

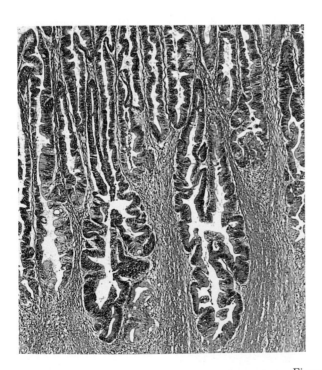

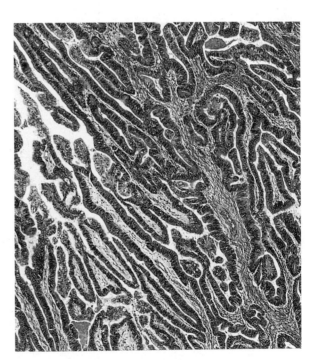

Figure 20-20
GRADUAL EVOLUTION OF INVASIVE CARCINOMA WITHIN AN AMPULLARY ADENOMA
Left: Deep aspect of the lesion shown on figure 20-18 consists of invasive carcinoma extending into the muscularis propria;
individual infiltrative glands are present.
Right: Sections from the central portion of the tumor display intermediate features between those of the adenoma and the
invasive carcinoma, emphasizing the gradual nature of the morphologic transition. The exact point at which the tumor becomes
invasive is unclear.

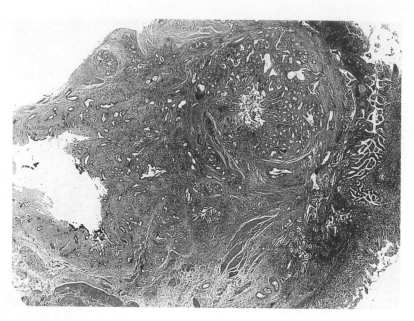

Figure 20-21
PANCREATOBILIARY TYPE
AMPULLARY ADENOCARCINOMA
This pancreatobiliary type ampullary adenocarcinoma has an intra-ampullary location and consists of well-formed glands in a densely sclerotic stroma surrounding the lumina of the ampulla and distal common bile duct.

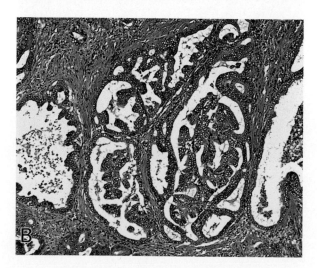

Figure 20-22
PANCREATOBILIARY TYPE ADENOCARCINOMA
A: The tumor consists of simple or branching glands surrounded by a markedly fibrotic and desmoplastic stroma. The glands are lined by a single layer of cells, in this case with abundant apical mucinous cytoplasm.
B: Some glands contain micropapillary formations.
C: Severe nuclear atypia in the presence of architecturally well-formed glands is a characteristic feature of this tumor.

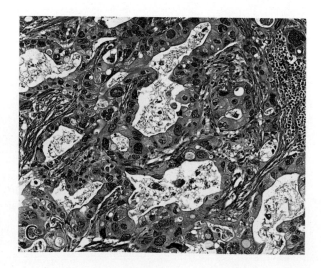

cells are found. The juxtaposition of very well-formed glands and bizarre individual tumor cells is common (fig. 20-23). Perineural invasion is common; vascular invasion is less frequent.

Some ampullary tumors exhibit mixed features of both intestinal and pancreatobiliary type adenocarcinomas. The distinction between the two patterns becomes more difficult in less differentiated examples. These tumors should be classified as intestinal type unless the pancreatobiliary pattern predominates (105).

Because the invasive component of pancreatobiliary type ampullary carcinoma may exhibit papillary formations, especially in better differentiated examples, many authors have designated these tumors as "papillary carcinomas" (102,113). This term may cause confusion, however, because its use for tumors of the bile ducts and pancreas generally refers to tumors with an exophytic, noninvasive growth pattern. If "papillary carcinoma" is used to refer to invasive carcinomas, the specific descriptor "invasive" must be used (see below).

Well-differentiated pancreatobiliary type carcinomas exhibiting remarkably well-formed simple glands may be difficult to distinguish from non-neoplastic periampullary ductules (fig. 20-24). Areas of residual adenoma or flat carcinoma in situ may be associated with pancreatobiliary type adenocarcinomas.

Some ampullary adenocarcinomas may be too poorly differentiated to permit subclassification. In our material, 4 of 129 (3 percent) adenocarcinomas were regarded as "poorly differentiated." There were no differences in clinical or gross features relative to other ampullary adenocarcinomas. Histologically, poorly differentiated adenocarcinomas grow in solid sheets and nests, often resulting in a highly cellular appearance under low-power microscopy (fig. 20-25). The cells vary in size, generally with marked nuclear atypia and abundant mitoses. Necrosis is often present. Gland formation, although focal and often poorly developed, is present, distinguishing these tumors from poorly differentiated carcinomas. Mucicarmine stains the glandular spaces and may also reveal intracellular mucin. Poorly differentiated adenocarcinoma also resembles high-grade neuroendocrine carcinoma, large cell type, a tumor which may also have focal glandular differentiation. Immunohistochemical stain

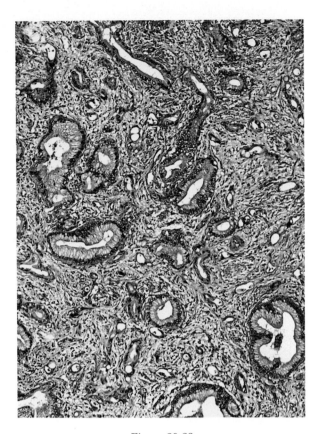

Figure 20-23
PANCREATOBILIARY ADENOCARCINOMA
Pancreatobiliary adenocarcinoma exhibits juxtaposed well-formed glands and individual markedly atypical tumor cells.

ing for neuroendocrine markers (chromogranin, synaptophysin, and neuron-specific enolase) is negative in most cells of poorly differentiated adenocarcinomas; however, scattered positive cells may be present as they are in other types of ampullary adenocarcinoma.

Immunohistochemical Staining

Endocrine cells are commonly found in typical ampullary adenocarcinomas. Although they may not be evident by routine microscopy, immunohistochemical staining for chromogranin reveals scattered endocrine cells in 33 percent of cases, and occasionally they are numerous (fig. 20-26). They are more common in intestinal type or mucinous adenocarcinomas than in pancreatobiliary type tumors (110), and are more frequent in better differentiated examples. The distribution of endocrine cells is random; in some cases

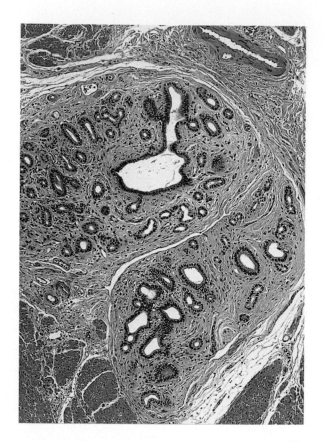 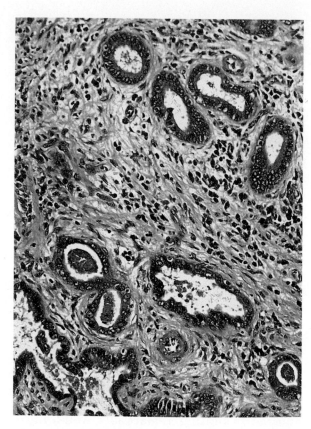

Figure 20-24

NON-NEOPLASTIC PERIAMPULLARY DUCTULES IN WELL-DIFFERENTIATED PANCREATOBILIARY TYPE
ADENOCARCINOMA

Left: Periampullary ductules have a lobular configuration, with central branched, ectatic ductules surrounded by smaller tubular ductules.

Right: Side by side comparison of benign ductules (top) and well-differentiated adenocarcinoma (bottom) emphasizes the cytologic uniformity of the former and the subtle variation in nuclear morphology from cell to cell in the latter.

they are scattered evenly throughout the tumor whereas in other cases they are clustered. These cells are indeed neoplastic, since they are not concentrated in portions of the tumor near the lumen of the duodenum or within the head of the pancreas, regions where residual entrapped non-neoplastic endocrine cells might be expected. In fact, endocrine cells may even be found in metastatic deposits, effectively excluding the possibility of entrapment.

Although well-developed Paneth cell differentiation is common in ampullary adenomas, fully granulated Paneth cells are abundant in only rare cases of invasive adenocarcinoma (fig. 20-27) (107). However, scattered cells with small numbers of granules may be detected in intestinal type carcinomas (especially in well-differentiated examples) at a greater frequency than in

their colorectal counterparts (101). Paneth cells are not detected in pancreatobiliary type carcinomas (110). Immunohistochemical staining for muramidase is helpful in identifying Paneth cell differentiation (107) and is at least focally positive in 80 percent of intestinal type tumors (110).

Staining of normal ampullary or duodenal mucosa for monoclonal carcinoembryonic antigen (CEA) reveals only focal, minimal staining of luminal membranes in occasional cases. In adenomas there is increased intensity of the luminal membrane (paralleling the distribution of the glycocalyx), with faint cytoplasmic staining as well. With increasing dysplasia, the intensity of the cytoplasmic staining increases. In invasive carcinomas there is a diffuse, intense cytoplasmic reaction for CEA, often with diffusion of the reaction product into the stroma

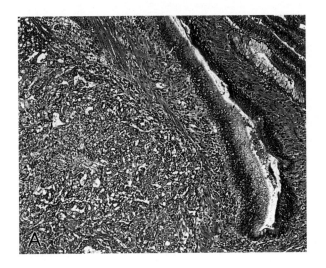

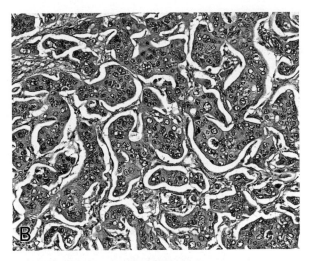

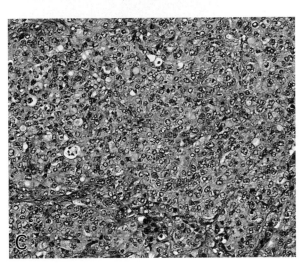

Figure 20-25
POORLY DIFFERENTIATED ADENOCARCINOMA

A: At low power, this poorly differentiated adenocarcinoma is highly cellular and contains minimal stroma. This example is associated with an intestinal type adenoma (right).

B: The poorly differentiated adenocarcinoma exhibits a nesting growth pattern, with marked nuclear pleomorphism and rare luminal formations.

C: This example has a sheet-like growth pattern, with extreme nuclear atypia, individual cell necrosis, and abundant mitoses.

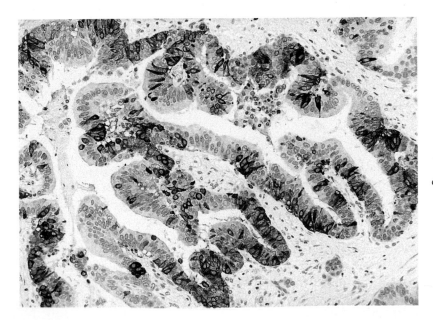

Figure 20-26
ENDOCRINE CELLS IN
AMPULLARY ADENOCARCINOMAS
Abundant chromogranin-positive cells are present in this adenocarcinoma.

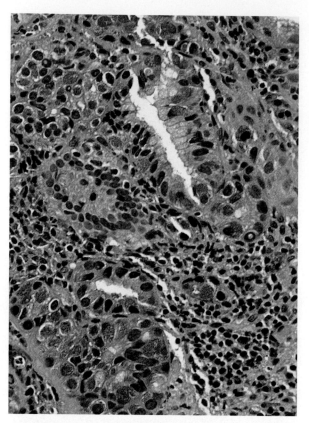

Figure 20-27
PANETH CELL DIFFERENTIATION IN
INTESTINAL TYPE ADENOCARCINOMA
The Paneth cells are characterized by coarsely granular
eosinophilic cytoplasm.

(104,110,112,114). Approximately 75 percent of invasive carcinomas show moderate to intense staining. Intestinal type adenocarcinomas are more likely to stain than pancreatobiliary type, as are well and moderately differentiated tumors (103); poorly differentiated tumors exhibit focal or no staining in 50 percent of cases. Most ampullary carcinomas also stain for the carbohydrate antigen CA19-9 (114,115).

Antibodies against DUPAN-2 recognize a glycoprotein expressed by pancreatic ductal cells but absent in intestinal epithelium. Overall, 58 percent of invasive ampullary carcinomas and 25 percent of adenomas express DUPAN-2. Pancreatobiliary type carcinomas are more frequently positive (88 percent of cases) than intestinal type tumors (42 percent of cases). There is no relationship to grade.

Ultrastructural Features

By electron microscopy, intestinal type adenocarcinomas resemble their more common large bowel counterparts. In well- and moderately differentiated examples, the cells have well-formed lumens lined by tall microvilli that are covered by a glycocalyx (fig. 20-28). Long rootlets extend from the base of the microvilli into the apical cytoplasm. The nuclei are basally situated and mucigen granules may be detected in the cytoplasm (fig. 20-28). A basement membrane surrounds each gland or nest of cells. The more poorly differentiated examples may exhibit loss of polarity. Luminal spaces are not as well formed and the microvilli and mucigen granules may be more sparse.

The ultrastructural features of pancreatobiliary type ampullary carcinomas have not been described.

UNUSUAL HISTOLOGIC TYPES OF AMPULLARY CARCINOMA

Papillary Carcinoma (Noninvasive)

Noninvasive papillary carcinomas of the ampulla are exophytic tumors arising in the intraampullary mucosa and resembling the nonintestinal, pancreatobiliary types of papillary neoplasms of the pancreatic or bile ducts. Although pancreatobiliary type papillary carcinomas are probably related to intestinal type adenomas and both represent precursors to invasive carcinoma, they differ histologically and presumably reflect origin from different portions of the periampullary epithelium.

Terminology for these papillary tumors is not standardized and reflects that used for analogous tumors affecting the adjacent epithelia of the duodenum as well as the pancreatic and bile ducts. In the pancreas and bile ducts these pancreatobiliary type exophytic tumors have been classified in a single group, despite the intestinal features of most cases, as intraductal papillary-mucinous neoplasms in the pancreas (133,135, 140) and papillary carcinomas, papillary adenomas, or papillomatosis in the bile ducts. In the intestinal tract, increasing atypia within papillary adenomas does not justify the diagnosis of carcinoma and is designated as increasing degrees of dysplasia. In the pancreas and bile

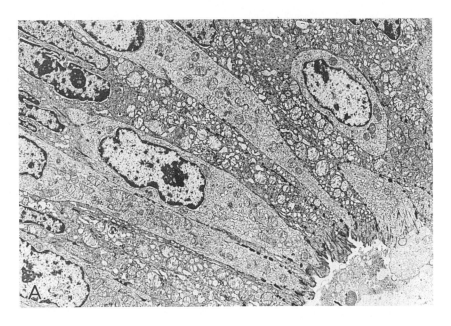

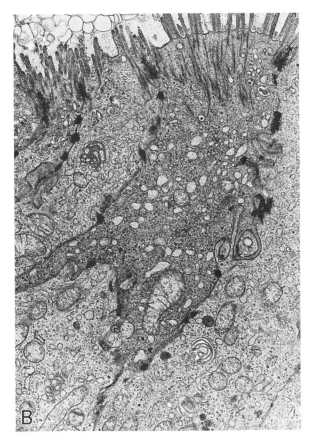

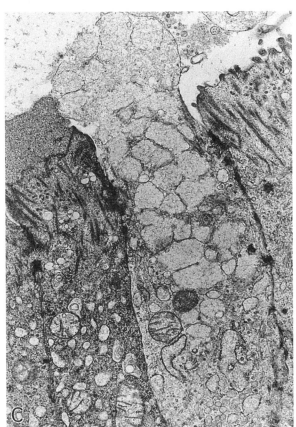

Figure 20-28

ULTRASTRUCTURAL APPEARANCE OF WELL-DIFFERENTIATED AMPULLARY ADENOCARCINOMA

A: The tumor cells are columnar and contain oval nuclei and abundant organelles.

B: Numerous long microvilli project from the apical surface.

C: A fine glycocalyx covers the microvilli, which have long intestinal type rootlets. Some cells contain abundant electron-lucent mucigen granules.

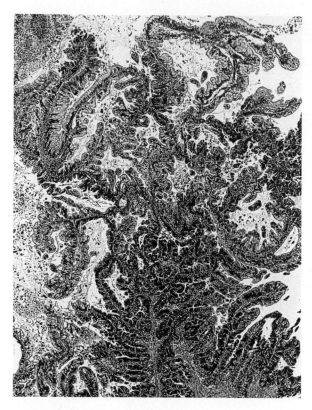

Figure 20-29
HISTOLOGIC APPEARANCE OF
NONINVASIVE PAPILLARY CARCINOMA
At low power this papillary carcinoma shows markedly complex, branching papillae with secondary micropapillae formation.

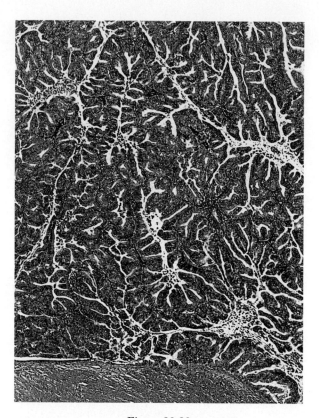

Figure 20-30
HISTOLOGIC APPEARANCE OF
NONINVASIVE PAPILLARY CARCINOMA
Same tumor as shown in figure 20-29. Note the absence of stromal invasion.

ducts, however, exophytic tumors with marked cytoarchitectural atypia (even focally), are designated as papillary carcinoma (or intraductal papillary-mucinous carcinoma). Analogous terminology may be used for exophytic ampullary tumors with pancreatobiliary features. Since all of the pancreatobiliary type papillary tumors we have observed in the ampulla have had at least focal (and usually widespread) cytoarchitectural atypia, the term papillary carcinoma is used. If there is invasive carcinoma as well, that component should be designated separately.

Pancreatobiliary type papillary carcinomas are uncommon in the ampulla. In our material 11 of 93 (12 percent) invasive carcinomas had residual foci of pancreatobiliary type papillary carcinoma. Only 2 of 36 (6 percent) predominantly exophytic ampullary neoplasms (i.e., less than 50 percent composed of invasive carcinoma) were pancreatobiliary type papillary carcino-

mas; the remainder were intestinal type adenomas. In fact, examples without invasion are exceedingly rare, and we have not seen a case.

Noninvasive papillary carcinoma does not invade the stroma, and therefore, could be regarded as in situ carcinoma. However, it is very common to find an invasive adenocarcinoma associated with papillary carcinoma of the ampulla. Since the invasive carcinoma may be focal, a thorough search must be carried out, including microscopic examination of the entire tumor. We have observed one case with lymph node metastasis in which only a 0.2 cm focus of invasive carcinoma was found.

In contrast to intestinal type papillary adenomas, pancreatobiliary type papillary carcinomas have a predominantly intra-ampullary location. The papillae are complex and branching, and are lined by moderately to markedly atypical cells (figs. 20-29, 26-30). Rather than the tall columnar

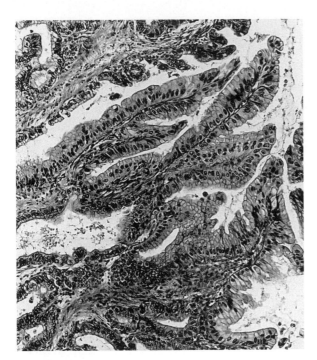
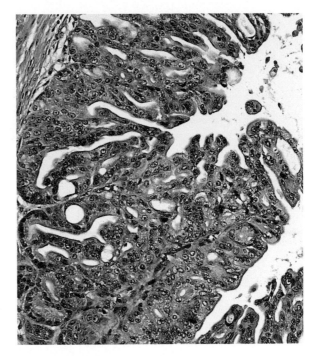

Figure 20-31
HISTOLOGIC APPEARANCE OF NONINVASIVE PAPILLARY CARCINOMA
Left: At higher magnification, the papillae in the tumor seen in figure 20-30 lack the features of intestinal type adenomas. Instead, single layers of cuboidal to low columnar cells with round, markedly atypical nuclei are seen.
Right: In other areas the cells are truly stratified and intraepithelial lumina and micropapillary formations are present.

cells with oval, pseudostratified nuclei which characterize intestinal type adenomas, the lining of papillary carcinoma consists of cuboidal to low columnar cells with round nuclei predominantly arranged in a single layer (fig. 20-31, left). When multiple cell layers are present, the cells are truly stratified. Other features common to intestinal type tumors, such as Paneth cells and goblet cells, are lacking, although an endocrine cell component is often present. The architectural complexity is marked, with intraepithelial lumina giving rise to a cribriform pattern. Micropapillary structures lacking fibrovascular cores may also be present (fig. 20-31, right). In some cases, features of both intestinal type adenoma and intraductal papillary carcinoma coexist in different regions of the same tumor. One case exhibited oncocytic cytoplasm (fig. 20-32) and resembled pancreatic tumors reported as intraductal oncocytic papillary neoplasms (116). Ampullary papillary carcinomas may extensively involve the pancreatic and biliary ducts (118,124,135); therefore, it may be impossible to determine with certainty where a tumor originated.

Generally, the invasive carcinoma accompanying pancreatobiliary type papillary carcinoma shows a tubular pattern of growth indistinguishable from the invasive carcinoma arising in association with intestinal type adenomas. Poorly differentiated adenocarcinomas and mucinous carcinomas also occur (fig. 20-33). The invasive component may form papillae (invasive papillary carcinoma), a finding more commonly associated with pancreatobiliary type papillary carcinoma than with intestinal type adenoma. It is important to distinguish invasive papillary carcinoma (or invasive carcinoma with papillary features) from the noninvasive papillary carcinomas defined herein, which essentially represent in situ carcinomas. The term "papillary carcinoma" has been used frequently in the literature (often in contradistinction to "intestinal type carcinoma" [134]) without specific reference to the presence or absence of invasion (117,145, 146); in some cases the term apparently referred to the gross configuration, meaning exophytic (121). In one study, ampullary carcinomas were

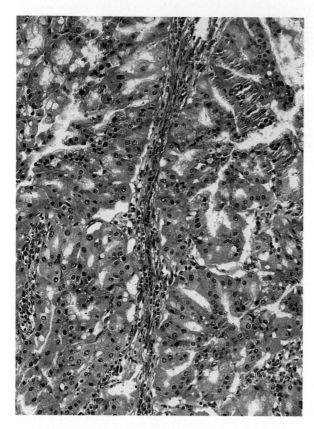

Figure 20-32
NONINVASIVE PAPILLARY CARCINOMA
The neoplastic cells have abundant oncocytic cytoplasm.

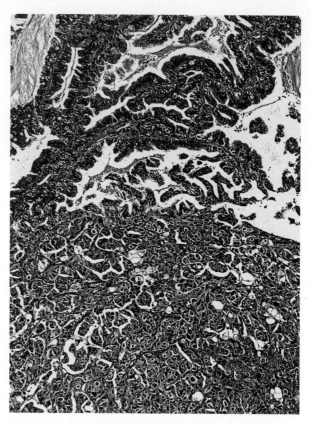

Figure 20-33
POORLY DIFFERENTIATED CARCINOMA
ARISING IN ASSOCIATION WITH
NONINVASIVE PAPILLARY CARCINOMA

divided into papillary (16 percent) and infiltrating (84 percent) types (127).

The distinction between papillary carcinoma (noninvasive) and intestinal type adenoma with severe dysplasia or carcinoma in situ is, in part, semantic and reflects the difficulty of having different terminology for analogous tumors in the tubular gastrointestinal tract and pancreatobiliary system. Although the morphology of severely dysplastic areas within intestinal type adenomas overlaps with that of pancreatobiliary type papillary carcinomas, there are some distinctions. Areas of residual intestinal type adenoma with low-grade dysplasia are more frequent and widespread in intestinal adenomas with severe dysplasia, and distinct foci with sharply contrasting degrees of atypia are found (fig. 20-34). Although a spectrum of atypia may exist in pancreatobiliary type papillary carcinomas, there is usually a gradual transition, and areas of typical intestinal type adenoma with low-grade dysplasia are uncommon. Foci of severe dysplasia or carcinoma in situ are usually more limited in intestinal type adenomas, whereas an entire papillary carcinoma frequently appears cytologically malignant. In addition, pancreatobiliary type papillary carcinomas do not exhibit the typical cribriformed glands with pseudostratified nuclei found in foci of severe dysplasia in intestinal adenomas.

Invasive Papillary Carcinoma

Most papillary carcinomas of the ampulla are exophytic tumors with sufficient cytoarchitectural atypia to be regarded as malignant. Based on their histologic features, these tumors are referred to as intestinal type papillary adenoma with severe dysplasia or carcinoma in situ, or pancreatobiliary type papillary carcinoma (see above); invasive carcinoma may be associated with either type

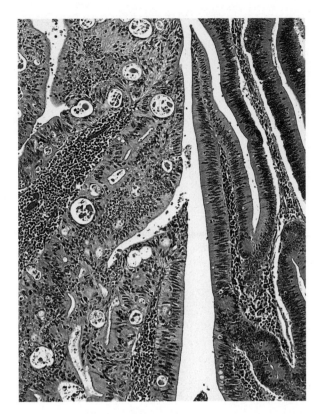

Figure 20-34
DYSPLASIA IN PAPILLARY ADENOMA
A focus of severe dysplasia within an intestinal type papillary adenoma may be nearly indistinguishable from a pancreatobiliary type papillary carcinoma. Often, the severely dysplastic region (left) sharply contrasts with adjacent foci showing only mild dysplasia (right).

and in most cases exhibits a tubular growth pattern. Invasive papillary adenocarcinomas are infiltrating carcinomas which predominantly form papillary or micropapillary structures in the invasive component.

Invasive papillary adenocarcinomas constitute less than 10 percent of ampullary carcinomas, although a focal papillary growth pattern is common in other types of ampullary adenocarcinoma, especially the pancreatobiliary type. Two thirds of cases are associated with an intestinal type adenoma or another preinvasive lesion.

Invasive papillary carcinomas may exhibit grossly visible papillary structures and often have a soft, friable consistency. Histologically, the majority of the tumor consists of complex, branching papillary structures with fibrovascular cores or micropapillary formations lacking fibrovascular cores (fig. 20-35). Foci of gland

formation or solid areas may be present. The cells lining the papillae may resemble those of either intestinal or pancreatobiliary type adenocarcinoma, since the diagnosis of invasive papillary carcinoma is based on the architecture of the tumor rather than on the cytologic appearance.

Mucinous (Colloid) Carcinoma

Mucinous (colloid) carcinomas consist predominantly (more than 50 percent) of pools of extracellular mucin in which the neoplastic cells are suspended. Less than 10 percent of ampullary carcinomas are mucinous (139,145); however, focal mucinous areas are found in 20 percent of intestinal type adenocarcinomas. Mucinous areas are rare in pancreatobiliary type adenocarcinomas. An adenomatous component is present in 80 percent of mucinous carcinomas. In some cases the tumor may be predominantly adenoma, with a minor invasive component of mucinous carcinoma.

Grossly, ampullary mucinous carcinomas resemble mucinous carcinomas occurring in other sites: the cut surface is gelatinous and exudes sticky gray-white mucin. In our material, 27 percent of mucinous carcinomas had a periampullary duodenal gross configuration, more than any other tumor type. Histologically, thin fibrous septa surround lakes of basophilic mucin which contain the tumor cells, either free floating or adherent to the peripheral stroma (figs. 20-36, 20-37). The cells are arranged in nests, strips, and cribriform structures; some individual cells may also be present, often with a signet ring cell appearance. Cytologically, the cells are generally moderately differentiated, although on occasion they form a well-organized columnar layer, with basal pseudostratified nuclei and apical mucin-rich cytoplasm, simulating adenomatous epithelium. There may be transitions to nonmucinous areas which are generally tubular or papillary, resembling intestinal type adenocarcinoma.

In some cases there is a relatively small amount of neoplastic epithelium within the mucin pools. In areas, acellular mucin may be seen dissecting into the stroma or within lymph nodes. As with mucinous tumors elsewhere, it is necessary to identify the epithelium to confirm that the mucin represents disseminated carcinoma, although in most cases, serial sections or immunohistochemical stains for keratin reveal tumor cells.

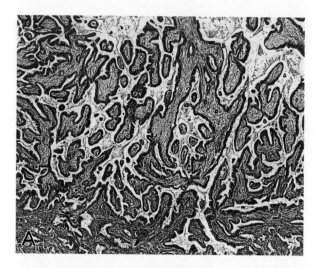

Figure 20-35
INVASIVE PAPILLARY CARCINOMA
A: At low power, abundant well-formed papillary structures are present.
B: Higher power reveals a desmoplastic stroma associated with irregularly shaped papillae lined by markedly atypical cells.
C: The papillary carcinoma extends into the duodenal muscularis propria.

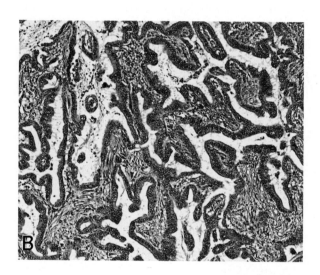

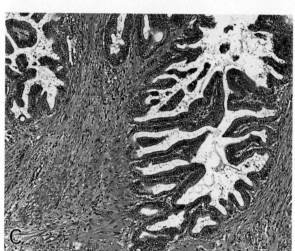

Figure 20-36
HISTOLOGIC APPEARANCE
OF AMPULLARY
MUCINOUS CARCINOMA
At low power, pools of mucin separated by thin fibrous septa contain widely spaced clusters of tumor cells. A residual intestinal type adenoma is present (right).

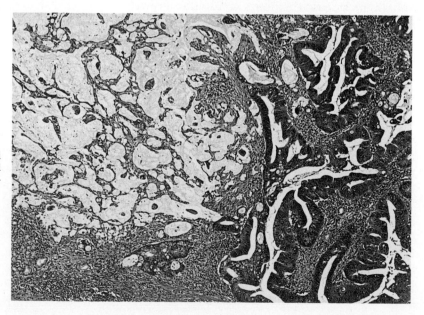

Signet Ring Cell Carcinoma

Although mucinous carcinomas commonly contain signet ring cells within pools of extracellular mucin, diffusely infiltrating signet ring cell carcinomas are rare in the ampulla. Only one case of a pure signet ring cell carcinoma has been reported in this location (126); we have observed three others. Seifert et al. (139) found one signet ring cell carcinoma among 35 cases, and Blackman and Nash (120) mentioned a signet ring cell component in 2 of 7 "anaplastic" carcinomas among 24 adenocarcinomas of the duodenum and ampulla. However, these diagnoses were based on endoscopic biopsies, so the extent of the signet ring cell component was not known. The patients have been adults (34 to 83 years; mean, 61 years) and the clinical presentation did not differ from that of other ampullary carcinomas. All of the cases were of the mixed ulcerated type, and no residual adenomatous elements were identified.

Histologically, the tumors display small, undifferentiated individual cells and classic signet ring cells (fig. 20-38), with a diffuse growth pattern and minimal gland formation. The resemblance to diffuse type gastric adenocarcinoma has been noted (120). In one case (126), there was a significant endocrine cell component, with 20 percent of the cells staining for chromogranin.

A minor component of signet ring cells may be observed in otherwise typical adenocarcinoma, especially when poorly differentiated. In order to classify an ampullary carcinoma as signet ring cell type, more than 50 percent of the tumor must exhibit signet ring cells or have a diffuse growth pattern.

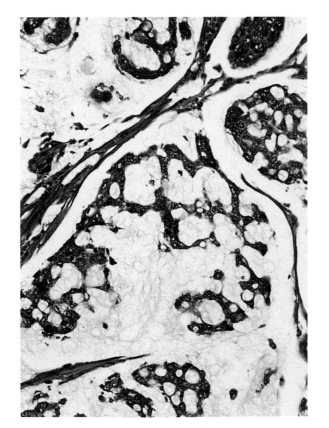 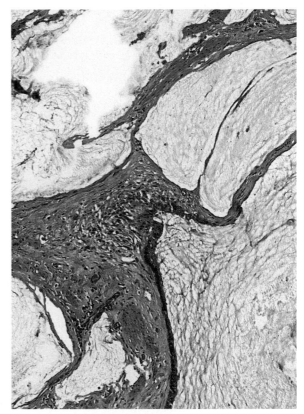

Figure 20-37
MUCINOUS CARCINOMA
Left: Mucinous carcinoma in which the neoplastic cells are arranged in cribriformed nests.
Right: The neoplastic epithelium is sparse.

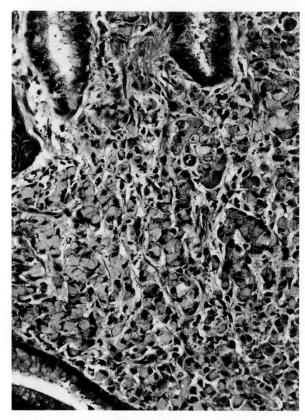

Figure 20-38
SIGNET RING CELL CARCINOMA
The entire tumor is composed of classic signet ring cells which are interposed between periampullary duodenal glands with minimal stromal reaction.

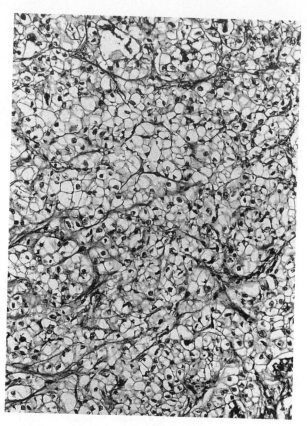

Figure 20-39
CLEAR CELL CARCINOMA OF THE AMPULLA
The tumor has a solid, nesting appearance, with polygonal clear cells separated by a fine fibrovascular stroma.

Clear Cell Carcinoma

A minor component of clear cells may be present in ampullary adenocarcinomas of intestinal or pancreatobiliary type. In rare instances, an ampullary carcinoma is composed predominantly of clear cells, resembling the clear cell carcinomas of the gallbladder and extrahepatic bile ducts (119,143). In the single case we have observed, the tumor had a polypoid intra-ampullary gross configuration, and there was minimal invasion into the submucosa. The cells were polygonal and arranged in solid sheets and cribriformed nests, the cytoplasm was clear throughout, and the nuclei were uniform and hyperchromatic (figs. 20-39, 2-40). Other than the presence of focal mucin, the resemblance to renal cell carcinoma was striking. Lymph node metastases were present and the patient died of tumor 7 months after resection.

Adenocarcinoma with Hepatoid Differentiation

Two ampullary intestinal adenocarcinomas with hepatoid features have been reported (125, 138). Both tumors resembled hepatoid carcinomas of other sites, with sheets of polygonal cells having eosinophilic cytoplasm, similar to hepatocytes (fig. 20-41). Focal luminal formations and bile secretion were present, and one case had superimposed clear cell changes (125). Immunohistochemical positivity for alpha-fetoprotein and CEA (in a canalicular pattern) was found (fig. 20-42) (125,138).

Adenosquamous Carcinoma

Adenosquamous carcinomas exhibit both glandular and squamous differentiation, and comprise 1 to 3 percent of ampullary carcinomas (Table 20-4) (144,146). The gross appearance is not distinctive.

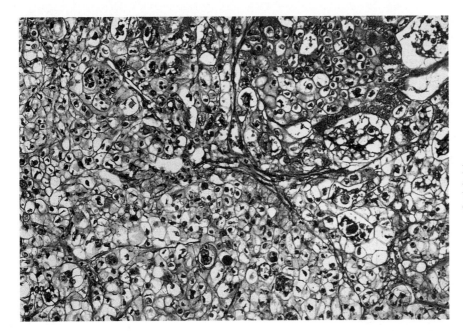

Figure 20-40
CLEAR CELL CARCINOMA
OF THE AMPULLA

Focal luminal and intracellular basophilic mucin is identifiable and helpful in separating this tumor from metastatic renal cell carcinoma.

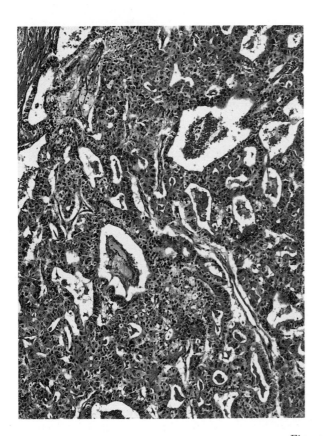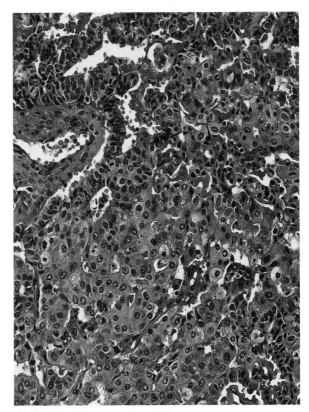

Figure 20-41
AMPULLARY CARCINOMA WITH HEPATOID FEATURES

Left: The tumor cells are arranged in nests punctuated by glandular formation.

Right: At high power, there is abundant eosinophilic cytoplasm and round nuclei with prominent nucleoli, closely resembling hepatocytes.

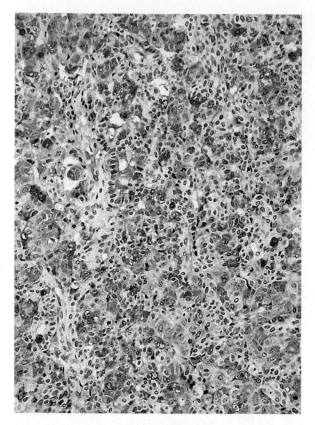

Figure 20-42
AMPULLARY CARCINOMA WITH
HEPATOID FEATURES

Immunohistochemical staining of the tumor cells in figure 20-41 shows diffuse alpha-fetoprotein positivity. (Courtesy of Dr. Yasushi Sato, Yamaguchi, Japan.)

Preexisting adenomas may be identified. Microscopically, the two components are intermingled, with gradual or abrupt transitions (fig. 20-43A). The proportion of each component may vary considerably. By convention, the squamous component should be significant (greater than 25 percent) before a diagnosis of adenosquamous carcinoma is made, although a tumor composed almost entirely of squamous elements is considered adenosquamous if even focal glandular differentiation is found. Keratinization is generally present in the squamous areas, as well as polygonal cells with abundant eosinophilic cytoplasm (fig. 20-43B,C). The glandular component may exhibit well-formed luminal spaces or may be more solid, with mucin only identified by special staining. When well-formed glands are present, they generally resemble those of pancreatobiliary type adenocarcinoma. Most adenosquamous carcinomas of the ampulla are moderately to poorly differentiated. Mucicarmine stains the glandular component and should be used whenever a putative "pure" squamous cell carcinoma of this region is found.

Squamous Cell Carcinoma

Pure squamous cell carcinomas are extraordinarily rare in the ampulla: there was only 1 in 836 carcinomas reported to the SEER Program. Most tumors with a predominantly squamous appearance are adenosquamous carcinomas when thoroughly sampled. In some cases, mucin stains may be necessary to identify the glandular differentiation.

Small Cell Carcinoma

Small cell carcinomas occur rarely in the ampulla: only 10 cases have been reported (122, 129,130,132,136,141,147). Because small cell carcinoma is not present in most of the series on ampullary carcinomas, the relative frequency is uncertain but is clearly less than 5 percent (122,130,147). We found only 1 case among 143 ampullary carcinomas (Table 20-4).

Patients with ampullary small cell carcinoma are between 53 and 86 years of age, with a mean age of 69. The majority are males. Presenting symptoms are similar to those of other ampullary carcinomas, including jaundice, weight loss, and abdominal pain (147). No paraneoplastic syndromes associated with small cell carcinoma have been described.

Grossly, ampullary small cell carcinomas may be polypoid or ulcerated. In three cases an overlying villous adenoma was present (122,132), analogous to the similar association which may be seen with small cell carcinomas of the colorectum (131). Histologically, the tumors have a diffuse growth pattern in most areas (fig. 20-44A), although focal nesting or trabecular patterns may occur. In cases associated with a villous adenoma, the transition to the carcinoma is abrupt (fig. 20-44B). Most of the tumors cells closely resemble those of pulmonary small cell carcinoma, with minimal cytoplasm, indistinct cell borders, and polygonal nuclei having finely dispersed chromatin and inconspicuous nucleoli (fig. 20-44C). Necrosis is usually plentiful and

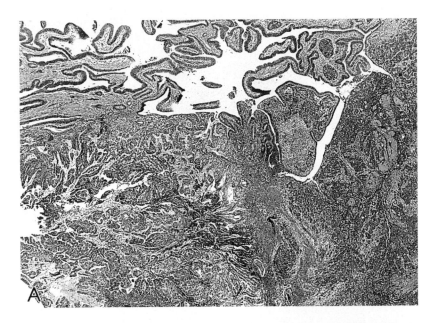

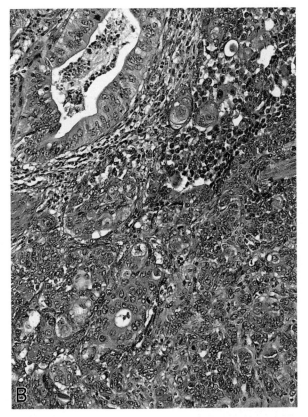

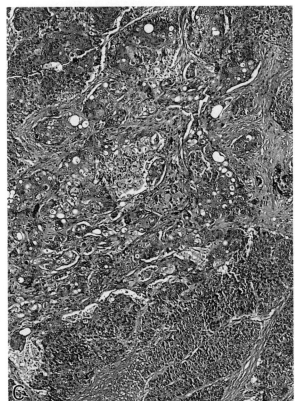

Figure 20-43
ADENOSQUAMOUS CARCINOMA

A: An overlying intestinal type adenoma is present. The glandular component (lower left) abuts the more solid squamous elements (lower right).

B: At higher power, the solid nests of squamous cells with focal keratin pearls contrast sharply with the well-formed glandular elements of the tumor (lower left).

C: Poorly differentiated adenosquamous carcinoma. Nests of small cells surround islands of keratinizing squamous cells exhibiting more abundant eosinophilic cytoplasm. In some areas, individual cells show keratinization.

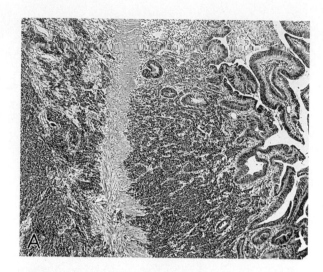

Figure 20-44
SMALL CELL CARCINOMA OF THE AMPULLA
ARISING IN TUBULOVILLOUS ADENOMA

A: At low power, the carcinoma has a diffuse, infiltrative growth pattern. Note the overlying intestinal type adenoma.

B: Although the small cell carcinoma abuts the residual adenoma, the transition is abrupt.

C: Cytologically, ampullary small cell carcinoma resembles its pulmonary counterpart, with minimal cytoplasm, polygonal nuclei with finely stippled chromatin, and indistinct nucleoli.

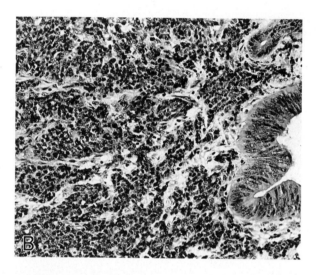

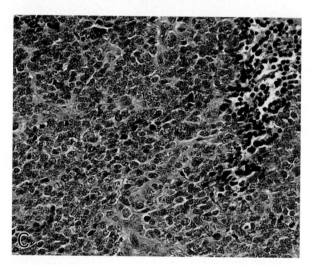

mitotic figures are innumerable. As is common with extrapulmonary small cell carcinomas, there may be regions with larger cells or focally prominent nucleoli; in general, these features are acceptable as long as the overall cytoarchitectural pattern fits that of small cell carcinoma. In one case we observed areas of glandular and squamous differentiation, a phenomenon described in small cell carcinomas from other locations, including the gallbladder and extrahepatic bile ducts.

The neuroendocrine nature of ampullary small cell carcinoma is confirmed by immunohistochemistry and electron microscopy. Most cases are focally positive for general endocrine markers such as chromogranin or neuron-specific enolase. Although vasoactive intestinal polypeptide was detected in one case (141), specific peptides are not usually found. Neurosecretory granules may be identified ultrastructurally, often within cytoplasmic processes (141). In histologically typical cases, however, it is not necessary to confirm the neuroendocrine nature of the tumor to establish the diagnosis of small cell carcinoma.

The differential diagnosis includes other neuroendocrine tumors, lymphoma, and poorly differentiated carcinoma. Carcinoid tumors can be distinguished by a more widespread organoid growth pattern and larger cells with more abundant cytoplasm, more evident nucleoli, a relatively low mitotic rate, and paucity of necrosis. In general, there is more diffuse positivity for general neuroendocrine markers in carcinoid tumors, although this features may be of little use in the individual case. The lower proliferative rate of carcinoid tumors is reflected in a relatively small percentage of cells being positive immunohistochemically for proliferation markers such as Ki-67 (MIB-1); the latter stain may help distinguish carcinoid from small cell carcinoma, which displays positivity in the majority of cells, especially when only small biopsies are available. Large cell neuroendocrine carcinomas share with small cell carcinomas a high mitotic rate and plentiful necrosis but are distinguished by a more marked organoid growth pattern, larger cells, and round nuclei having prominent nucleoli.

Immunohistochemical positivity for keratin, a marker uniformly present in small cell carcinoma, and negative staining for lymphoid markers help exclude lymphoma. Poorly differentiated carcinomas often share a diffuse growth pattern, absent gland formation, and relatively small cells with small cell carcinoma. However, the nuclear features differ and neuroendocrine differentiation is not seen. Finally, the possibility of a metastasis from an occult pulmonary primary should always be considered.

Large Cell Neuroendocrine Carcinoma

Although most reported high-grade neuroendocrine carcinomas of the ampulla have been small cell carcinomas, some cases resemble the recently characterized large cell neuroendocrine carcinoma of the lung (142). Only four large cell neuroendocrine carcinomas of the ampulla have been reported (123,132), although it is possible that other cases have been regarded as carcinoid tumors in the past. Grossly, large cell neuroendocrine carcinomas are large, deeply invasive tumors with a fleshy appearance and abundant necrosis (fig. 20-45). They grow as nests and sheets of cells (fig. 20-46). The cell size is intermediate to large and there is moderate cytoplasm. The nuclei are round with clumped chromatin and frequently prominent nucleoli. In keeping with their high-grade nature, there is a brisk mitotic rate and plentiful necrosis. Like small cell carcinoma, an associated adenoma may be seen. Focal glandular differentiation also occurs. Keratin and endocrine markers including chromogranin, synaptophysin, and neuron-specific enolase are positive (fig. 20-47); CEA may also be detected. Neurosecretory granules are detectable by electron microscopy (fig. 20-48). Both the intensity of the

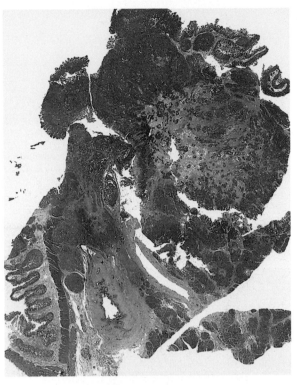

Figure 20-45
LARGE CELL NEUROENDOCRINE
CARCINOMA OF THE AMPULLA
A microscopic whole mount section reveals a highly cellular tumor with abundant areas of necrosis.

immunohistochemical staining for neuroendocrine markers as well as the abundance of neurosecretory granules identified ultrastructurally may be less than in carcinoid tumors.

The differential diagnosis is largely with carcinoid tumors. Although the architectural features overlap, large cell neuroendocrine carcinomas have more mitoses (greater than 15 in 10 high-power fields) and more extensive necrosis than carcinoid tumors. The features distinguishing large cell neuroendocrine carcinoma from small cell carcinoma are discussed above.

In some cases, poorly differentiated carcinomas may be indistinguishable from large cell neuroendocrine carcinomas. Two of the five poorly differentiated carcinomas in our material had neuroendocrine features that could not be confirmed immunohistochemically. Unlike small cell carcinoma, however, proof of neuroendocrine differentiation is necessary for the diagnosis of large cell neuroendocrine carcinoma. Until the clinical and

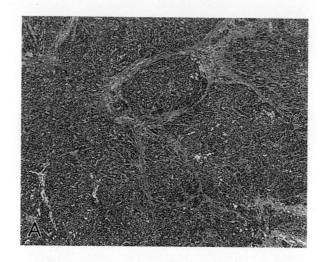

Figure 20-46
MICROSCOPIC APPEARANCE OF
LARGE CELL NEUROENDOCRINE CARCINOMA

A: At low power, the cells are arranged in nests, superficially resembling a carcinoid tumor.

B: There is abundant necrosis.

C: The tumor cells are large with moderate amounts of cytoplasm, round vesicular nuclei, and prominent nucleoli. Numerous mitotic figures are present.

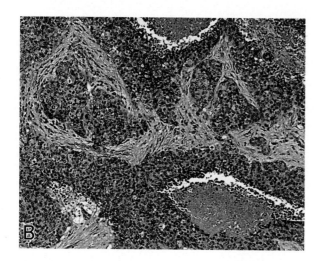

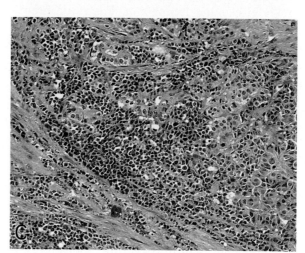

Figure 20-47
LARGE CELL
NEUROENDOCRINE CARCINOMA

Staining for chromogranin reveals nests of intensely positive cells, with faint staining in the majority.

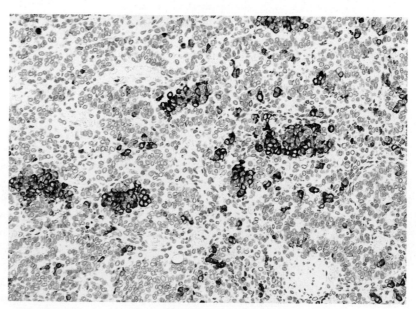

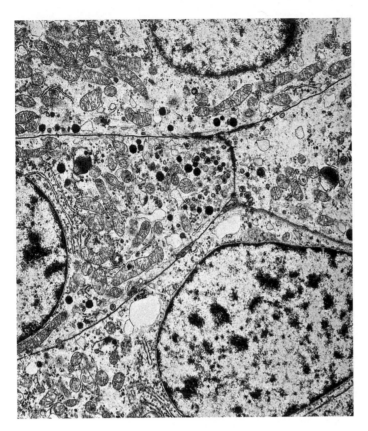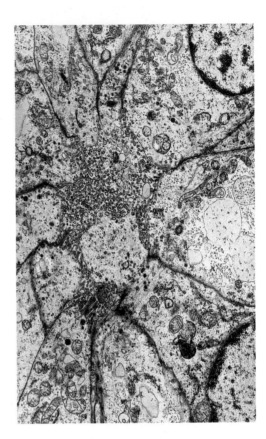

Figure 20-48
LARGE CELL NEUROENDOCRINE CARCINOMA

Left: Neurosecretory granules are found in large cell neuroendocrine carcinoma by electron microscopy. The cells are polygonal with moderate numbers of organelles.

Right: Evidence of focal glandular differentiation is present as lumen formation.

pathologic features of these rare tumors are better understood, it is reasonable to keep the cases with proven neuroendocrine differentiation separate from those without, although recognizing that they may not actually represent different entities.

Undifferentiated Carcinoma

One of the least common ampullary carcinomas, undifferentiated carcinoma, exhibits no histologic features of glandular or other differentiation (137), often appearing sarcomatoid instead. Only five undifferentiated carcinomas were found among 140 cases (3.6 percent) in our material. The clinical and gross features are not distinctive.

Several histologic subtypes of undifferentiated carcinoma exist. In most cases, the cells have an epithelial appearance and are arranged in sheets, with a diffuse growth pattern (fig. 20-49). The

tumors are cellular and have minimal fibrous stroma. The cells are intermediate in size and have little cytoplasm. Necrosis is abundant and mitotic figures are innumerable. No glandular spaces or signet ring cells are identifiable; mucin stains are negative. In some cases, a nesting growth pattern may result in the appearance of a high-grade neuroendocrine carcinoma (generally large cell type); however, immunohistochemical stains for neuroendocrine markers are negative, but positive for keratin.

Other cases represent undifferentiated carcinoma, spindle cell type (sarcomatoid carcinoma). There may be transitions to more epithelioid areas, and components of adenocarcinoma may also be found. The spindle cells are arranged in fascicles and have pleomorphic nuclei; giant anaplastic cells may be seen (fig. 20-50). Because of the similarity

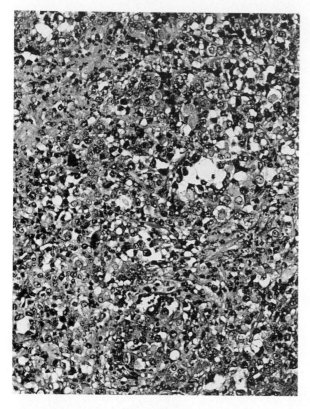

Figure 20-49
UNDIFFERENTIATED CARCINOMA OF THE AMPULLA
These tumors show no histologic evidence of glandular, squamous, or other differentiation. Highly atypical epithelioid cells are arranged in sheets and vague nests. Although the cytology may suggest a high-grade neuroendocrine carcinoma, immunohistochemical stains for neuroendocrine markers are negative.

with sarcomas, immunohistochemistry may be necessary to confirm the epithelial nature of the tumor. Stains for keratin or epithelial membrane antigen are generally positive, and coexpression of vimentin is often found. If heterologous bone or cartilage are present, the designation "carcinosarcoma" is appropriate.

Finally, we have observed two cases of undifferentiated carcinoma with numerous osteoclast-like giant cells involving the ampulla. The histologic appearance resembled that of similar tumors of the gallbladder, bile ducts, or pancreas (119,131a): the neoplastic cells were discohesive, pleomorphic and epithelioid to spindled, and lacked any architectural pattern (fig. 26-51). The osteoclast-like giant cells scattered throughout the tumor are regarded as non-neoplastic (128). Associated foci of adenocarcinoma may be present (fig. 20-51B).

HISTOLOGIC GRADING

Ampullary carcinomas can be graded as well, moderately, and poorly differentiated or undifferentiated using the same criteria used for gallbladder and extrahepatic bile duct carcinomas. Generally, a moderately or poorly differentiated carcinoma has a gradual transition from gland-forming areas to solid areas; infiltrating nests of cells may be intermixed with well-formed glands. Occasionally, a carcinoma may exhibit a biphasic appearance,

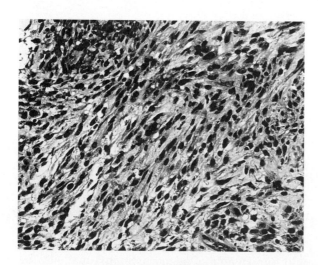

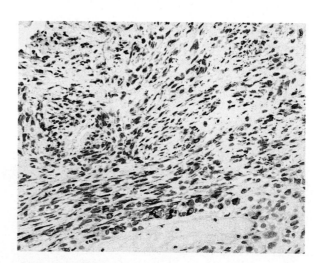

Figure 20-50
UNDIFFERENTIATED CARCINOMA OF THE AMPULLA
Left: Undifferentiated carcinoma with a spindle cell pattern.
Right: Immunohistochemical staining for keratin confirms the epithelial nature of the tumor.

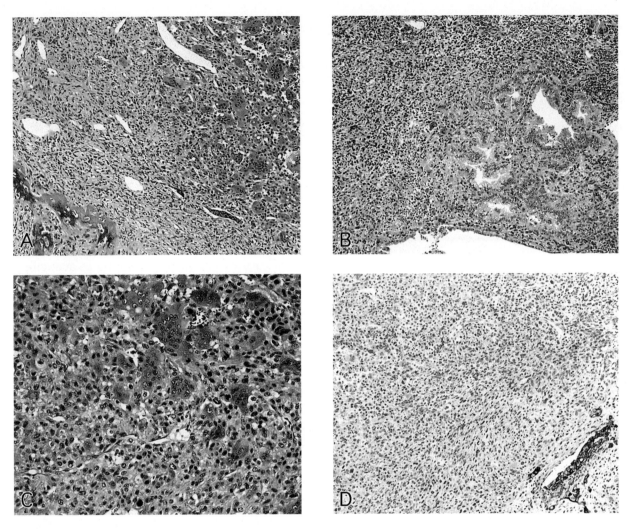

Figure 20-51

UNDIFFERENTIATED CARCINOMA WITH OSTEOCLAST-LIKE GIANT CELLS INVOLVING THE AMPULLA

A: The tumor is composed of sheets of atypical polygonal cells with numerous osteoclast-like giant cells. A focus of metaplastic bone formation is present (lower right).

B: A focus of adenocarcinoma.

C: At higher power, the osteoclast-like cells resemble their non-neoplastic counterparts. The tumor cells show marked nuclear atypia and abundant mitoses.

D: Immunohistochemical staining for keratin highlights the adenocarcinomatous component (lower right); the tumor cells also show faint staining.

with a poorly or undifferentiated component separated from a well- or moderately differentiated area (fig. 20-52). In such cases, the two components should be described separately, although the more poorly differentiated component would be expected to determine the behavior of the tumor.

Well-differentiated carcinomas are uncommon, representing less than 10 percent of cases, 65 percent are moderately differentiated, while 25 percent are poorly differentiated or undifferentiated (148,149).

MOLECULAR PATHOLOGY

p53

Abnormalities in the p53 tumor suppressor gene are among the most common molecular abnormalities identified in human cancers, and ampullary carcinomas are no exception. Mutations have been found in exons 5, 6, and 7 with roughly equal frequency in 70 percent of cases (160). Immunohistochemistry to detect abnormally

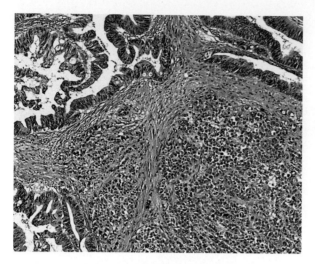

Figure 20-52
AMPULLARY ADENOCARCINOMA
WITH BIPHASIC APPEARANCE
The tumor exhibits a well-differentiated, intestinal type adenocarcinoma component as well as a separate component of poorly differentiated adenocarcinoma.

stable mutant proteins may be negative in cases having nonsense mutations, although cases with an abnormally stable wild type p53 protein are positive. The proportion of cases showing immunohistochemical staining for p53 has varied widely, from 30 to 94 percent of invasive ampullary carcinomas (160,162,164,168). Although some authors have suggested that the p53 mutation is a relatively late event in carcinogenesis, present only in invasive carcinomas and more prevalent in higher stage tumors (160), others have found nuclear accumulation in adenomas, largely in areas of moderate to severe dysplasia (162). In more than 80 percent of cases there is concordance of immunohistochemical staining for p53 between areas of adenoma and invasive carcinoma within the same tumor; only rarely is p53 positive in the adenoma and not in the invasive component (162). There is no relationship between grade and p53 abnormalities (164). Intestinal type adenocarcinomas more commonly have p53 abnormalities than do those of pancreatobiliary type (162).

K-*ras*

Mutations in the K-*ras* oncogene are prevalent in gastrointestinal carcinomas. The frequency of K-*ras* mutations, the relative proportion involving each codon, and the specific nucleotide substitutions most commonly involved vary with the site of the tumor. K-*ras* oncogene mutations have been reported in 13 to 100 percent of ampullary carcinomas in various studies (152,154,155,156,158, 160,161,163,167); overall, 59 of 156 (38 percent) of the analyzed tumors have shown mutations. The majority of the mutations involve codon 12; codon 13 mutations are present in 12 percent of cases (155). The frequency and specific types of mutations are similar to those found in colorectal carcinomas (153,166). K-*ras* mutation does not correlate with histologic type, grade, or stage of disease, although larger tumors are more likely to have mutations (155).

K-*ras* mutations are also found in adenomas (152,154,155), even at the level of mild dysplasia (155), suggesting that this mutation is an early event in the development of ampullary carcinoma. The concordance rate for mutations in adenomas and associated invasive carcinomas is high (93 percent), although some adenomas show mutations in the absence of mutations in the invasive tumor, and occasionally different mutations are found in the two components (155). One adenoma was found to have a codon 12 N-*ras* mutation (161).

Growth Factors

Overexpression of the epidermal growth factor receptor (EGFR) has been proposed to result in increased proliferation in tumors. EGFR is overexpressed in 50 to 65 percent of invasive ampullary carcinomas (159) and is increasingly expressed in adenomas with increasing dysplasia. Pancreatobiliary type carcinomas are more likely to overexpress EGFR than are intestinal type tumors. Related growth factor receptors c-erbB-2 and c-erbB-3 are also overexpressed in ampullary carcinoma (165). Both of the ligands for the EGFR, epidermal growth factor and transforming growth factor alpha, are also overexpressed in ampullary carcinomas (151,159).

Other Factors

Adenomatous polyposis coli (*APC*) gene mutations are important in the development of colorectal carcinoma in patients with familial polyposis and in sporadic cases. *APC* gene mutations have also been found in ampullary adenomas of

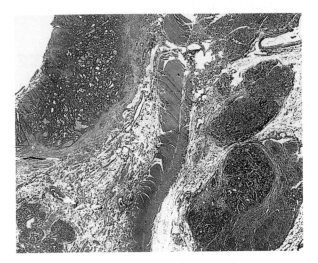

Figure 20-53
SUPERFICIAL AMPULLARY CARCINOMA
Superficially invasive ampullary carcinomas limited to the sphincter of Oddi generally do not develop metastases; however, this example has a peripancreatic lymph node metastasis (lower right).

patients with familial polyposis, with different mutations identified in different adenomas (150,154); the frequency of these mutations in ampullary carcinoma is less than in colorectal carcinoma (154). Allelic loss from chromosome 5, another genetic alteration found in colorectal adenocarcinoma, has also been reported in ampullary carcinoma (157). A recent study has concluded that MIB1 index and DNA ploidy are important factors in carcinoma of the ampulla of Vater (162).

BEHAVIOR

Spread

Local spread proceeds from the mucosa of the papilla or ampullary channel (which may be expanded if a preexisting adenoma is present) through the sphincter of Oddi (or duodenal muscularis mucosa) into the duodenal submucosa, muscularis propria, and finally the underlying pancreas or periduodenal soft tissue. At the time of resection, 12.5 percent of tumors are limited to the mucosa or the sphincter of Oddi, 30 percent have extended into duodenal submucosa, 12.5 percent have involved the duodenal muscularis propria, and 45 percent have penetrated the muscularis or extended into the pancreas (193). Lymphatic and blood vessel invasion are seen in 35 to 80 percent of cases, whereas perineural invasion is less common (179,193); regional lymph node metastases are found in 30 to 55 percent of resected ampullary carcinomas (179,186,193,202). Although tumors limited to the mucosa or sphincter of Oddi almost never metastasize, those that invade the submucosa involve lymph nodes in 42 percent of cases (fig. 20-53) (193).

Following surgical resection, both local recurrence and metastatic spread may occur. Recurrence may involve the tumor bed or the para-aortic lymphatics (203). Nodal involvement is most common in the peripancreatic lymph nodes and is more likely to be limited to this region in ampullary than in pancreatic carcinoma (183). Metastases other than those to regional nodes are most commonly found in the liver, followed by the peritoneum, lungs, and pleura (172,183,195, 203). Ampullary carcinomas generally spread in a halsteadian manner, with nodal metastases appearing first, followed by liver metastases, and subsequently distant dissemination.

Staging

The AJCC/UICC TNM staging system (196) is used for ampullary carcinomas (fig. 20-54). The T classification depends on the extent of primary tumor invasion and requires assessment of extension through the ampulla into the duodenal wall or beyond that into the head of the pancreas. If the pancreas is invaded, the extent of invasion (in centimeters) must be known to distinguish T3 from T4. In our material, 21 percent of resected cases were classified T1, 29 percent were T2, 49 percent were T3, and 1 percent were T4. Although the invasive carcinoma may be contained within the mucosa, usually as carcinoma arising in an adenoma, less than 10 percent of ampullary carcinomas do not invade the underlying tissues (169).

Regional lymph nodes include superior and inferior pancreatic (head region only), anterior and posterior pancreatoduodenal, pyloric, proximal mesenteric, and common bile duct lymph node groups. Thirty to 55 percent of resected tumors are classified N1. A greater proportion of pancreatobiliary type tumors, neuroendocrine carcinomas, and poorly differentiated carcinomas involve lymph nodes. Metastases to lymph nodes outside the regional groups are staged as metastatic disease (M1), as are metastases to

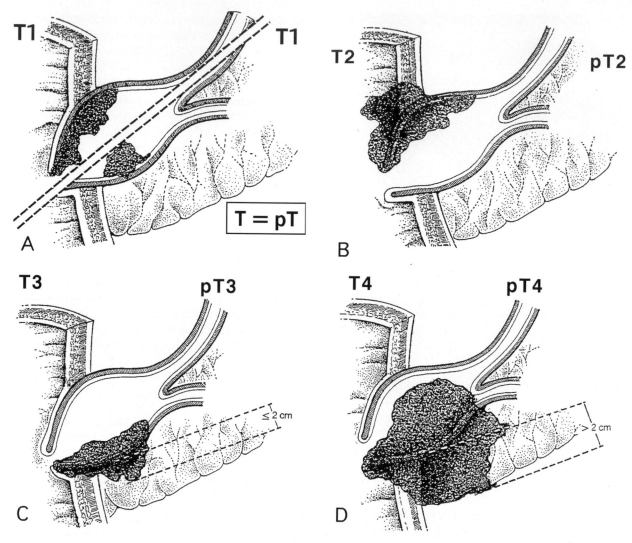

Figure 20-54
AJCC/UICC TNM STAGING SYSTEM FOR AMPULLARY CARCINOMA

The T classification (A–D) is based on the extent of invasion of the primary tumor.

A: T1 tumors are limited to the ampulla.

B: T2 tumors invade the duodenal wall but not the pancreas or peripancreatic soft tissues.

C: Invasion into the duodenal wall may include the submucosa or muscularis propria. In T3 tumors, there is invasion into the pancreas for a distance of up to 2 cm.

D: Peripancreatic soft tissue invasion may also occur in T3 tumors. T4 tumors invade more than 2 cm into the pancreas or into other adjacent organs.

any other sites. The TNM stage groupings are shown in Table 20-5.

The distinction between a duodenal and an ampullary site of origin, which may be impossible to determine in some cases, has implications for staging. In duodenal carcinoma, any invasion of the pancreas is classified as T4 whereas in ampullary carcinoma invasion less than 2 cm is classified as stage T3.

Outcome

Based on the data from the SEER Program, the median survival period for all patients with ampullary carcinoma is 23.2 months, the 5-year relative survival rate is 33.6 percent, and the 10-year relative survival rate is 28.4 percent. For patients presenting with liver metastases, the median survival period is 8 months (172). Following

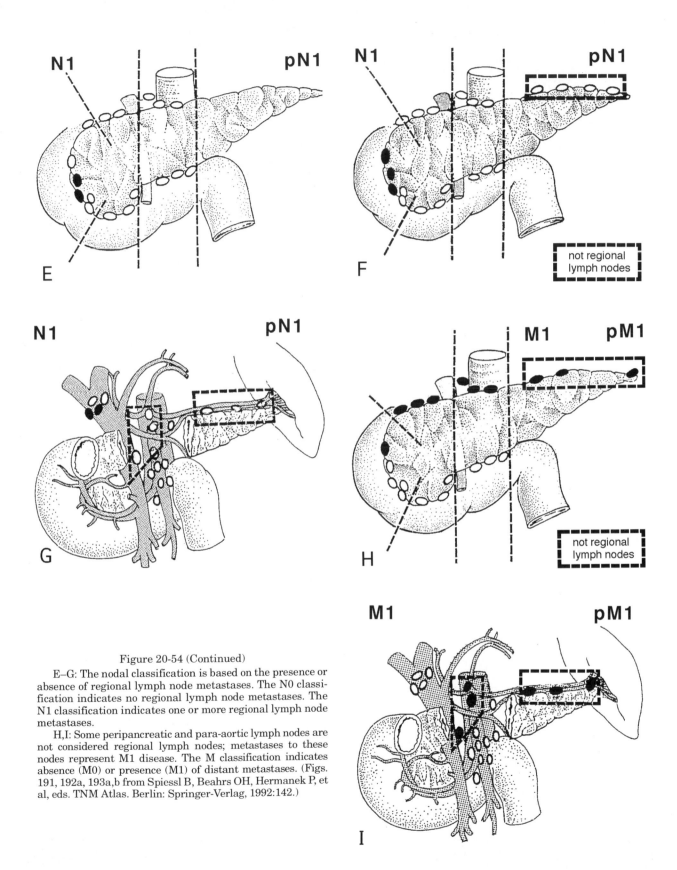

Figure 20-54 (Continued)

E–G: The nodal classification is based on the presence or absence of regional lymph node metastases. The N0 classification indicates no regional lymph node metastases. The N1 classification indicates one or more regional lymph node metastases.

H,I: Some peripancreatic and para-aortic lymph nodes are not considered regional lymph nodes; metastases to these nodes represent M1 disease. The M classification indicates absence (M0) or presence (M1) of distant metastases. (Figs. 191, 192a, 193a,b from Spiessl B, Beahrs OH, Hermanek P, et al, eds. TNM Atlas. Berlin: Springer-Verlag, 1992:142.)

Table 20-5

TNM STAGE GROUPINGS FOR CARCINOMA OF THE AMPULLA OF VATER*

Stage	TNM		
I	T1	N0	M0
II	T2	N0	M0
	T3	N0	M0
III	T1	N1	M0
	T2	N1	M0
	T3	N1	M0
IV	any T	any N	M1

*See reference 196.

Table 20-6

POSTRESECTION SURVIVAL OF PATIENTS WITH AMPULLARY CARCINOMA: REPORTED SERIES

First Author (Reference)	Year	No. of Cases	5-Year Survival (%)
Warren (202)	1975	112	32
Makipour (184)	1976	23	17
Wise (205)	1976	47	23
Akwari (169)	1977	87	34
Nakase (190)	1977	459	6
Schlippert (192)	1978	38	10
Treadwell (200)	1978	19	32
Forrest (176)	1979	34	24
Williams (204)	1979	33	27
Cohen (173)	1982	22	30
Herter (178)	1982	44	28
Walsh (201)	1982	44	16
Kellum (181)	1983	17	35
Jones (180)	1985	40	32
Tarazi (199)	1986	59	37
Crist (174)	1987	19	36
Neoptolomos (191)	1987	28	56
Hayes (177)	1988	31	53
Delcore (175)	1989	23	60
Michelassi (187)	1989	25	29
Martin (185)	1990	23	43
Mori (189)	1990	26	50
Shutze (194)	1990	24	61
Bakkevold (171)	1993	24	20
Matory (186)	1993	55	43
Willett (203)	1993	41	55
Sperti (195)	1994	31	56
Allema (170)	1995	67	50
Shirai (193)	1995	40	45
Klempnauer (182)	1995	85	38
Talamini (198)	1997	106	38
Howe (179)	1997	101	46

surgical resection, the 5-year survival rate has ranged from 6 to 61 percent in different series, with an average of 35 percent. However, in studies reported since 1990, this rate has increased to 50 percent, reflecting both improvements in surgical technique (174) and earlier diagnosis (Table 20-6). Median survival after resection is 49 to 59 months (179,198). Survival continues to decrease after 5 years, with approximately one third of 5-year survivors dying before 10 years (195).

A comparison of the survival rates for patients with ampullary carcinoma and those with carcinomas of the head of pancreas, extrahepatic bile ducts, and duodenum is shown in figure 20-55. The postresection survival curves for ampullary and duodenal carcinomas are similar. The overall survival of patients with periampullary carcinomas, while poor, is better than the survival of those with pancreatic carcinomas (171,179,182), in part due to the greater resectability rate of ampullary carcinomas. Although pancreatic ductal adenocarcinomas are resectable in only 10 to 25 percent of cases, 70 to 80 percent of ampullary carcinomas are resectable (Table 20-1) (179,187,188,190,197). However, it appears that earlier stage at presentation alone does not explain the relatively favorable prognosis of patients with ampullary carcinoma (179,182). Even when only stage I patients are considered, the survival of those with ampullary carcinoma is more favorable than those with pancreatic carcinoma (171). Comparative survival curves for patients with and without nodal metastases from carcinomas of the ampulla and pancreas resected at Memorial Sloan-Kettering

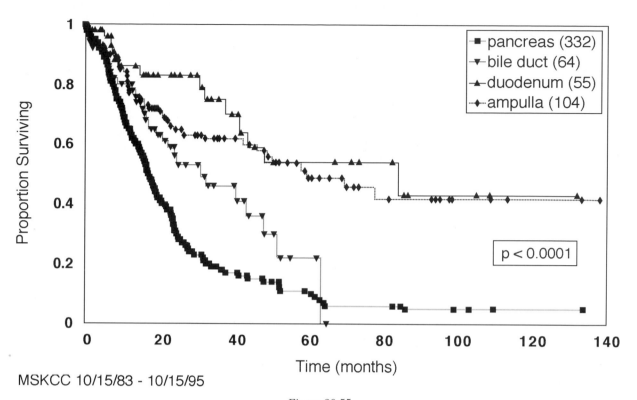

MSKCC 10/15/83 - 10/15/95

Figure 20-55
COMPARATIVE SURVIVAL OF PATIENTS WITH CARCINOMAS OF THE PANCREAS,
COMMON BILE DUCT, DUODENUM, AND AMPULLA FOLLOWING RESECTION
Patients with duodenal and ampullary carcinomas survive longer than those with bile duct or pancreas cancers, and the difference is statistically significant. Data from Memorial Sloan-Kettering Cancer Center.

Cancer Center are shown in figure 20-56. The survival of patients with ampullary carcinomas is better than that of patients with pancreatic carcinoma even in the presence of nodal metastases; in fact, ampullary carcinoma patients with lymph node metastases survive somewhat longer than pancreatic carcinoma patients without nodal disease. These data show that ampullary carcinomas are inherently less aggressive than pancreatic carcinomas and emphasize the importance of distinguishing these two tumor types.

Prognostic Factors

Although various studies have come to differing conclusions regarding some potential prognostic factors in ampullary carcinoma, stage is consistently correlated with survival. A comparison of survival rates for patients with localized, regional, and distant disease based on the data from the SEER Program is shown in figure 20-57. The median, 5- and 10-year survival figures for these patients are shown in Table 20-7.

Most studies have evaluated the impact of prognostic factors after surgical resection. Resectability itself is a favorable prognostic factor since patients with resectable tumors have more limited disease. The difference in 5-year survival between resected patients (approximately 50 percent) and nonresected patients (approximately 10 percent) is dramatic (225,227), although occasional patients do experience long-term survival following only biliary bypass procedures. The presence of tumor at the surgical margins is associated with a worse prognosis (207,217,224).

Of 30 patients, those with stages I and II disease exhibited similar survival curves, much better than for those with stages III and IV disease, whose curves were also similar (209,234). Mori et al. (226) found a 5-year survival rate of 100

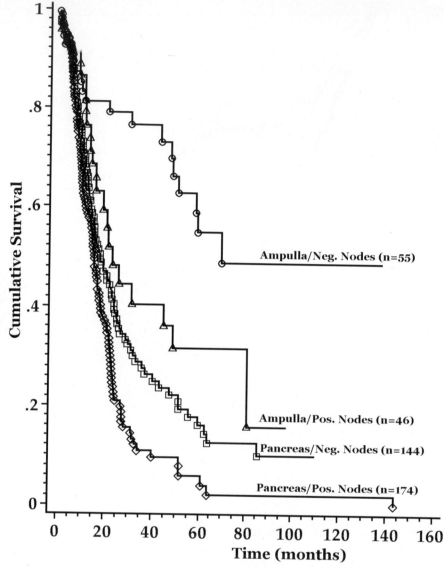

Figure 20-56
COMPARATIVE SURVIVAL
OF PATIENTS WITH
AMPULLARY AND
PANCREATIC CARCINOMAS
FOLLOWING RESECTION,
STRATIFIED FOR
NODAL STATUS

Patients with ampullary carcinoma survive longer than those with pancreatic carcinoma, even in the presence of positive lymph nodes. The difference is statistically significant. Data are from Memorial Sloan-Kettering Cancer Center.

percent for those with stage I, 65 percent for those with stage II, and 15 percent for those with stage III carcinoma (only one stage IV patient was present in this series of resected patients). The primary tumor stage (T classification) alone is not significantly predictive of survival by multivariate analysis in most cases (217,221), except for patients with T1 tumors who have a better prognosis. These findings reflect the fact that lymph node metastases may develop even from relatively early stage tumors. Further subdivision of depth of invasion with separation of intramucosal invasion from invasion of the sphincter of Oddi, and duodenal submucosal invasion

from invasion of muscularis propria (229), does not significantly improve the prognostic power of the TNM T classification. Patients with tumors limited to the mucosa or sphincter of Oddi have an 80 percent 5-year survival, those with invasion of duodenal submucosa or muscularis propria have a 50 to 60 percent rate, while only 27 to 29 percent of those with extension into periduodenal soft tissue or head of pancreas live 5 years (229).

"Early" ampullary carcinoma, analogous to early gastric carcinoma, can be defined as tumor limited to the mucosa or invading only into the sphincter of Oddi (229,235,238). Most early ampullary carcinomas consist predominantly of

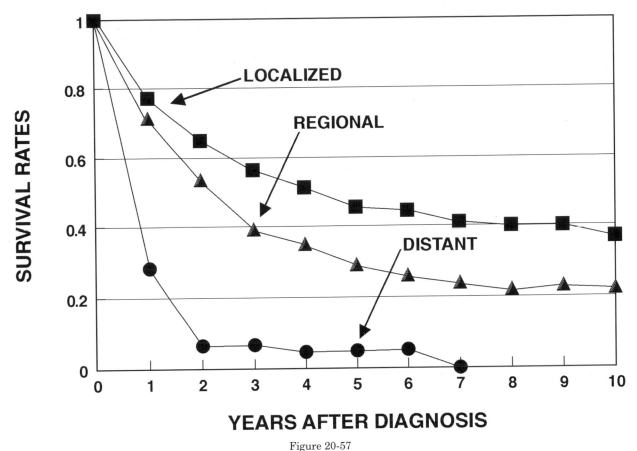

Figure 20-57

TEN-YEAR SURVIVAL RATES FOR CANCERS OF THE AMPULLA OF VATER ACCORDING TO STAGE OF DISEASE

All grades and histologic types are included. The data are taken from the Surveillance, Epidemiology, and End Results Program, National Cancer Institute, for the years 1981–1990.

intestinal type adenomas or pancreatobiliary type papillary carcinomas with only focal invasive carcinoma (fig. 20-58). Less commonly, an early carcinoma arises de novo or from foci of flat carcinoma in situ; these tumors may be nearly inapparent on endoscopic or gross examination (fig. 20-59).

The relationship of lymph node status to survival is controversial: although some reports found no statistically different postresection survival between node-positive and node-negative patients with ampullary carcinoma (207,225), most authors have reported a significantly worse survival for those with positive nodes (206,210,211,213,215, 217,222,230,231,233,237), and patients with more than two involved lymph nodes have a particularly poor prognosis (227). Comparative 5-year survival figures for node-positive and node-negative patients from selected clinical studies are shown in Table 20-8. Figure 20-60 shows the survival

Table 20-7

SURVIVAL OF PATIENTS WITH AMPULLARY CARCINOMA BY STAGE BASED ON DATA FROM THE SEER PROGRAM

	Median (Mos.)	5-Year Survival* (%)	10-Year Survival* (%)
Localized	37.3	50.9	44.2
Regional	25.3	28.3	24.1
Distant	7.8	5.9	0

*Relative survival rates.

curves based on data from Memorial Sloan-Kettering Cancer Center. One study reported no difference in survival with or without surgical resection in node-positive patients (231).

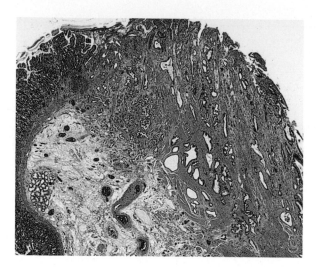

Figure 20-58
EARLY AMPULLARY CARCINOMA ARISING
IN THE ABSENCE OF AN
EXOPHYTIC PREINVASIVE LESION
The tumor extends through the sphincter of Oddi.

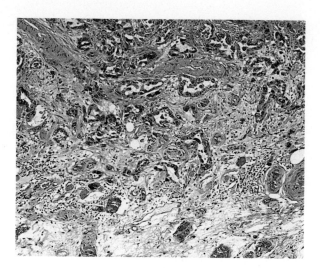

Figure 20-59
EARLY AMPULLARY CARCINOMA ARISING
IN THE ABSENCE OF AN
EXOPHYTIC PREINVASIVE LESION
Higher magnification of tumor shown in figure 20-58
depicts pancreatobiliary features.

Histologic grade has been found to correlate with depth of invasion and lymph node status. Although the close relationship of survival with grade found by some authors was not independent of other prognostic factors, the observation that high-grade carcinomas are associated with a poor 5-year survival rate (206,233) may be helpful in preoperative planning. In addition, some authors have found grade to be of independent prognostic significance (226).

The combination of histologic grade and stage of the tumor provides a powerful prognostic parameter (226). Willett et al. (236) classified patients following resection into low-risk and high-risk groups: low-risk patients had well- or moderately differentiated tumors limited to the ampulla or duodenum (pT1 or pT2), uninvolved resection margins, and no nodal metastases, whereas patients with poorly differentiated tumors, invasion of the pancreas, involved margins, or nodal metastases were considered high risk. The low-risk patients had a 5-year survival rate of 80 percent, compared to 38 percent for the high-risk group.

Patients with ampullary carcinomas with a mixed ulcerated gross configuration have a worse prognosis than those with other gross types (225, 235), perhaps because these tumors tend to be larger and more deeply invasive (238). It has

Table 20-8

**FIVE-YEAR SURVIVAL RATE AFTER
RESECTION OF AMPULLARY
CARCINOMA BASED ON
LYMPH NODE INVOLVEMENT**

Author (Ref.)	Year	Positive Nodes	Negative Nodes
Warren (202)	1975	10%	40%
Akwari (206)	1977	16%	41%
Martin (223)	1990	0%	67%
Shutze (230)	1990	50%	78%
Sperti (233)	1994	0%	65%
Howe (216)	1997	29%	57%

been reported that carcinomas with a residual adenomatous component have a better prognosis than those without (239), although tumors lacking such a component also tend to be of higher stage.

The influence of histologic type on prognosis is difficult to assess both because of variations in terminology as well as the rarity of carcinomas other than the intestinal and pancreatobiliary types. The outcome of intestinal type tumors is somewhat more favorable than that of the

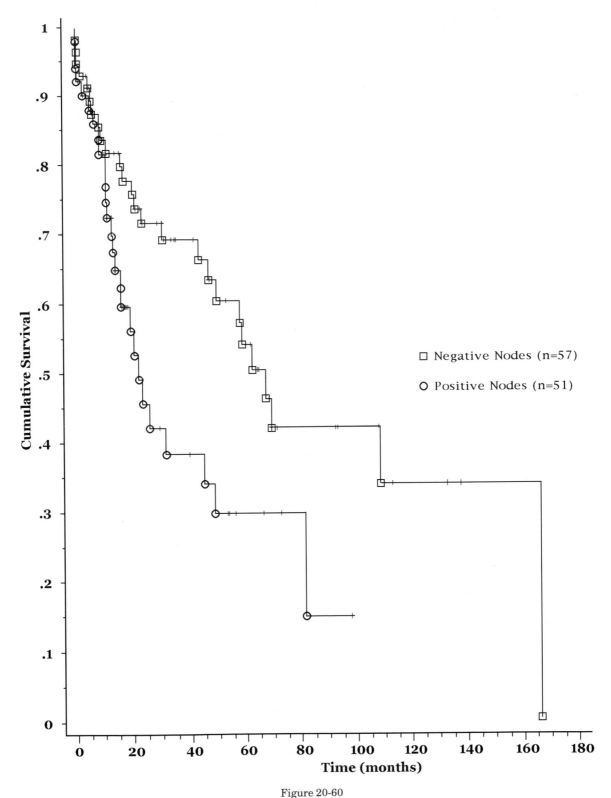

Figure 20-60
SURVIVAL FOLLOWING RESECTION OF
AMPULLARY CARCINOMAS WITH NEGATIVE AND POSITIVE LYMPH NODES
The difference in survival is statistically significant (p=0.012). The data are from Memorial Sloan-Kettering Cancer Center.

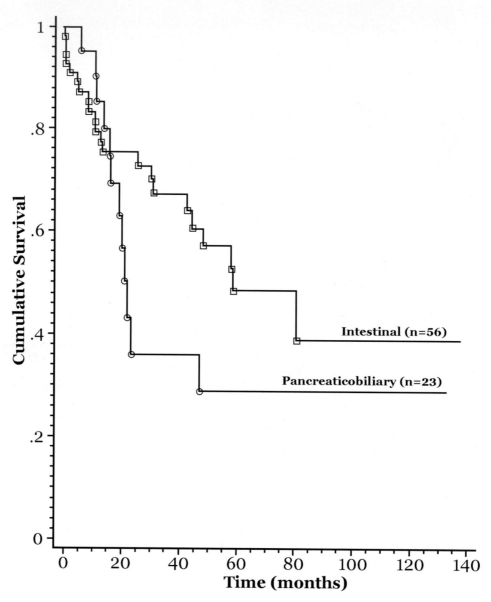

Figure 20-61
SURVIVAL FOLLOWING RESECTION OF INTESTINAL AND
PANCREATOBILIARY TYPE AMPULLARY ADENOCARCINOMAS

Although patients with pancreatobiliary type adenocarcinomas have a median survival of 22.5 months (versus 59.6 months for those with intestinal type adenocarcinomas), the trend towards more aggressive behavior does not reach statistical significance (p=0.23). Data are from Memorial Sloan Kettering Cancer Center.

pancreatobiliary type (fig. 20-61) (217,220). Mucinous (colloid) carcinomas have a somewhat less favorable prognosis; in our cases, the post-resection median survival period was 37 months compared to 59 months for the entire group (217). Because "papillary carcinoma" has often been used without specific indication of whether the tumor also contained an invasive component, it is difficult to interpret studies showing a more favorable survival rate for patients with papillary carcinoma (206,222). Patients with papillary carcinomas lacking stromal invasion have an excellent prognosis. The clinical course of small cell carcinoma is highly aggressive, with most patients dying within 1 year of presentation. The clinical course of large cell neuroendocrine carcinoma is also aggressive, although perhaps not equaling that of small cell carcinoma (214).

The presence of vascular or lymphatic invasion correlates with other indicators of poor prognosis and is not of independent prognostic significance (225).

As assessed by flow cytometry, 60 percent of ampullary carcinomas are aneuploid (228,232). Aneuploid carcinomas behave more aggressively than diploid tumors (228,232), and ploidy has been suggested to be an independent prognostic factor more powerful than stage of disease (232). The possibility has been raised of using ploidy analysis of endoscopic biopsies to identify higher risk patients preoperatively (232), although the frequent finding of heterogeneity in DNA content in different regions of ampullary carcinomas indicates that multiple samples should be studied (234). Patients whose tumors have a larger mean nuclear volume, as measured stereometrically, also have a worse outcome (208).

The proliferative rate may be measured as S-phase fraction by flow cytometry or immunohistochemical staining for proliferation-associated antigens such as Ki-67. In ampullary carcinoma the proliferative rate correlates with other prognostic indices such as tumor stage (218,233) but is not an independent predictor of survival.

Tumors producing sulphomucins may be more aggressive than those producing sialomucins (212). CA19-9-positive tumors are more aggressive (219). There is no difference in survival between those with tumors with or without K-*ras* mutations (216).

REFERENCES

General

1. Baczako K, Buchler M, Beger HG, Kirkpatrick CJ, Haferkamp O. Morphogenesis and possible precursor lesions of invasive carcinoma of the papilla of Vater: epithelial dysplasia and adenoma. Hum Pathol 1985;16:305–10.
2. Blackman E, Nash SV. Diagnosis of duodenal and ampullary epithelial neoplasms by endoscopic biopsy: a clinicopathologic and immunohistochemical study. Hum Pathol 1985;16:901–10.
3. Jones BA, Langer B, Taylor BR, Girotti M. Periampullary tumors: which ones should be resected? Am J Surg 1985;149:46–52.
4. Kellum JM, Clark J, Miller HH. Pancreatoduodenectomy for resectable malignant periampullary tumors. Surg Gyn Obstet 1983;157:362–6.
5. Martin FM, Rossi RL, Dorrucci V, Silverman ML, Braasch JW. Clinical and pathologic correlations in patients with periampullary tumors. Arch Surg 1990;125:723–6.
6. Scarpa A, Capelli P, Zamboni G, et al. Neoplasia of the ampulla of Vater Ki-ras and p53 mutations. Am J Pathol 1993;142:1163–72.
7. Warren KW, Choe DS, Plaza J, Relihan M. Results of radical resection for periampullary cancer. Ann Surg 1975;181:534–40.
8. Wise L, Pizzimbono C, Dehner LP. Periampullary cancer. A clinicopathologic study of sixty-two patients. Am J Surg 1976;131:141–8.

Epidemiology

9. Baczako K, Buchler M, Beger HG, Kirkpatrick CJ, Haferkamp O. Morphogenesis and possible precursor lesions of invasive carcinoma of the papilla of Vater: epithelial dysplasia and adenoma. Hum Pathol 1985;16:305–10.
10. Cattell RB, Pyrtek LJ. Premalignant lesions of the ampulla of Vater. Surg Gyn Obstet 1949;90:21–30.
11. Kimura W, Ohtsubo K. Incidence, sites of origin, and immunohistochemical and histochemical characteristics of atypical epithelium and minute carcinoma of the papilla of Vater. Cancer 1988;61:1394–402.
12. Longmire WP Jr. Periampullary tumours. J R Coll Surg Edinb 1973;18:131–6.

Associated Conditions

13. Alexander JR, Andrews JM, Buchi KN, Lee RG, Becker JM, Burt RW. High prevalence of adenomatous polyps of the duodenal papilla in familial adenomatous polyposis. Dig Dis Sci 1989;34:167–70.

14. Baczako K, Buchler M, Beger HG, Kirkpatrick CJ, Haferkamp O. Morphogenesis and possible precursor lesions of invasive carcinoma of the papilla of Vater: epithelial dysplasia and adenoma. Hum Pathol 1985;16:305–10.

15. Brandt-Rauf PW, Fallon LF. Ampullary cancer in chemical workers. Brit J Ind Med 1987;44:569–70.

16. Cabot RC. Case records of the Massachusetts General Hospital, case 21601. N Engl J Med 1935;212:263–7.

17. Catford J, Prosser IM, Zeegen R, Naik E. Carcinoma of the ampulla of Vater in a haemophiliac patient. Postgrad Med J 1976;52:92–5.

18. Cattell RB, Pyrtek LJ. Premalignant lesions of the ampulla of Vater. Surg Gyn Obstet 1949;90:21–30.

19. Cohen JR, Kuchta N, Geller N, Shires T, Dineen P. Pancreaticoduodenectomy. A 40 year experience. Ann Surg 1982;195:608–17.

20. Colarian J, Pietruk T, LaFave L, Calzada R. Adenocarcinoma of the ampulla of Vater associated with neurofibromatosis [Letter]. J Clin Gastroenterol 1990;12:118–19.

21. Ekbom A, Yuen J, Karlsson BM, McLaughlin JK, Adami HO. Risk of pancreatic and periampullary cancer following cholecystectomy. A population-based cohort study. Dig Dis Sci 1996;41:387–91.

22. Fava M, Foradori G, Cruz F, Guzman S. Papillomatosis of the common bile duct associated with ampullary carcinoma. AJR Am J Roentgenol 1991;156:405–6.

23. Gouma DJ, Obertop H, Vismans J, Willebrand D, Soeters PB. Progression of a benign epithelial ampullary tumor to adenocarcinoma. Surgery 1987;101:501–4.

24. Harned RK, Williams SM. Familial polyposis coli and periampullary malignancy. Dis Colon Rectum 1982;25:227–9.

25. Hatch EE, Curtis RE, Boice JD, Fraumeni JF. Malignant neoplasms associated with cancer of the ampulla of Vater [Letter]. Br J Cancer 1992;66:1204.

26. Hayes DH, Bolton JS, Willis GW, Bowen JC. Carcinoma of the ampulla of Vater. Ann Surg 1987;206:572–7.

27. Jagelman DG, DeCosse JJ, Bussey HJ. Upper gastrointestinal cancer in familial adenomatous polyposis. Lancet 1988;8595:1149–51.

28. Jones TR, Nance FC. Periampullary malignancy in Gardner's syndrome. Ann Surg 1977;185:565–73.

29. Kimura W, Ohtsubo K. Incidence, sites of origin, and immunohistochemical and histochemical characteristics of atypical epithelium and minute carcinoma of the papilla of Vater. Cancer 1988;61:1394–402.

30. Klein A, Clemens J, Cameron J. Periampullary neoplasms in von Recklinghausen's disease. Surgery 1989;106:815–9.

31. Komorowski RA, Tresp MG, Wilson SD. Pancreaticobiliary involvement in familial polyposis coli/Gardner's syndrome. Dis Colon Rectum 1986;29:55–8.

32. Kozuka S, Tsubone M, Yamaguchi A, Hachishuka K. Adenomatous residue in cancerous papilla of Vater. Gut 1981;22:1031–4.

33. Lynch HT, Smyrk TC, Lanspa SJ, et al. Upper gastrointestinal manifestations in families with hereditary flat adenoma syndrome. Cancer 1993;71:2709–14.

34. Mao C, Huang Y, Howard JM. Carcinoma of the ampulla of Vater and mesenteric fibromatosis (desmoid tumor) associated with Gardner's syndrome: problems in management. Pancreas 1995;10:239–45.

35. Neoptolemos JP, Talbot IC, Shaw DC, Carr-Locke DL. Long-term survival after resection of ampullary carcinoma is associated independently with tumor grade and a new staging classification that assesses local invasiveness. Cancer 1988;61:1403–7.

36. Nishihara K, Tsuneyoshi M, Shimura H, Yasunami Y. Three synchronous carcinomas of the papilla of Vater, common bile duct and pancreas. Pathol Int 1994;44:325–32.

37. Noda Y, Watanabe H, Iida M, et al. Histologic follow-up of ampullary adenomas in patients with familial adenomatosis coli. Cancer 1992;70:1847–56.

38. Offerhaus GJ, Giardiello FM, Krush AJ, et al. The risk of upper gastrointestinal cancer in familial adenomatous polyposis. Gastroenterology 1992;102:1980–82.

39. Pauli RM, Pauli ME, Hall JG. Gardner syndrome and periampullary malignancy. Am J Med Genet 1980;6:205–19.

40. Robertson JF, Boyle P, Imrie CW. Patients with ampullary carcinoma are prone to other malignant tumours. Br J Cancer 1988;58:216–8.

41. Sahel J, Bastid C, Choux R. Biliary ascariasis combined with a villous tumor of the papilla. Diagnostic and therapeutic value of endoscopy. Endoscopy 1987;19:243–5.

42. Schlippert W, Lucke D, Anuras S, Christensen J. Carcinoma of the papilla of Vater. A review of fifty-seven cases. Am J Surg 1978;135:763–70.

43. Seifert E, Schulte F, Stolte M. Adenoma and carcinoma of the duodenum and papilla of Vater: a clinicopathologic study. Am J Gastroenterol 1992;87:37–42.

44. Shemesh E, Bat L. A prospective evaluation of the upper gastrointestinal tract and periampullary region in patients with Gardner syndrome. Am J Gastroenterol 1985;80:825–7.

45. Shirai Y, Tsukada K, Ohtani T, et al. Carcinoma of the ampulla of Vater: histopathologic analysis of tumor spread in Whipple pancreatoduodenectomy specimens. World J Surg 1995;19:102–7.

46. Stolte M, Pscherer C. Adenoma-carcinoma sequence in the papilla of Vater. Scand J Gastroenterol 1996;31:376–82.

47. Talbot IC, Neoptolemos JP, Shaw DE, Carr-Locke DL. The histopathology and staging of carcinoma of the ampulla of Vater. Histopathology 1988;12:155–65.

48. Transveldt E, Keith RG, Fonger J, Fisher MM. Annular pancreas with coexistent ampullary carcinoma in an elderly woman. Can J Surg 1982;25:687–8.

49. Vayopoulos G, Constanopoulos C, Fotiou C, Kaklamanis PH, Fessas PH. Dermatomyositis/polymyositis and carcinoma of the ampulla of Vater [Letter]. Ann Rheum Dis 1987;46:945–6.

50. Williams JA, Cubilla A, Maclean BJ, Fortner JG. Twenty-two year experience with periampullary carcinoma at Memorial Sloan–Kettering Cancer Center. Am J Surg 1979;138:662–5.

51. Wormsley, KG, Logan WF, Sorrell VF, Cole GC. Neurofibromatosis with pancreatic duct obstruction and steatorrhoea. Postgrad Med J 1967;43:432–5.

52. Yamaguchi K, Enjoji M. Adenoma of the ampulla of Vater: putative precancerous lesion. Gut 1991;32:1558–61.

53. Yamashita H, Higashijima H, Fukushima K, et al. Carcinoma of the ampulla of Vater synchronously associated with early gastric cancer—a report of two cases. Eur J Surg Oncol 1995;21:427–34.

54. Yamauchi H, Nitta A, Kakizaki K, Imamura M, Namiki T, Ichinohasama R. Different distribution of CA19-9 in carcinomas arising in the papilla of Vater. An immunohistochemical study. Tohoku J Exp Med 1993;170:235–44.

55. Yoshida J, Morisaki T, Yamaguchi K, et al. Carcinoma in adenoma of the ampulla of Vater synchronous with cancer of the sigmoid colon. Dig Dis Sci 1990;35:271–5.

Clinical Features

56. Akwari OE, van Heerden JA, Adson MA, Baggenstoss AH. Radical pancreatoduodenectomy for cancer of the papilla of Vater. Arch Surg 1977;112:451–6.

57. Baczako K, Buchler M, Beger HG, Kirkpatrick CJ, Haferkamp O. Morphogenesis and possible precursor lesions of invasive carcinoma of the papilla of Vater: epithelial dysplasia and adenoma. Hum Pathol 1985;16:305–10.

58. Bakkevold KE, Arnesjo B, Kambestad B. Carcinoma of the pancreas and papilla of Vater: presenting symptoms, signs, and diagnosis related to stage and tumour site. A prospective multicentre trial in 472 patients. Scand J Gastroenterol 1992;27:317–25.

59. Jones BA, Langer B, Taylor BR, Girotti M. Periampullary tumors: which ones should be resected? Am J Surg 1985;149:46–52.

60. Makipour H, Cooperman A, Danzi JT, Farmer RG. Carcinoma of the ampulla of Vater: review of 38 cases with emphasis on treatment and prognostic factors. Ann Surg 1976;183:341–4.

61. Neoptolemos JP, Talbot IC, Carr-Locke DL, et al. Treatment and outcome in 52 consecutive cases of ampullary carcinoma. Br J Surg 1987;74:957–61.

62. Ponchon T, Berger F, Chavaillon A, Bory R, Lambert R. Contribution of endoscopy to diagnosis and treatment of tumors of the ampulla of Vater. Cancer 1989;64:161–7.

63. Schlippert W, Lucke D, Anuras S, Christensen J. Carcinoma of the papilla of Vater. A review of fifty-seven cases. Am J Surg 1978;135:763–70.

64. Treadwell TA, Jimenez-Chapa JF, White RR. Carcinoma of the ampulla of Vater. South Med 1978;71:365–7.

65. Walsh DB, Eckhauser FE, Cronenwett JL, Turcotte JG, Lindenauer SM. Adenocarcinoma of the ampulla of Vater. Diagnosis and treatment. Ann Surg 1982;195:152–7.

66. Williams JA, Cubilla A, Maclean B, Fortner JG. Twenty-two year experience with periampullary carcinoma at Memorial Sloan-Kettering Cancer Center. Am J Surg 1979;138:662–5.

67. Wise L, Pizzimbono C, Dehner LP. Periampullary cancer. A clinicopathologic study of sixty-two patients. Am J Surg 1976;131:141–8.

Laboratory Findings

68. Akwari OE, van Heerden JA, Adson MA, Baggenstoss AH. Radical pancreatoduodenectomy for cancer of the papilla of Vater. Arch Surg 1977;112:451–6.

69. Lee YT, Tatter D. Carcinoma of the pancreas and periampullary structures. Arch Pathol Lab Med 1984;108:584–7.

70. Ponchon T, Berger F, Chavaillon A, Bory R, Lambert R. Contribution of endoscopy to diagnosis and treatment of tumors of the ampulla of Vater. Cancer 1989;64:161–7.

71. Sato Y, Tominaga H, Tangoku A, Hamanaka Y, Yamashita Y, Suzuki T. Alpha-fetoprotein-producing cancer of the ampulla of Vater. Hepatogastroenterology 1992;39:566–9.

72. Walsh DB, Eckhauser FE, Cronenwett JL, Turcotte JG, Lindenauer SM. Adenocarcinoma of the ampulla of Vater. Diagnosis and treatment. Ann Surg 1982;195:152–7.

73. Wise L, Pizzimbono C, Dehner LP. Periampullary cancer. A clinicopathologic study of sixty-two patients. Am J Surg 1976;131:141–8.

Diagnostic Considerations

74. Blackman E, Nash SV. Diagnosis of duodenal and ampullary epithelial neoplasms by endoscopic biopsy: a clinicopathologic and immunohistochemical study. Hum Pathol 1985;16:901–10.

75. Bourgeois N, Dunham F, Verhest A, Cremer M. Endoscopic biopsies of the papilla of Vater at the time of endoscopic sphincterotomy: difficulties in interpretation. Gastrointest Endo 1984;30:163–6.

76. Buck JL, Elsayed AM. Ampullary tumors: radiologic-pathologic correlation. Radiographics 1993;13:193–212.

77. Buice WS, Walker LG Jr. The role of intra-operative biopsy in the treatment of resectable neoplasms of the pancreas and periampullary region. Am Surg 1989;55:307–10.

78. Conlon KC, Dougherty E, Klimstra DS, Coit DG, Turnbull AS, Brennan MF. The value of minimal access surgery in the staging of patients with potentially resectable peripancreatic malignancy. Ann Surg 1996;223:134–40.

79. Earnhardt RC, McQuone SJ, Minasi JS, Feldman PS, Jones RS, Hanks JB. Intraoperative fine needle aspiration of pancreatic and extrahepatic biliary masses. Surg Gynecol Obstet 1993;177:147–52.

80. Fockens P. The role of endoscopic ultrasonography in the biliary tract: ampullary tumors. Endoscopy 1994;26:803–5.

81. Geng JZ, Qin PR, Hui LD, Po PD. CT guided fine needle aspiration biopsy of biliopancreatic lesions: report of 30 cases. Jpn J Surg 1987;17:461–4.

82. Hall TJ, Blackstone MO, Cooper MJ, Hughes RG, Moossa AR. Prospective evaluation of endoscopic retrograde cholangiopancreatography in the diagnosis of periampullary cancers. Ann Surg 1978;187:313–7.

83. Howe JR, Klimstra DS, Moccia RD, Conlon KC, Brennan MF. Factors predictive of survival in ampullary carcinoma: results in 123 patients between 1983–1995. Ann Surg 1998;228:87–94.

84. Huibregtse K, Tytgat GN. Carcinoma of the ampulla of Vater: the endoscopic approach. Endoscopy 1988;20:223–6.

85. Inamoto K, Tanaka S, Yamazaki H, Suzuki E, Ishikawa Y. Computed tomography of carcinoma of the ampulla of Vater. ROFO Fortschr Geb Rontgenstr Nuklearmed 1982;136:689–93.

86. Khandelwal KC, Merchant NH, Udani RJ, Sharma OP, Goel S. CT staging of pancreatic and periampullary carcinoma. Indian J Cancer 1992;29:66–70.

87. Komorowski RA, Beggs BK, Geenan JE, Venu RP. Assessment of ampulla of Vater pathology. An endoscopic approach. Am J Surg Pathol 1991;15:1188–96.

88. Lim JH, Lee DH, Ko YT, Yoon Y. Carcinoma of the ampulla of Vater: sonographic and CT diagnosis. Abdom Imaging 1993;18:237–41.

89. Mukai H, Nakajima M, Yasuda K, Mizuno S, Kawai K. Evaluation of endoscopic ultrasonography in the pre-operative staging of carcinoma of the ampulla of Vater and common bile duct. Gastrointest Endosc 1992;38:676–83.

90. Nix GA, Van Overbeeke IC, Wilson JH, Ten Kate FJ. ER diagnosis of tumors in the region of the head of the pancreas. Analysis of criteria and computer-aided diagnosis. Dig Dis Sci 1988;33:577–86.

91. Ponchon T, Berger F, Chavaillon A, Bory R, Lambert R. Contribution of endoscopy to diagnosis and treatment of tumors of the ampulla of Vater. Cancer 1989;64:161–7.

92. Rosch T, Braig C, Gain T, et al. Staging of pancreatic and ampullary carcinoma by endoscopic ultrasonography. Comparison with conventional sonography, computed tomography, and angiography. Gastroenterology 1992;102:188–99.

93. Stolte M, Pscherer C. Adenoma-carcinoma sequence in the papilla of Vater. Scand J Gastroenterol 1996;31:376–82.

94. Witte S. Brush cytology of the papilla of Vater. Scand J Gastroenterol 1979;54:55–8.

95. Yamaguchi K, Enjoji M, Kitamura K. Endoscopic biopsy has limited accuracy in diagnosis of ampullary tumors. Gastrointest Endosc 1990;36:588–92.

Pathologic Features

96. Akwari OE, van Heerden JA, Adson MA, Baggenstoss AH. Radical pancreatoduodenectomy for cancer of the papilla of Vater. Arch Surg 1977;112:451–6.

97. Cubilla AL, Fitzgerald PJ. Surgical pathology aspects of cancer of the ampulla-head of pancreas region. Monogr Pathol 1980;21:67–81.

98. Tasaka K. Carcinoma in the region of the duodenal papilla. A histopathologic study (author's transl). Fukuoka Igaku Zasshi 1977;68:20–44.

99. Wise L, Pizzimbono C, Dehner LP. Periampullary cancer. A clinicopathologic study of sixty-two patients. Am J Surg 1976;131:141–8.

100. Yamaguchi K, Enjoji M. Carcinoma of the ampulla of Vater. A clinicopathologic study and pathologic staging of 109 cases of carcinoma and 5 cases of adenoma. Cancer 1987;59:506–15.

Microscopic Features

101. Attanoos R, Williams GT. Epithelial and neuroendocrine tumors of the duodenum. Semin Diag Pathol 1991;8:149–62.

102. Baczako K, Buchler M, Beger HG, Kirkpatrick CJ, Haferkamp O. Morphogenesis and possible precursor lesions of invasive carcinoma of the papilla of Vater: epithelial dysplasia and adenoma. Hum Pathol 1985;16:305–10.

103. Batge B, Bosslet K, Sellacek HH, Kern HF, Kloppel G. Monoclonal antibodies against CEA-related components discriminate between pancreatic duct type carcinomas and nonneoplastic duct lesions as well as nonduct type neoplasias. Virchows Arch [A] 1986;408:361–74.

104. Blackman E, Nash SV. Diagnosis of duodenal and ampullary epithelial neoplasms by endoscopic biopsy: a clinicopathologic and immunohistochemical study. Hum Pathol 1985;16:901–10.

105. Chareton B, Coiffic J, Landen S, Bardaxoglove E, Campion JP, Launois B. Diagnosis and therapy for ampullary tumors: 63 cases. World J Surg 1996;20:707–12.

106. Dawson PJ, Connolly MM. Influence of site of origin and mucin production on survival in ampullary carcinoma. Ann Surg 1989;210:173–9.

107. Ferrell LD, Beckstead JH. Paneth-like cells in an adenoma and adenocarcinoma in the ampulla of Vater. Arch Pathol Lab Med 1991;115:956–8.

108. Howe JR, Klimstra DS, Moccia RD, Conlon KC, Brennan MF. Factors predictive of survival in ampullary carcinoma: results in 123 patients between 1983–1995. Ann Surg 1998;228:87–94.

109. Kimura W, Futakawa N, Yamagata S, et al. Different clinicopathologic findings in two histologic types of carcinoma of papilla of Vater. Jpn J Cancer Res 1994;85:161–6.

110. Kimura W, Ohtsubo K. Incidence, sites of origin, and immunohistochemical and histochemical characteristics of atypical epithelium and minute carcinoma of the papilla of Vater. Cancer 1988;61:1394–402..

111. Malik AK, Bhaskar KV, Wig JD. Periampullary carcinoma with special reference to their mucin characteristics—a pathologic study of 53 cases. Indian J Pathol Microbiol 1992;35:81–7.

112. Maxwell P, Davis RI, Sloan JM. Carcinoembryonic antigen (CEA) in benign and malignant epithelium of the gallbladder, extrahepatic bile ducts, and ampulla of Vater. J Pathol 1993;170:73–6.

113. Talbot IC, Neoptolemos JP, Shaw DE, Carr-Locke DL. The histopathology and staging of carcinoma of the ampulla of Vater. Histopathology 1988;12:155–65.

114. Yamaguchi K, Enjoji M, Tsumeyoshi M. Pancreatoduodenal carcinoma: a clinicopathologic study of 304 patients and immunohistochemical observation for CEA and CA19.9. J Surg Oncol 1991;47:148–54.

115. Yamauchi H, Nitta A, Kakizaki K, Imamura M, Namiki T, Ichinohasama R. Different distribution of CA19-9 in carcinomas arising in the papilla of Vater. An immunohistochemical study. Tohoku J Exp Med 1993;170:235–44.

Unusual Histologic Types of Ampullary Carcinoma

116. Adsay NV, Adair CF, Heffess CS, Klimstra DS. Intraductal oncocytic papillary neoplasms of the pancreas. Am J Surg Pathol 1996;20:980–94.

117. Akwari OE, van Heerden JA, Adson MA, Baggenstoss AH. Radical pancreatoduodenectomy for cancer of the papilla of Vater. Arch Surg 1977;112:451–6.

118. Albores-Saavedra J, Henson DE, Milchgrub S. Intraductal papillary carcinoma of the main pancreatic duct. Int J Pathol 1994;16:223–4.

119. Albores-Saavedra J, Molberg K, Henson DE. Unusual malignant epithelial tumors of the gallbladder. Semin Diag Pathol 1996;13:326–38.

120. Blackman E, Nash SV. Diagnosis of duodenal and ampullary epithelial neoplasms by endoscopic biopsy: a clinicopathologic and immunohistochemical study. Hum Pathol 1985;16:901–10.

121. Blumgart LH, Kennedy A. Carcinoma of the ampulla of Vater and duodenum. Br J Surg 1973;60:33–40.

122. Dawson PJ, Connolly MM. Influence of site of origin and mucin production on survival in ampullary carcinoma. Ann Surg 1989;210:173–9.

123. Emory RE Jr, Emory TS, Goellner JR, Grant CS, Nagorney DM. Neuroendocrine ampullary tumors: spectrum of disease including the first report of a neuroendocrine carcinoma of non-small cell type. Surgery 1994;115:762–6.

124. Fava M, Foradori G, Cruz F, Guzman S. Papillomatosis of the common bile duct associated with ampullary carcinoma. AJR Am J Roentgenol 1991;156:405–6.

125. Gardiner GW, Lajoie G, Keith R. Hepatoid adenocarcinoma of the papilla of Vater. Histopathology 1992;20:541–4.

126. Gardner HA, Matthews J, Ciano PS. A signet-ring cell carcinoma of the ampulla of Vater. Arch Pathol Lab Med 1990;114:1071–2.

127. Hayes DH, Bolton JS, Willis GW, Bowen JC. Carcinoma of the ampulla of Vater. Ann Surg 1987;206:572–7.

128. Klimstra DS, Rosai JR. Osteoclastic giant cell tumor of the pancreas. Critical commentary. Path Res Pract 1993;189:232–3.

129. Lee CS, Machet D, Rode J. Small cell carcinoma of the ampulla of Vater. Cancer 1992;70:1502–4.

130. Michelassi F, Erroi F, Dawson PJ, et al. Experience with 647 consecutive tumors of the duodenum, ampulla, head of the pancreas, and distal common bile duct. Ann Surg 1989;210:544–56.

131. Mills SE, Allen MS Jr, Cohen AR. Small cell undifferentiated carcinoma of the colon. A clinicopathological study of five cases and their association with colonic adenomas. Am J Surg Pathol 1983;7:643–51.

131a. Molberg KH, Heffess C, Delgado R, Albores-Saavedra J. Undifferentiated carcinoma with osteoclast-like giant cells of the pancreas and periampullary region. Cancer 1998;82:1279–87.

132. Mori K, Ikei S, Yamane T, et al. Pathological factors influencing survival of the ampulla of Vater carcinoma. Eur J Surg Oncol 1990;16:183–8.

133. Nagai E, Ueki T, Chijiwa K, Tanaka M, Tsuneyoshi M. Intraductal papillary mucinous neoplasms of the pancreas associated with so-called mucinous ductal ectasia. Am J Surg Pathol 1995;19:576–89.

134. Neoptolemos JP, Talbot IC, Shaw DC, Carr-Locke DL. Long-term survival after resection of ampullary carcinoma is associated independently with tumor grade and a new staging classification that assesses local invasiveness. Cancer 1988;61:1403–7.

135. Nishihara K, Tsuneyoshi M, Shimura H, Yasunami Y. Three synchronous carcinomas of the papilla of Vater, common bile duct and pancreas. Pathol Int 1994;44:325–32.

136. Sarker AB, Hoshida SY, Akagi S, et al. An immunohistochemical and ultrastructural study of case of small cell neuroendocrine carcinoma in the ampullary region of the duodenum. Acta Pathol Jpn 1992;42:529–35.

137. Sato T, Yamamoto K, Ouchi A, Imaoka Y, Tokumura H, Matsushiro T. Undifferentiated carcinoma of the duodenal ampulla. J Gastroenterol 1995;30:517–9.

138. Sato Y, Tominaga H, Tangoku A, Hamanaka Y, Yamashita Y, Suzuki T. Alpha-fetoprotein-producing cancer of the ampulla of Vater. Hepatogastroenterology 1992;39:566–9.

139. Seifert E, Schulte F, Stolte M. Adenoma and carcinoma of the duodenum and papilla of Vater: a clinicopathologic study. Am J Gastroenterol 1992;87:37–42.

140. Sessa F, Solcia E, Capella C, et al. Intraductal papillary mucinous tumours represent a distinct group of pancreatic neoplasms: an investigation of tumour cell differentiation and K-ras, p53, and c-erbB-2 abnormalities in 26 patients. Virchows Arch 1994;425:357–67.

141. Swanson PE, Dykoski PA, Wick MR, Snover DC. Primary duodenal small-cell neuroendocrine carcinoma with production of vasoactive intestinal polypeptide. Arch Pathol Lab Med 1986;110:317–20.

142. Travis WD, Linnoila RI, Tsokos MG, et al. Neuroendocrine tumors of the lung with proposed criteria for large-cell neuroendocrine carcinoma. An ultrastructural, immunohistochemical, and flow cytometric study of 35 cases. Am J Surg Pathol 1991;15:529–53.

143. Vardaman C, Albores-Saavedra J. Clear cell carcinoma of the gallbladder and extrahepatic bile ducts. Am J Surg Pathol 1995;19:91–9.

144. Warren KW, Choe DS, Plaza J, Relihan M. Results of radical resection for periampullary cancer. 1975;181:534–40.

145. Wise L, Pizzimbono C, Dehner LP. Periampullary cancer. A clinicopathologic study of sixty-two patients. Am J Surg 1976;131:141–8.

146. Yamaguchi K, Enjoji M. Carcinoma of the ampulla of Vater. A clinicopathologic study and pathologic staging of 109 cases of carcinoma and 5 cases of adenoma. Cancer 1987;59:506–15.

147. Zamboni G, Franzin G, Bonetti F, et al. Small-cell neuroendocrine carcinoma of the ampullary region. A clinicopathologic, immunohistochemical, and ultrastructural study of three cases. Am J Surg Pathol 1990;14:703–13.

Histologic Grading

148. Baczako K, Buchler M, Beger HG, Kirkpatrick CJ, Haferkamp O. Morphogenesis and possible precursor lesions of invasive carcinoma of the papilla of Vater: epithelial dysplasia and adenoma. Hum Pathol 1985;16:305–10.

149. Howe JR, Klimstra DS, Moccia RD, Conlon KC, Brennan MF. Factors predictive of survival in ampullary carcinoma: results in 123 patients between 1983–1995. Ann Surg 1998;228:87–94.

Molecular Biologic Considerations

150. Bapat B, Odze R, Mitri A, Berk T, Ward M, Gallinger S. Identification of somatic APC gene mutations in periampullary adenomas in a patient with familial adenomatous polyposis (FAP). Hum Mol Gen 1993;2:1957–9.

151. Bulow S, Olsen PS, Poulsen SS, Kirkegaard P. Is epidermal growth factor involved in development of duodenal polyps in familial polyposis coli? Am J Gastroenterol 1988;83:404–6.

152. Chung CH, Wilentz RE, Polak MM, et al. Clinical significance of K-ras oncogene activation in ampullary neoplasms. J Clin Pathol 1996;49:460–4.

153. Finkelstein SD, Sayegh R, Christensen S, Swalsky PA. Genotypic classification of colorectal adenocarcinoma. Biologic behavior correlates with k-ras-2 mutation type. Cancer 1993;71:3827–38.

154. Gallinger S, Vivona AA, Odze RD, et al. Somatic APC and K-ras codon 12 mutations in periampullary adenomas and carcinomas from familial adenomatous polyposis patients. Oncogene 1995;10:1875–8.

155. Howe JR, Klimstra DS, Cordon-Cardo C, Paty PB, Park P, Brennan MF. K-ras mutation in adenomas and carcinomas of the ampulla of Vater. Clin Can Res 1997;3:129–33.

156. Malats N, Porta M, Pinol JL, Corominas JM, Rifa J, Real FX. Ki-ras mutations as a prognostic factor in extrahepatic bile system cancer. PANK-ras I project investigators. J Clin Oncol 1995;13:1679–86.

157. Michelassi F, Erroi F, Dawson PJ, et al. Experience with 647 consecutive tumors of the duodenum, ampulla, head of the pancreas, and distal common bile duct. Ann Surg 1989;210:544–56.

158. Motojima K, Tsunoda T, Kanematsu ST, Nagata Y, Urano T, Shiku H. Distinguishing pancreatic carcinoma from other periampullary carcinomas by analysis of mutations in the Kirsten-ras oncogene. Ann Surg 1991;214:657–62.

159. Resnick MB, Gallinger S, Wang HH, Odze RD. Growth factor expression and proliferation kinetics in periampullary neoplasms in familial adenomatous polyposis. Cancer 1995;76:187–94.

160. Scarpa A, Capelli P, Zamboni G, Oda T, Mukai K, Bonetti F. Neoplasia of the ampulla of Vater Ki-ras and p53 mutations. Am J Pathol 1993;142:1163–72.

161. Scarpa A, Zamboni G, Achille A, et al. Ras-family gene mutations in neoplasia of the ampulla of Vater. Int J Cancer 1994;59:39–42.

162. Shyr YM, Su CH, Li AF, et al. Prognostic value of MIB1, index and DNA ploidy in resectable ampulla of Vater carcinoma. Ann Surg 1999;229:523–7.

163. Stork P, Loda M, Bosari S, Wiley B, Poppenhusen K, Wolfe H. Detection of K-ras mutations in pancreatic and hepatic neoplasms by non-isotopic mismatched polymerase chain reaction. Oncogene 1991;6:857–62.

164. Teh M, Wee A, Raju GC. An immunohistochemical study of p53 protein in gallbladder and extrahepatic bile duct/ampullary carcinomas. Cancer 1994;74:1542–5.

165. Vaidya P, Kawarada Y, Higashiguchi T, Yoshida T, Sakakura T, Yatani R. Overexpression of different members of the type I growth factor receptor family and their association with cell proliferation in periampullary carcinoma. J Pathol 1996;178:140–5.

166. Vogelstein B, Fearon ER, Hamilton SR, et al. Genetic alterations during colorectal tumor development. N Engl J Med 1988;319:252–32.

167. Watanabe M, Asaka M, Tanaka J, Kurosawa M, Kasai M, Miyazaki T. Point mutation of K-ras gene codon 12 in biliary tract tumors. Gastroenterology 1994;107:1147–53.

168. Younes M, Riley S, Genta RM, Mosharaf M, Mody DR. p53 protein accumulation in tumors of the ampulla of Vater. Cancer 1995;76:1150–4.

Behavior

169. Akwari OE, van Heerden JA, Adson MA, Baggenstoss AH. Radical pancreatoduodenectomy for cancer of the papilla of Vater. Arch Surg 1977;112:451–6.

170. Allema JH, Reinders ME, van Gulik TM, et al. Results of pancreaticoduodenectomy for ampullary carcinoma and analysis of prognostic factors for survival. Surgery 1995;117:247–53.

171. Bakkevold KE, Kambestad B. Long-term survival following radical and palliative treatment of patients with carcinoma of the pancreas and papilla of Vater—the prognostic factors influencing the long-term results. A prospective multicentre study. Eur J Surg Oncol 1993;19:147–61.

172. Barton RM, Copeland EM III. Carcinoma of the ampulla of Vater. Surg Gyn Obs 1983;156:297–301.

173. Cohen JR, Kuchta N, Geller N, Shires T, Dineen P. Pancreaticoduodenectomy. A 40 year experience. Ann Surg 1982;195:608–17.

174. Crist DW, Sitzmann JV, Cameron JL. Improved hospital morbidity, mortality and survival after the Whipple procedure. Ann Surg 1987;206:358–65.

175. Delcore R Jr, Connor CS, Thomas JH, Friesen SR, Hermreck AS. Significance of tumor spread in adenocarcinoma of the ampulla of Vater. Am J Surg 1989;158:593–7.

176. Forrest JF, Longmire WP. Carcinoma of the pancreas and periampullary region. A study of 279 patients. Ann Surg 1979;189:129–38.
177. Hayes DH, Bolton JS, Willis GW, Bowen JC. Carcinoma of the ampulla of Vater. Ann Surg 1988;205:572–7.
178. Herter FP, Cooperman AM, Ahlborn TN, Antinori C. Surgical experience with pancreatic and periampullary cancer. Ann Surg 1982;195:274–81.
179. Howe JR, Klimstra DS, Moccia RD, Conlon KC, Brennan MF. Factors predictive of survival in ampullary carcinoma: results in 123 patients between 1983–1995. Ann Surg 1998;228:87–94.
180. Jones BA, Langer B, Taylor BR, Girotti M. Periampullary tumors: which ones should be resected. Am J Surg 1985;149:46–52.
181. Kellum JM, Clark J, Miller HH. Pancreatoduodenectomy for resectable malignant periampullary tumors. Surg Gynecol Obstet 1983;157:362–6.
182. Klempnauer J, Ridder GJ, Pichlmayr R. Prognostic factors after resection of ampullary carcinomas: multivariate survival analysis in comparison with ductal cancer of the pancreatic head. Br J Surg 1995;82:1686–91.
183. Lee YT, Tatter D. Carcinoma of the pancreas and periampullary structures. Arch Pathol Lab Med 1984;108:584–7.
184. Makipour H, Cooperman A, Danzi JT, Farmer RG. Carcinoma of the ampulla of Vater: review of 38 cases with emphasis on treatment and prognostic factors. Ann Surg 1976;183:341–4.
185. Martin FM, Rossi RL, Dorrucci V, Silverman ML, Braasch JW. Clinical and pathologic correlations in patients with periampullary tumors. Arch Surg 1990;125:723–6.
186. Matory YL, Gaynor J, Brennan M. Carcinoma of the ampulla of Vater. Surg Gynecol Obstet 1993;177:366–70.
187. Michelassi F, Erroi F, Dawson PJ, et al. Experience with 647 consecutive tumors of the duodenum, ampulla, head of the pancreas, and distal common bile duct. Ann Surg 1989;210:544–56.
188. Monge JJ, Judd ES, Gage RP. Radical pancreatoduodenectomy: a 22 year experience with the complications, mortality rate and survival rate. Ann Surg 1964;160:711–22.
189. Mori K, Ikei S, Yamane T, et al. Pathological factors influencing survival of carcinoma of the ampulla of Vater. Eur J Surg Oncol 1990;16:183–8.
190. Nakase A, Matsumoto Y, Uchida K, Honjo I. Surgical treatment of cancer of the pancreas and the periampullary region: cumulative results in 57 institutions in Japan. Ann Surg 1977;185:52–7.
191. Neoptolemos JP, Talbot IC, Carr-Locke DL, et al. Treatment and outcome in 52 consecutive cases of ampullary carcinoma. Br J Surg 1987;74:957–61.
192. Schlippert W, Lucke D, Anuras S, Christensen J. Carcinoma of the papilla of Vater. A review of fifty-seven cases. Am J Surg 1978;135:763–70.
193. Shirai Y, Tsukada K, Ohtani T, et al. Carcinoma of the ampulla of Vater: histopathologic analysis of tumor spread in Whipple pancreatoduodenectomy specimens. World J Surg 1995;19:102–7.
194. Shutze WP, Sack J, Aldrete JS. Long-term follow-up of 24 patients undergoing radical resection for ampullary carcinoma, 1953–1988. Cancer 1990;66:1717–20.
195. Sperti C, Pasquali C, Piccoli A, Sernagiotto C, Pedrazzoli S. Radical resection for ampullary carcinoma: long-term results. Br J Surg 1994;81:668–71.
196. Spiessl B, Beahrs OH, Hermanek P, et al, eds. TNM Atlas. Berlin: Springer-Verlag, 1992.
197. Stephenson LW, Blackstone EH, Aldrete JS. Radical resection for periampullary carcinomas. Results in 53 patients. Arch Surg 1977;112:245–9.
198. Talamini MA, Moesinger RC, Pitt HA, et al. Adenocarcinoma of the ampulla of Vater. A 28 year experience. Ann Surg 1997;225:590–600.
199. Tarazi RY, Hermann RE, Vogt DP, et al. Results of surgical treatment of periampullary tumors: a thirty-five year experience. Surgery 1986;100:716–23.
200. Treadwell TA, Jimenez-Chapa JF, White RR. Carcinoma of the ampulla of Vater. South Med 1978;71:365–7.
201. Walsh DB, Eckhauser FE, Cronenwett JL, Turcotte JG, Lindenauer SM. Adenocarcinoma of the ampulla of Vater. Diagnosis and treatment. Ann Surg 1982;195:152–7.
202. Warren KW, Choe DS, Plaza J, Relihan M. Results of radical resection for periampullary cancer. Ann Surg 1975;181:534–40.
203. Willett CG, Warshaw AL, Convery K, Compton CC. Patterns of failure after pancreaticoduodenectomy for ampullary carcinoma. Surg Gynecol Obstet 1993;176:33–8.
204. Williams JA, Cubilla A, Maclean B, Fortner JG. Twenty-two year experience with periampullary carcinoma at Memorial Sloan-Kettering Cancer Center. Am J Surg 1979;138:662–5.
205. Wise L, Pizzimbono C, Dehner LP. Periampullary cancer. A clinicopathologic study of sixty-two patients. Am J Surg 1976;131:141–8.

Prognostic Factors

206. Akwari OE, van Heerden JA, Adson MA, Baggenstoss AH. Radical pancreatoduodenectomy for cancer of the papilla of Vater. Arch Surg 1977;112:451–6.
207. Allema JH, Reinders ME, van Gulik TM, et al. Results of pancreaticoduodenectomy for ampullary carcinoma and analysis of prognostic factors for survival. Surgery 1995;117:247–53.
208. Artacho-Perula E, Roldan-Villalobos R, Lopez-Rubio F, Vaamonde-Lemos R. Stereological estimates of nuclear volume in carcinoma of the ampulla of Vater. Histopathology 1992;21:241–8.
209. Bakkevold KE, Kambestad B. Long-term survival following radical and palliative treatment of patients with carcinoma of the pancreas and papilla of Vater– the prognostic factors influencing the long-term results. A prospective multicentre study. Eur J Surg Oncol 1993;19:147–61.
210. Bakkevold KE, Kambestad B. Staging of carcinoma of the pancreas and ampulla of Vater. Tumor (T), lymph node (N), and distant metastases (M) as prognostic factors. Int J Pancreatol 1995;17:249–59.
211. Barton RM, Copeland EM III. Carcinoma of the ampulla of Vater. Surg Gyn Obs 1983;156:297–301.
212. Dawson PJ, Connolly MM. Influence of site of origin and mucin production on survival in ampullary carcinoma. Ann Surg 1989;210:173–9.

213. Delcore R Jr, Connor CS, Thomas JH, Friesen SR, Hermreck AS. Significance of tumor spread in adenocarcinoma of the ampulla of Vater. Am J Surg 1989;158:593–7.

214. Emory RE Jr, Emory TS, Goellner JR, Grant CS, Nagorney DM. Neuroendocrine ampullary tumors: spectrum of disease including the first report of a neuroendocrine carcinoma of non-small cell type. Surgery 1994;115:762–6.

215. Hayes DH, Bolton JS, Willis GW, Bowen JC. Carcinoma of the ampulla of Vater. Ann Surg 1988;205:572–7.

216. Howe JR, Klimstra DS, Cordon-Cardo C, Paty PB, Park PY, Brennan MF. K-ras mutation in adenomas and carcinomas of the ampulla of Vater. Clin Cancer Res 1997;3:129–33.

217. Howe JR, Klimstra DS, Moccia RD, Conlon KC, Brennan MF. Factors predictive of survival in ampullary carcinoma: results in 123 patients between 1983–1995. Ann Surg 1998;228:87–94.

218. Isozaki H, Okajima K, Ichinona T, et al. The significance of proliferating cell nuclear antigen (PCNA) expression in cancer of the ampulla of Vater in terms of prognosis. Surg Today 1994;24:494–9.

219. Kamisawa T, Fukayama M, Koike M, et al. Carcinoma of the ampulla of Vater: expression of cancer-associated antigens inversely correlated with prognosis. Am J Gastroenterol 1988;83:1118–23.

220. Kimura W, Futakawa N, Yamagata S, et al. Different clinicopathologic findings in two histologic types of carcinoma of papilla of Vater. Jpn J Cancer Res 1994;85:161–6.

221. Klempnauer J, Ridder GJ, Pichlmayr R. Prognostic factors after resection of ampullary carcinomas: multivariate survival analysis in comparison with ductal cancer of the pancreatic head. Br J Surg 1995;82:1686–91.

222. Makipour H, Cooperman A, Danzi JT, Farmer RG. Carcinoma of the ampulla of Vater: Review of 38 cases with emphasis on treatment and prognostic factors. Ann Surg 1976;183:341–4.

223. Martin FM, Rossi RL, Dorrucci V, Silverman ML, Braasch JW. Clinical and pathologic correlations in patients with periampullary tumors. Arch Surg 1990;125:723–6.

224. Matory YL, Gaynor J, Brennan M. Carcinoma of the ampulla of Vater. Surg Gynecol Obstet 1993;177:366–70.

225. Mori K, Ikei S, Yamane T, et al. Pathological factors influencing survival of carcinoma of the ampulla of Vater. Eur J Surg Oncol 1990;16:183–8.

226. Neoptolemos JP, Talbot IC, Carr-Locke DL, et al. Treatment and outcome in 52 consecutive cases of ampullary carcinoma. Br J Surg 1987;74:957–61.

227. Roder JD, Schneider PM, Stein HJ, Siewert JR. Number of lymph node metastases is significantly associated with survival in patients with radically resected carcinoma of the ampulla of Vater. Br J Surg 1995;82:1693–6.

228. Sciallero S, Giaretti W, Geido E, et al. DNA aneuploidy is an independent factor of poor prognosis in pancreatic and peripancreatic cancer. Int J Pancreatol 1993;14:21–8.

229. Shirai Y, Tsukada K, Ohtani T, et al. Carcinoma of the ampulla of Vater: histopathologic analysis of tumor spread in Whipple pancreatoduodenectomy specimens. World J Surg 1995;19:102–7.

230. Shutze WP, Sack J, Aldrete JS. Long-term follow-up of 24 patients undergoing radical resection for ampullary carcinoma, 1953–1988. Cancer 1990;66:1717–20.

231. Shyr YM, Su CH, Lo SS, Wang HC, Lui WY. Is pancreatoduodenectomy justified for periampullary cancers with regional lymph node involvement. Am Surg 1995;61:288–93.

232. Shyr YM, Su CH, Wu LH, Liu AF, Chiu JH, Lui WY. DNA ploidy as a major prognostic factor in resectable ampulla of Vater cancers. J Surg Oncol 1993;53:220–5.

233. Sperti C, Pasquali C, Piccoli A, Sernagiotto C, Pedrazzoli S. Radical resection for ampullary carcinoma: long-term results. Br J Surg 1994;81:668–71.

234. Suto T, Sasaki K, Sugai T, Kanno S, Saito K. Heterogeneity in the nuclear DNA content of cells in carcinomas of the biliary tract and pancreas. Cancer 1993;72:2920–8.

235 Tajiri H, Yoshimori M, Nakamura K, et al. A clinicopathologic study of carcinoma of the papilla of Vater. Jpn J Clin Oncol 1984;14:667–77.

236. Willett CG, Warshaw AL, Convery K, Compton CC. Patterns of failure after pancreaticoduodenectomy for ampullary carcinoma. Surg Gynecol Obstet 1993;176:33–8.

237. Wise L, Pizzimbono C, Dehner LP. Periampullary cancer. A clinicopathologic study of sixty-two patients. Am J Surg 1976;131:141–8.

238. Yamaguchi K, Enjoji M. Carcinoma of the ampulla of Vater. A clinicopathologic study and pathologic staging of 109 cases of carcinoma and 5 cases of adenoma. Cancer 1987;59:506–15.

239. Yamauchi H, Nitta A, Kakizaki K, Imamura M, Namiki T, Ichinohasama R. Different distribution of CA19-9 in carcinomas arising in the papilla of Vater. An immunohistochemical study. Tohoku J Exp Med 1993;170:235–44.

✧✧✧

21
ENDOCRINE TUMORS AND RELATED NEOPLASMS
OF THE AMPULLARY REGION

Endocrine neoplasms of the ampulla and peri-ampullary duodenum have a broad morphologic and biologic spectrum. Most can be classified as carcinoid tumors, although variants have been defined based on their morphologic appearance and association with specific clinical syndromes. The ampullary region is the origin of less than 5 percent of intestinal endocrine tumors and less than 30 percent of those involving the upper small intestine (1–3). Although malignant, most of these tumors are indolent and regarded as low grade. High-grade endocrine tumors (small cell carcinoma and large cell neuroendocrine carcinoma) also occur in the periampullary region, although they are rare.

CARCINOID TUMORS

Carcinoid tumors constitute only 3.1 percent of ampullary epithelial neoplasms in our material. A recent review identified only 85 carcinoid tumors of the ampulla (18a). Most ampullary carcinoid tumors exhibit insular and glandular features, often with psammoma body formation (18a).

Clinical Features. Most patients with carcinoid tumors of the ampulla are in the fifth or sixth decades, and there is a male predominance (12,22). The frequently reported association with neurofibromatosis (5,6,9,15,16,26) is largely for glandular carcinoids producing somatostatin; however, there have also been a few cases of nonglandular carcinoid tumors in patients with neurofibromatosis (13,14,17). These tumors also frequently produce somatostatin. A second association with ampullary and more commonly duodenal carcinoid tumors is the Zollinger-Ellison syndrome, often as part of multiple endocrine neoplasia (MEN) 1. The tumors associated with this syndrome are gastrin-producing carcinoids or "gastrinomas." The carcinoid syndrome is rarely seen with carcinoid tumors of the ampulla, and it usually occurs in the presence of liver metastases (12). Patients with nonsyndromic ampullary carcinoid tumors present with the same symptoms as do those with other ampullary

neoplasms: jaundice (12,19,22) or obstructive pancreatitis (11).

Although it is difficult to predict which carcinoid tumors will give rise to metastases, the prognosis has some relation to tumor size and depth of penetration (24). Increased mitoses (more than 5 per 10 high-power fields) have also been associated with a less favorable outcome (18). One third to half of patients develop lymph node or liver metastases; however, the tumors are slow growing and survival for many years is possible even in the presence of multiple liver metastases (4,12). The 5-year survival rate is 90 percent (12).

Pathologic Findings. Grossly, carcinoid tumors of the ampulla are submucosal nodules, usually less than 2 cm, and centered in the periampullary submucosa or surrounding the intraduodenal portion of the distal bile duct. The overlying mucosa may be intact or ulcerated over larger examples (fig. 21-1). Nests of tumor cells may extend into the mucosa. The tumors are generally circumscribed but not encapsulated.

Histologically, the typical patterns of foregut carcinoid tumors are represented: nesting, cribriform, and trabecular patterns are characteristically present and frequently mixed (fig. 21-2). The cells are uniform and the cell borders are poorly defined. Moderate amounts of cytoplasm and round nuclei with stippled chromatin are typical. In most cases there are few mitoses (1 to 2 per 10 high-power fields) and minimal or no necrosis (7). In the region of the distal pancreatic and bile ducts and common channel, periductal ductules may be entrapped within the tumor (fig. 21-3).

Silver staining reveals argyrophilia in most ampullary and duodenal carcinoid tumors; only about 10 percent are argentaffin positive (7). Immunohistochemically, positive staining for endocrine markers such as chromogranin, synaptophysin, Leu-7, and neuron-specific enolase is seen in more than 90 percent of cases (fig. 21-4). In most instances the staining is diffuse and strong, with staining for chromogranin generally the most intense and reliable. Specific peptides are also commonly found; only 10 percent of cases do

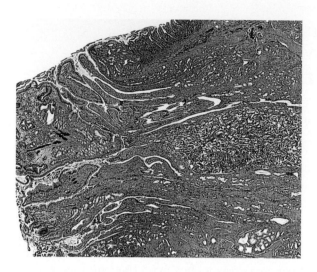
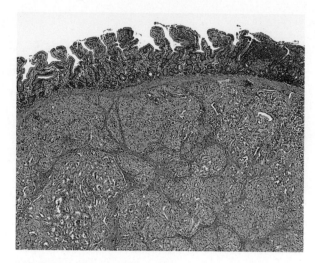

Figure 21-1
AMPULLARY CARCINOID TUMOR
Left: In this minute example, the tumor compresses the intra-ampullary portion of the distal common bile duct.
Right: This example is sharply circumscribed and underlies an intact duodenal mucosa.

Figure 21-2
CARCINOID TUMOR
The tumor cells are arranged in nests (A), trabeculae (B), or a cribriform pattern (C), with small luminal spaces punctuating the larger nests.

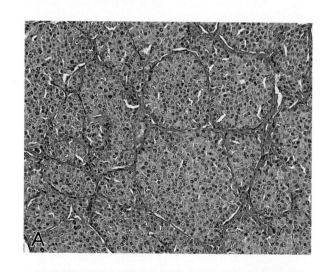
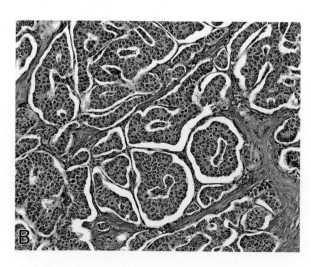
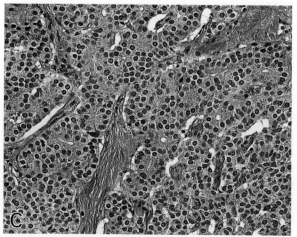

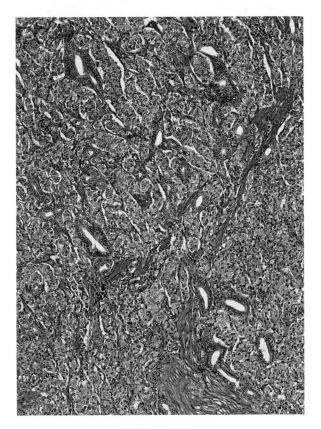

Figure 21-3
CARCINOID TUMOR

Periampullary ductules are commonly entrapped within carcinoid tumors and must be distinguished from true glandular formations by the neoplastic cells.

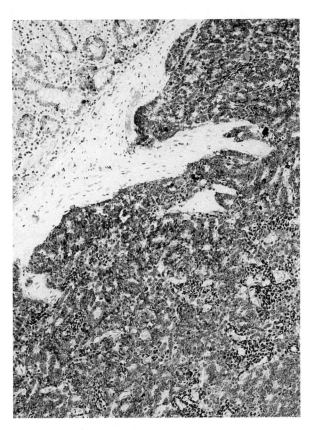

Figure 21-4
CHROMOGRANIN REACTIVITY
IN CARCINOID TUMOR

Immunohistochemical staining of an ampullary carcinoid for chromogranin reveals intense positivity of the tumor cells. Non-neoplastic endocrine cells of the overlying duodenal mucosa are also positive (top left).

not express any specific peptides at the immunohistochemical level (7). Somatostatin production is common, although usually in glandular carcinoid tumors. Most somatostatin-producing carcinoids occur in the ampullary region, especially if it is the only hormone produced by the tumor (7,10). Gastrin and serotonin may also be identified. When serotonin is detected, it is usually within a small percentage of the tumor cells (7). It is exceptional for carcinoid tumors of the ampulla not to express either somatostatin or gastrin (23). However, coexpression of more than one peptide is frequent, and widely scattered cells may contain other peptides such as calcitonin, pancreatic polypeptide, insulin, and vasoactive intestinal polypeptide (4,25). Most carcinoid tumors express keratin.

Carcinoid tumors of the ampulla most likely arise from endocrine cells located within the surrounding duodenal mucosa or even within the ampullary epithelium. In addition to serotonin, the two peptide hormones most consistently detected in the non-neoplastic duodenal mucosa are the same ones commonly found in ampullary carcinoid tumors: somatostatin and gastrin. Somatostatin-positive cells have also been found in the ampullary epithelium (7,8), perhaps in part explaining the ampullary predilection for somatostatin-producing carcinoids. The possibility that endocrine cells proliferate through hyperplastic, dysplastic, and finally neoplastic stages (as occurs in the stomach) is not well documented in the ampullary region. Endocrine cell hyperplasia has occasionally been associated with carcinoid tumors of the ampulla (21,25); endocrine cell micronests have been identified in nearly 5 percent of systematically examined major papillae (20).

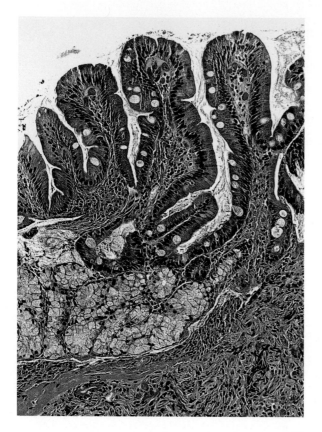 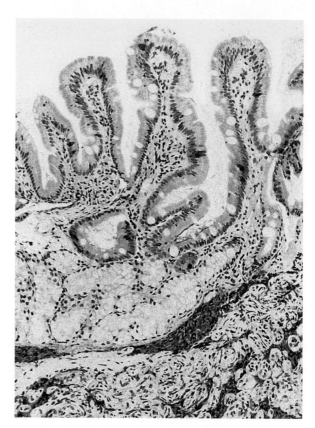

Figure 21-5
PERIAMPULLARY CARCINOID TUMOR

Left: Duodenal endoscopic biopsies of periampullary carcinoid tumors may reveal only small, indistinct nests of tumor within the mucosa and superficial submucosa by routine microscopy.

Right: Immunohistochemical staining for chromogranin highlights these tumor cell nests and is helpful in establishing the correct diagnosis.

Because of their submucosal location, carcinoid tumors may be missed on endoscopic biopsy; occasionally, only a few nests of tumor cells may be found among small intestinal glands (fig. 21-5, left). Immunohistochemical staining for chromogranin or other general endocrine markers is useful for establishing the endocrine nature of ampullary carcinoids, especially on small biopsies (fig. 21-5, right). Somatostatin-producing tumors however, have been noted to express chromogranin inconsistently (7).

Differential Diagnosis. The differential diagnosis includes higher grade neoplasms, such as adenocarcinomas with a solid or cribriform pattern and high-grade neuroendocrine carcinomas. These tumors exhibit more nuclear atypia and necrosis, and a higher mitotic rate than carcinoid tumors. One lesion that may be difficult to distinguish from carcinoid tumor is gangliocytic paraganglioma (see below), particularly on the basis of small biopsies which may not sample all patterns in the latter tumor. The presence of ganglion-like and Schwann cells mixed with carcinoid-like elements should suggest the diagnosis of gangliocytic paraganglioma.

Although the concept of an atypical carcinoid tumor is not well accepted outside of the lung, there are occasional tumors in the gastrointestinal tract, including the ampulla, which exhibit more mitoses than classic carcinoids, as well as punctate necrosis (fig. 21-6), but not to the extent of a high-grade neuroendocrine carcinoma (see chapter 20). Unfortunately, the rarity of these cases has prevented an assessment of their clinical behavior.

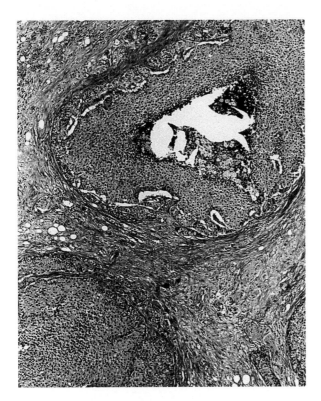 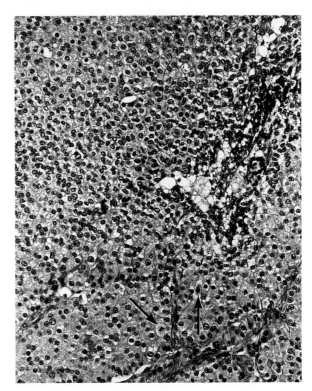

Figure 21-6
PERIAMPULLARY CARCINOID TUMOR WITH ATYPICAL FEATURES
Left: The tumor forms large nests with central, comedo-like necrosis.
Right: Although the tumor cells are not markedly pleomorphic, there are relatively abundant mitotic figures (arrows).

GLANDULAR CARCINOID TUMOR

Definition. Glandular carcinoid tumors are low-grade neuroendocrine tumors with a glandular growth pattern, which occur most commonly in the duodenum and the ampullary region. Ampullary carcinoids usually contain somatostatin and less frequently serotonin (18a). Psammomatous calcifications are often present within the glands, resulting in alternative terms such as *ampullary somatostatinoma, psammomatous carcinoid,* or *psammomatous somatostatinoma.* These tumors are usually not associated with the clinical features of somatostatin hypersecretion (28). Also, psammoma body formation is not invariable. Thus, glandular carcinoid tumor best reflects the most consistent features of these tumors.

Clinical Features. Glandular carcinoids affect both sexes equally and occur in middle aged adults. Blacks have an increased incidence (29). There is a strong association with neurofibromatosis (31,32,37,38,42), although the syndrome is not

invariably present (34,36,39). Pheochromocytoma, another manifestation of neurofibromatosis, has also been present in some patients (32,33,42).

It is uncommon for glandular carcinoids to produce the somatostatinoma syndrome (38), despite the common production of somatostatin. Only a few reported patients had endocrine symptoms attributable to the tumor (40,41). Thus, the presenting symptoms are usually similar to those of other ampullary neoplasms.

Glandular carcinoids are more likely than other ampullary carcinoids to metastasize; lymph node metastases occur in 50 to 70 percent of cases (30,34,41). Liver metastases are not infrequent. Death attributable to glandular and conventional carcinoids occur in about 20 percent of the cases (18a).

Pathologic Findings. Grossly, glandular carcinoids resemble other ampullary carcinoids, although they have a greater tendency to infiltrate (28). Most cases are exquisitely glandular, composed of large cribriform nests as well as single

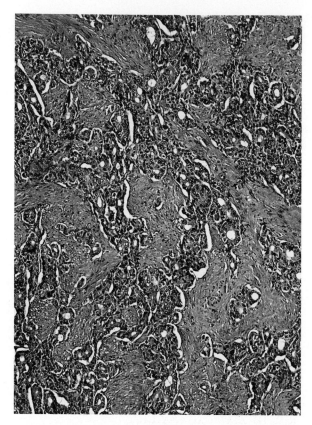

Figure 21-7
GLANDULAR CARCINOID TUMOR
In this example, small glands are present and a stromal component is relatively abundant.

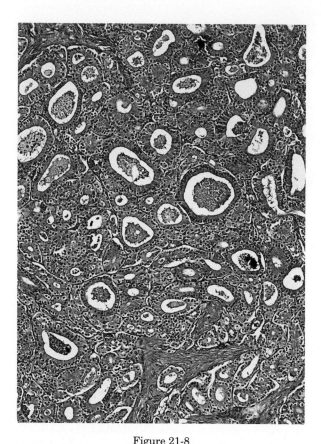

Figure 21-8
GLANDULAR CARCINOID TUMOR
In other regions, the glands are more ectatic and contain inspissated secretory material. (Figures 21-8 and 21-9 are from the same patient.)

glands infiltrating a fibrous stroma (fig. 21-7). In some tumors, however, insular and trabecular patterns predominate. Infiltration into the muscularis and underlying pancreas is common; often linear arrays of glands are seen between fascicles of smooth muscle (figs. 21-7, 21-8). The cells are cuboidal to low columnar and arranged in a single layer with basal round, uniform nuclei (fig. 21-9). Mitotic figures are rare. The cytoplasm is eosinophilic and granular. The luminal spaces are lined by a thick cuticular layer and frequently contain eosinophilic proteinaceous secretions and psammoma bodies (fig. 21-9). The psammoma bodies may form by calcium encrustation of the luminal secretions (35), although an intracellular origin has also been suggested (41). Although not all glandular carcinoid tumors contain psammoma bodies, most psammomatous carcinoids exhibit gland formation (28).

By silver staining techniques, glandular carcinoids are argentaffin negative, and argyrophilia is uncommon (27,31,34). Immunohistochemical stains for chromogranin and other general endocrine markers are positive (fig. 21-10, left). Most cases stain diffusely for somatostatin (fig. 21-10, right) and serotonin. Prosomatostatin is also detectable in some cases (36). Other peptides may be found, although generally not in somatostatin-positive tumors (28,30,31,41). Mucin is positive in the lumina (fig. 21-11); intracellular mucin is not detected. By electron microscopy, neurosecretory granules are usually abundant (fig. 21-12). Two populations of granules may be identified, one measuring 800 nm, the other 275 nm (30). A basement membrane surrounds the glands. True glandular lumina are lined by microvilli with rootlets, and a glycocalyx is present (35,39).

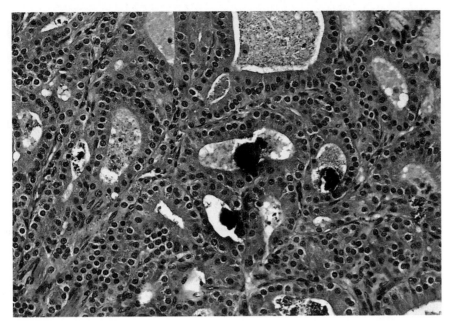

Figure 21-9
GLANDULAR
CARCINOID TUMOR
At high power, the glands exhibit sharply outlined lumina containing scattered psammoma bodies. The nuclei are round and uniform, and exhibit a stippled chromatin pattern typical of endocrine neoplasms. Moderate amounts of amphophilic to eosinophilic cytoplasm are present.

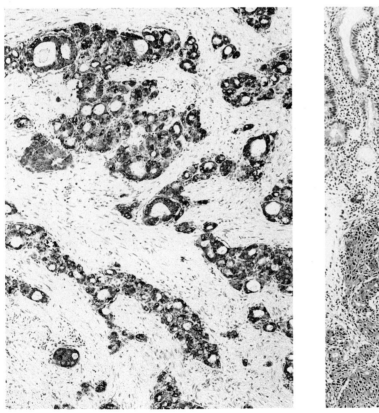
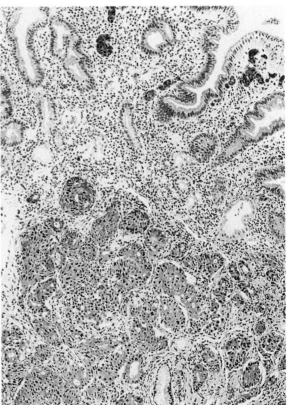

Figure 21-10
CHROMOGRANIN AND SOMATOSTATIN REACTIVITY IN CARCINOID TUMOR
Immunohistochemical staining of glandular carcinoid tumor shows positive reactivity for chromogranin (left), as well as somatostatin (right), hence the alternative name ampullary somatostatinoma. Note the small nests of tumor cells in the superficial mucosa.

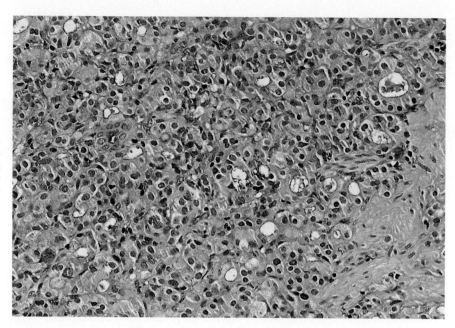

Figure 21-11
MUCIN-PRODUCING
GLANDULAR CARCINOID
Staining of a glandular carcinoid tumor with mucicarmine reveals ultraluminal mucin and staining of the luminal cell surfaces, although intracellular mucin is not detected.

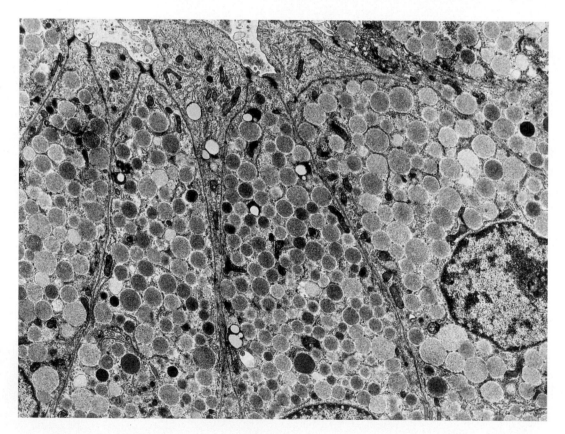

Figure 21-12
ULTRASTRUCTURAL APPEARANCE OF SOMATOSTATIN-PRODUCING GLANDULAR CARCINOID TUMOR
The tumor cells are filled with variably electron dense granules averaging 800 nm. The granule contents are surrounded by a thin halo beneath the limiting membrane. At their apical aspect, the tumor cells border a luminal space and are joined by tight junctions.

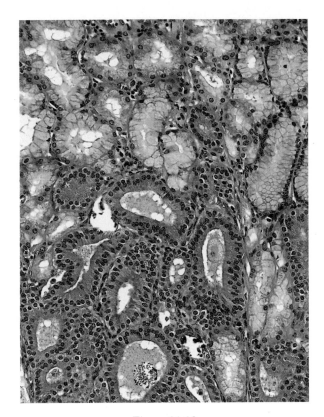

Figure 21-13
GLANDULAR CARCINOID TUMOR
INVOLVING THE DUODENAL SUBMUCOSA
Note the adjacent Brunner's glands (top), which bear some
cytoarchitectural similarity to those of the carcinoid tumor.

Differential Diagnosis. Glandular carcinoid tumors may be confused with well-differentiated adenocarcinomas. The presence of psammoma bodies and the absence of nuclear atypia, significant mitotic activity, and a desmoplastic stroma should suggest the correct diagnosis. Immunohistochemistry is confirmatory. Both the simple nature of the glands and the lack of atypia may suggest a Brunner gland proliferation (fig. 21-13), especially on endoscopic biopsy where the infiltrative nature of a glandular carcinoid may not be apparent. Again, immunohistochemistry may be necessary in questionable cases.

GASTRIN-PRODUCING CARCINOID TUMOR (GASTRINOMA)

Gastrin-producing carcinoid tumors may cause peptic ulcer disease due to persistent hypergastrinemia (Zollinger-Ellison syndrome).

Gastrinomas are also found in patients with MEN 1, who often have multiple duodenal and pancreatic endocrine tumors. Although the term "gastrinoma" is applied to a tumor associated with the clinical syndrome, nonsyndromic carcinoid tumors may also produce gastrin, which may be detected by immunohistochemistry. Conversely, gastrin production may not be demonstrable by immunohistochemistry in some tumors from patients with the Zollinger-Ellison syndrome. Since not all gastrin production is detected by routine immunohistochemistry (44), it may still be appropriate to designate these tumors as gastrinomas as long as one excludes the possibility of additional endocrine tumors being the source of the hypergastrinemia (e.g., in MEN 1 patients). Approximately half of gastrin-producing carcinoid tumors occur in the pancreas and half in the gastrointestinal tract, generally in the first and second parts of the duodenum (45). Duodenal gastrinomas in patients with MEN 1 are commonly multiple (43). Despite the common occurrence in the duodenum, gastrinomas of the ampulla are rare (46). Although clinically symptomatic cases may measure only a few millimeters, one third of duodenal gastrinomas metastasize (43,45,46), a rate which probably also applies to those tumors specifically involving the ampulla. The gross and microscopic features of gastrinomas are not significantly different from those of classic ampullary carcinoid tumors (fig. 21-14).

ADENOCARCINOID TUMOR

In the appendix, endocrine tumors with the architectural pattern of carcinoid tumors as well as intracellular mucin production are termed adenocarcinoid tumors or *goblet cell carcinoids* (47,52). Similar mixed endocrine/exocrine neoplasms also occur, although rarely, in the ampulla (49,50). Presenting symptoms are not different from those of other ampullary neoplasms. Although there is insufficient experience to estimate prognosis, adenocarcinoid tumors probably behave in a fashion intermediate between carcinoid tumors and adenocarcinomas (48,49).

Adenocarcinoid tumors are usually small (less than 2 cm in both reported cases) and situated in the submucosa. The consistency is firmer than for classic carcinoid tumors. Microscopically, the

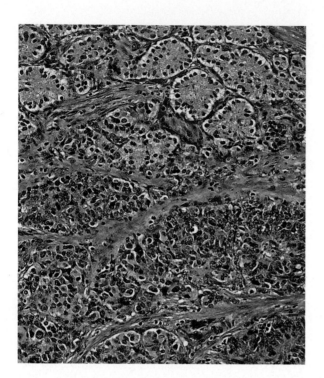 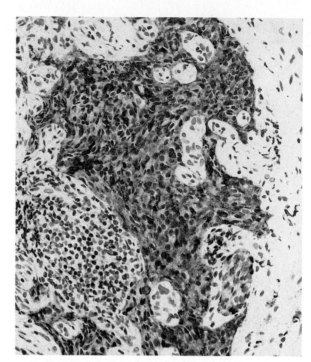

Figure 21-14
PERIAMPULLARY GASTRIN-PRODUCING CARCINOID TUMOR
Left: The histologic features are not significantly different from those of other carcinoid tumors.
Right: Neoplastic cells show positive immunohistochemical staining for gastrin.

cells grow in small nests and tubules with interspersed signet ring cells (figs. 21-15, 21-16). The stroma is relatively abundant. There is a moderate amount of cytoplasm which may exhibit a mucinous appearance in some cells. The nuclei are basally situated and uniform; mitoses are rare. Staining highlights the intracellular mucin in the signet ring cells as well as in other cells within the nests (figs. 21-15C, 21-16D). The tumor cells are also argyrophilic (fig. 21-16C). Carcinoembryonic antigen, chromogranin (figs. 21-15D, 21-16D), synaptophysin, and neuron-specific enolase are positive immunohistochemically. No specific peptides have been detected although serotonin was detected in one case (fig. 21-16E). In one case, electron microscopy revealed both mucigen granules and neurosecretory granules, although apparently not within the same cells (fig. 21-16D) (49).

Adenocarcinoid tumors must be distinguished from high-grade carcinomas showing both glandular and endocrine differentiation (51). Although these mixed adenocarcinoma/endocrine carcinomas also display composite features, they are more aggressive, similar to other ampullary carcinomas. It is not uncommon to detect minor degrees of endocrine differentiation in adenocarcinomas. Adenocarcinoid tumors should also be distinguished from signet ring cell adenocarcinoma. Although both may contain signet ring cells, the pattern of infiltration is more diffuse in signet ring cell adenocarcinoma, and a significant endocrine component is absent.

GANGLIOCYTIC PARAGANGLIOMA

Found almost exclusively in the periampullary region, gangliocytic paraganglioma contains three components: epithelioid (paraganglioma-like or carcinoid-like), ganglion cell–like, and nerve sheath elements. The first description of this lesion appears to be that of Dahl in 1957 (61), who included a duodenal tumor in a review of ganglioneuromas of the gastrointestinal tract. The description and illustrations of that case reveal a small focus of gland-like or "carcinoid-like" nests, in addition to the nerve sheath and ganglionic elements. The first recognition of

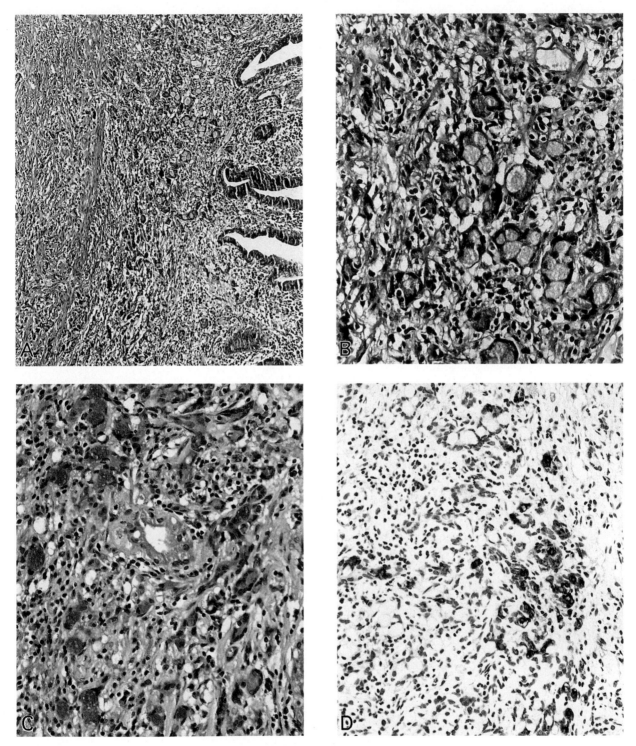

Figure 21-15
ADENOCARCINOID TUMOR OF THE AMPULLA

A: The tumor cells diffusely infiltrate in small nests and individual cells around adjacent duodenal glands.

B: At higher power, signet ring cells are present within the nests and individually.

C: There is mild cytologic atypia. Staining with mucicarmine highlights the intracellular mucin in the signet ring cells.

D: Immunohistochemical staining for chromogranin shows a significant proportion of the tumor cells to exhibit endocrine differentiation. (Courtesy of Dr. Brian West, New Haven, CT; this case has been previously reported [49].)

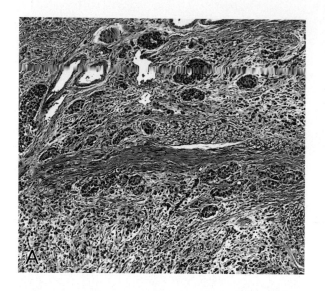

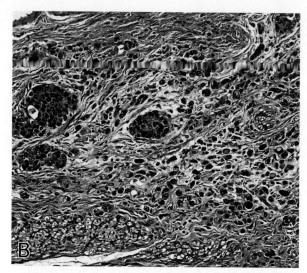

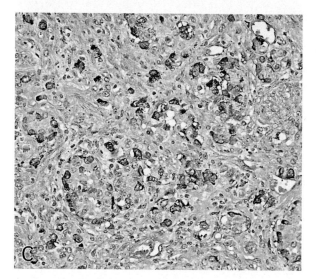

Figure 21-16
ADENOCARCINOID TUMOR OF THE AMPULLA

A: In this example, larger cell nests are present, resembling a typical carcinoid tumor; in addition, there are individual infiltrating cells.

B: The nuclei exhibit typical neuroendocrine features. Individual signet ring cells infiltrate the muscularis.

C: A Grimelius argyrophil stain demonstrates numerous neurosecretory granules within the tumor cells.

D: Double staining for chromogranin and periodic acid–Schiff shows the relationship between the endocrine and mucin-producing cells of this tumor.

E: Although individual nests contain both cell types, it is not possible to recognize both mucin and endocrine differentiation within the same cell. In this case, the neoplastic cells also produce immunohistochemically detectable serotonin.

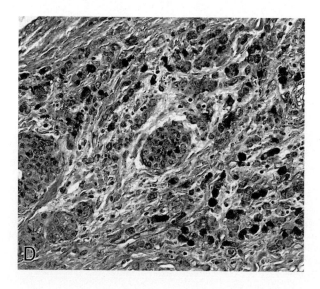

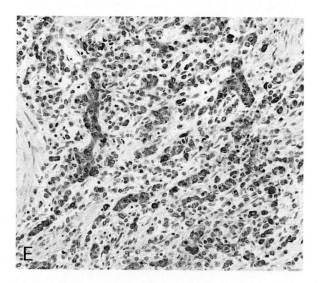

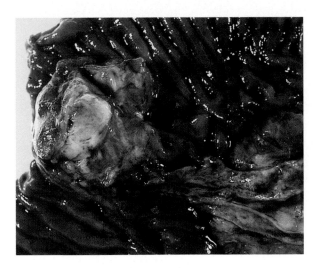

Figure 21-17
GROSS APPEARANCE OF
GANGLIOCYTIC PARAGANGLIOMA
This example is pedunculated, forming a polyp adjacent
to the ampulla. The tumor is tan and circumscribed, and
situated in the duodenal submucosa.

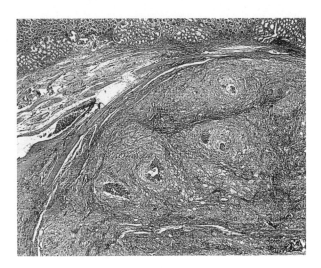

Figure 21-18
GANGLIOCYTIC PARAGANGLIOMA
At low power, this gangliocytic paraganglioma is circumscribed and centered within the submucosa; the overlying
duodenal mucosa is uninvolved.

gangliocytic paraganglioma as a distinct entity came in 1962 when nine cases were reported under the term "nonchromaffin paraganglioma" (85). The term gangliocytic paraganglioma was first used in 1971 in recognition of the ganglion cell component (70). Since then more than 100 cases have been reported, with complete descriptions of the histologic, immunohistochemical, ultrastructural, and clinical features. Some reports have used alternate terms including *paraganglioneuroma* (58,60,69).

Clinical Features. Gangliocytic paraganglioma is an uncommon tumor, representing only 1.2 percent of ampullary neoplasms in our material. Based on the number of reported cases it appears to be more common than ampullary carcinoid, although there may have been a tendency for a greater proportion of cases to be reported because of the unusual nature of the tumor. Gangliocytic paraganglioma can occur from the third to ninth decades; the mean age is 53 years (57,79, 81,85). The youngest patient was 15 years old (80). Males outnumber females by 1.7 to 1 (57,79,81,85). Most patients present with gastrointestinal hemorrhage and abdominal pain (79, 82,85) since the tumor, although generally in the periampullary duodenum, rarely obstructs the bile duct. Some cases have been associated with neu-

rofibromatosis (72,84), although the association is not nearly as strong as for glandular carcinoid tumor. Coexistent duodenal and pancreatic adenocarcinomas have been reported (53,59).

In general gangliocytic paraganglioma is regarded as benign. However, several that metastasized to regional lymph nodes have been reported (56,57,63,67,68). In most of these cases, only the epithelioid element was found in the metastasis. No deaths due to tumor have been recorded.

Gangliocytic paragangliomas occur in the second portion of the duodenum, generally near the ampulla. One case was associated with a duodenal diverticulum (62). The rarity of cases outside this region has made them the subject of case reports. Other locations include jejunum (54,57,79), pylorus (57), and elsewhere in the duodenum (75). Paragangliomas of the cauda equina may exhibit ganglionic differentiation (83) and resemble gangliocytic paraganglioma (81), but they do not exhibit true epithelial (carcinoid) differentiation and therefore are histogenetically different neoplasms.

Pathologic Findings. Grossly, gangliocytic paragangliomas may be sessile or pedunculated (fig. 21-17). They are centered in the submucosa (fig. 21-18); ulceration of the overlying mucosa is common. Most tumors measure 1 to 3 cm, although a 10 cm example has been reported (81). The tumors are tan to white and moderately firm in consistency.

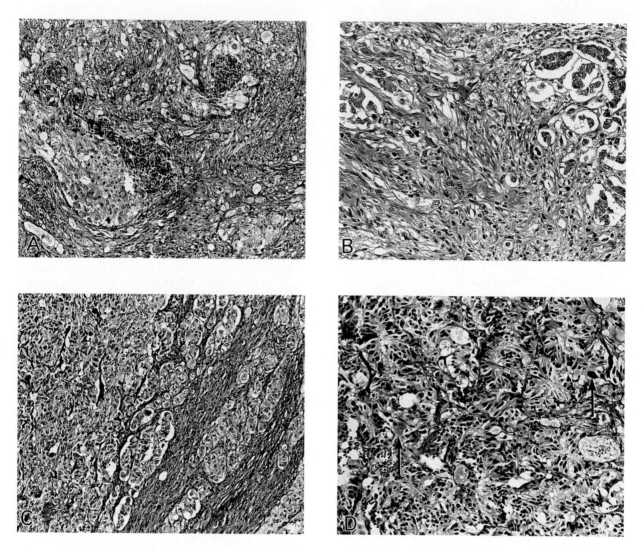

Figure 21-19
HISTOLOGIC APPEARANCE OF GANGLIOCYTIC PARAGANGLIOMA

A: The epithelioid cells are confined to small nests surrounded by an abundant spindle cell stroma (the nerve sheath elements) and the ganglion-like cells are present both individually and in larger aggregates.

B: The epithelioid cells form circumscribed nests resembling those of carcinoid tumors or paragangliomas and are easily distinguished from the other cell types.

C: In this example, the epithelioid cell component predominates, with minimal spindle cell elements.

D: This gangliocytic paraganglioma contains ganglion-like cells (arrows) and very few spindle cells.

The histologic appearance varies from case to case and between different regions of the same tumor. All three cell types, epithelioid, ganglion-like, and nerve sheath, are present in varying proportions (fig. 21-19). Some cases exhibit a predominance of the nerve sheath component, resembling a ganglioneuroma; others have largely epithelioid elements, resembling a paraganglioma or carcinoid tumor. Even when equal amounts of the different elements are present, they often are not evenly distributed throughout the lesion.

The epithelioid cells are arranged in nests or trabeculae surrounded by a rich microvasculature (fig. 21-20A). They have moderate amounts of amphophilic to eosinophilic cytoplasm and round nuclei with inconspicuous nucleoli. The appearance of the epithelioid cells may vary in different regions, resembling a paraganglioma in some areas and a carcinoid tumor in others.

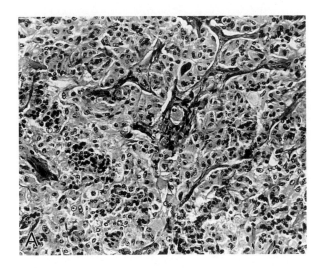

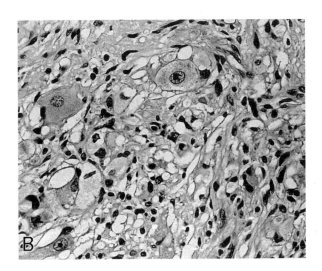

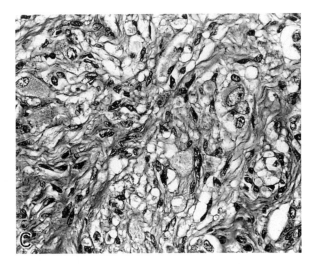

Figure 21-20
GANGLIOCYTIC PARAGANGLIOMA

A: The epithelioid cells vary in nuclear size and amount of cytoplasm.

B: The epithelioid cells are arranged in nests surrounded by a rich microvasculature. Larger cells with dense cytoplasm, open chromatin, and prominent nuclei are indistinguishable from the individual ganglion-like cells found between the spindle cells.

C: Some of the ganglion-like cells of this tumor are nearly indistinguishable from normal ganglion cells. The nerve sheath elements contain both Schwann cells with elongate, curved nuclei and vacuolated cytoplasm, as well as axons, which are inapparent by light microscopy.

The larger ganglion-like cells occur singly, mixed with nerve sheath elements, or in nests. Some resemble normal ganglion cells, having abundant granular cytoplasm and large open nuclei with prominent nucleoli (fig. 21-20B). Others show transitional epithelioid cells, with less cytoplasm and inconspicuous nucleoli. The spindled nerve sheath elements are indistinguishable from Schwann cells (fig. 21-20C). A neuronal component is also present mixed with the Schwann cells. The growth pattern of gangliocytic paraganglioma is infiltrative, with entrapment of smooth muscle or ductular structures. In some cases there is proliferation of the ductules with cytologic atypia, simulating a carcinoma (fig. 27-21). These ductules have been regarded to be heterotopic pancreatic tissue (57),

an interpretation that is especially attractive for those cases located away from the ampulla.

Immunohistochemical studies reveal expression of numerous antigens in gangliocytic paragangliomas (55,57,66,77). The epithelioid cell element is often (50 to 70 percent of cases) positive for keratin (fig. 21-22A) (57,59,63). General endocrine markers such as chromogranin, synaptophysin, and neuron-specific enolase are found in the majority of cases (fig. 21-22B). Specific peptides are also found, especially pancreatic polypeptide and somatostatin (fig. 21-22C,D). The reactivity for pancreatic polypeptide does not appear to be due to cross reactivity with polypeptide YY or with neuropeptide Y (55), peptides that are found in extrapancreatic intestinal endocrine cells (polypeptide YY) or in the brain and

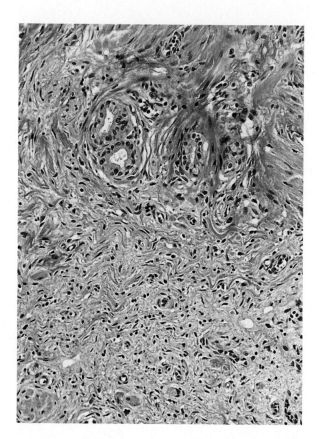 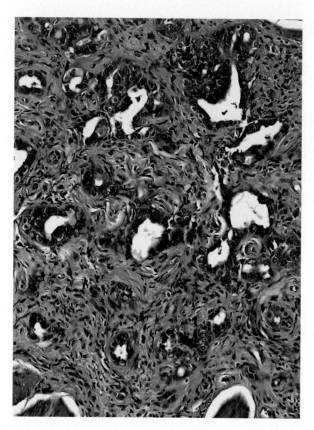

Figure 21-21
GANGLIOCYTIC PARAGANGLIOMA
Left: Small biliary type ductules are often entrapped within gangliocytic paraganglioma.
Right: In some examples, there may be proliferation of these ductules and cytologic atypia, suggesting a carcinoma arising in a gangliocytic paraganglioma.

peripheral nerves (neuropeptide Y) (77). In addition to serotonin, peptides such as gastrin, vasoactive intestinal polypeptide, and glucagon are occasionally found (65,77). The ganglion cells are negative for chromogranin and positive for neuron-specific enolase and synaptophysin (fig. 21-22B). The nerve sheath elements contain S-100 protein, reflecting the Schwann cell component (fig. 21-22E). Neurofilaments are often found within the neurons (fig. 21-22F). Neuron-specific enolase may also stain these cells. S-100 protein–positive cells may surround nests of epithelioid cells, resembling the sustentacular cells of paragangliomas (57).

By electron microscopy, the epithelioid cells are joined by small desmosomes and contain moderate amounts of mitochondria, rough endoplasmic reticulum, and myeloid figures (66). Neurosecretory granules, ranging from 150 to 400 nm, are abundant (fig. 21-23A). Aggregates of intermediate filaments may be present (64, 70). Other than being larger, having more abundant intermediate filaments, and more rough endoplasmic reticulum, the ganglionic cells are not specifically distinct from the epithelioid cells by electron microscopy (fig. 21-23B) (77,78,84). The nerve sheath elements consist of Schwann cells, with interdigitating cell processes, and well-developed basement membrane and axonal processes, with longitudinally oriented microtubules (fig. 21-23C,D) (80).

The origin and nature of gangliocytic paraganglioma remain obscure. The presence of keratin-positive components clearly relates the epithelioid cells more closely to carcinoid tumors than to paraganglioma. Furthermore, the finding of a consistently positive reaction for pancreatic polypeptide establishes a relationship to

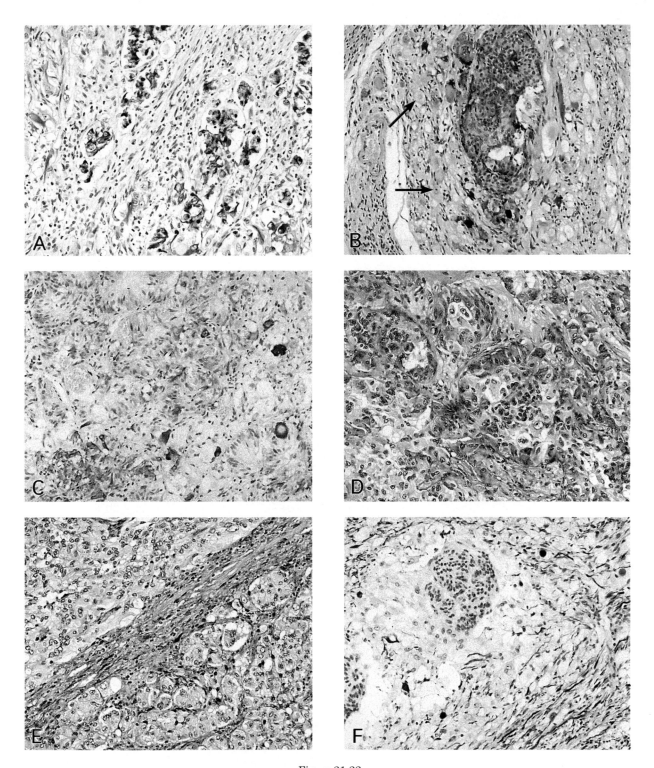

Figure 21-22

IMMUNOHISTOCHEMICAL STAINING OF GANGLIOCYTIC PARAGANGLIOMA

The epithelioid cells stain for cytokeratin (A). Chromogranin reactivity is seen in the epithelioid cells (B); however, the ganglion-like cells are not stained (arrows). The most common peptides identified in these tumors are somatostatin (C) and pancreatic polypeptide (D). The nerve sheath elements are positive for S-100 protein (E), reflecting the Schwann cell component. Note the presence of S-100 protein-positive cells surrounding epithelioid cell nests in a pattern similar to that of the sustentacular cells of paragangliomas (F). The nerve sheath elements also contain neurofilaments within the axonal component.

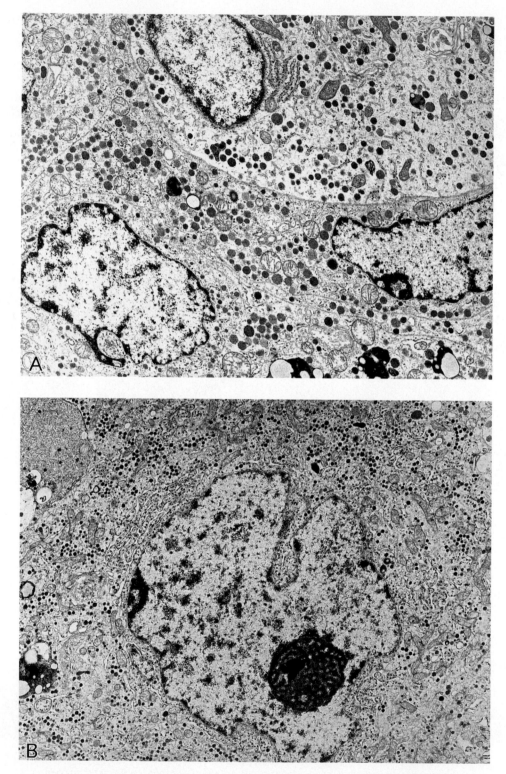

Figure 21-23
ULTRASTRUCTURAL APPEARANCE OF GANGLIOCYTIC PARAGANGLIOMA

A: The epithelioid cells contain numerous neurosecretory type granules.

B: Some larger cells containing nuclei with prominent nucleoli resemble the ganglion-like cells; this example contains abundant rough endoplasmic reticulum but in other ways resembles the epithelioid cells more than a true ganglion cell.

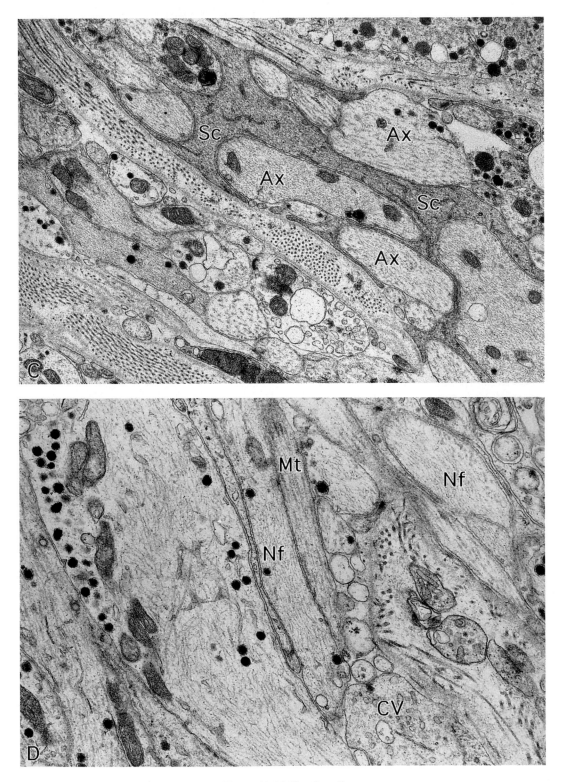

Figure 21-23 (Continued)

C,D: The spindle cell component contains Schwann cells and axons. The Schwann cells (Sc) have dense cytoplasm and elongate cell processes which surround the axons (Ax). A well-formed basement membrane surrounds the Schwann cells. The axons contain neurofilaments (Nf) as well as longitudinally orientated microtubules (Mt). They also contain dense core neurosecretory granules as well as rare clear vesicles (CV).

pancreatic endocrine cells. Thus, the tumor consists of both neuroectodermally derived elements (Schwann cells, neurons, and ganglion cells) as well as an endodermally derived component (carcinoid cells). Whether some of the epithelioid cells truly represent a paragangliomatous component is unclear; the absence of keratin in many areas and the presence of sustentacular-like cells would support a true paragangliomatous component.

Several theories about the histogenesis exist, none of which is entirely satisfactory. Origin from embryonic celiac ganglia (85) or Meissner's plexus (73) has been proposed. Some observers believe the tumor to be a hamartoma rather than a neoplasm (57). Others regard it as a paraganglioma with the ability to differentiate into other neuroectodermal elements (81). Considerable evidence points to a relationship between gangliocytic paraganglioma and the embryonic ventral pancreas (77). The location of most cases parallels the route of migration of the ventral pancreas; pancreatic polypeptide (consistently found in gangliocytic paraganglioma) is derived from the endocrine component of the ventral pancreas; and ductular structures of possible pancreatic origin are often found within the tumors. How is the neuroectodermal component explained in this model? It turns out that an embryologic structure known as the "sympathico-insular complex" may be seen in other animals (fig. 21-24) and in humans. These complexes, found in the pancreas, are composed of islet cells and branches of sympathetic nerves, including ganglion cells (86,87). Perhaps some maldevelopmental process involving sympathico-insular complexes within remnants of the ventral pancreas gives rise to gangliocytic paraganglioma (71,77). It may be that in some cases the epithelioid component becomes truly neoplastic, explaining the occasional nodal metastasis of this component.

There also may be a relationship between gangliocytic paraganglioma and glandular carcinoid tumor (76). They both occur almost exclusively in the periampullary region; glandular structures and psammoma bodies may be found (albeit rarely) in gangliocytic paraganglioma (57,74); small foci of nerve sheath and ganglion-like cells have been reported in otherwise typical glandular carcinoids (57,84); somatostatin is consistently identified in both lesions; and al-

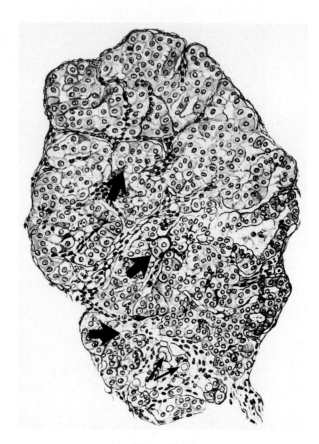

Figure 21-24
SO CALLED SYMPATHICO-INSULAR COMPLEX
OF THE EMBRYONIC PANCREAS
These complexes contain islet cells (large arrows) as well as branches of sympathetic nerves that contain ganglion cells (small arrows); thus, they exhibit a similar cellular composition to gangliocytic paragangliomas. (Fig. 11 from Perrone T, Sibley RK, Rosai J. Duodenal gangliocytic paraganglioma. An immunohistochemical and ultrastructural study and a hypothesis concerning its origin. Am J Surg Pathol 1985;9:31–41.)

though the association is not as convincing for gangliocytic paraganglioma, both tumors are associated with neurofibromatosis. If gangliocytic paragangliomas and glandular carcinoid tumors are indeed related neoplasms then it would seem reasonable to expect hybrid tumors with components of both lesions to exist. In fact, such a tumor has been reported (84). A 54-year-old woman with neurofibromatosis was found to have bilateral pheochromocytomas, and during surgical excision of those tumors, an incidental ampullary mass was excised. Components of glandular carcinoid with psammoma bodies and immunohistochemical positivity for somato-statin were found along with separate components of gangliocytic paraganglioma showing positivity for S-100 protein, neurofilaments, and pancreatic polypeptide.

Differential Diagnosis. The differential diagnosis of gangliocytic paraganglioma depends largely upon which component of a given tumor predominates. If the spindle cell component predominates, then other spindle cell neoplasms such as neurofibroma, ganglioneuroma, or gastrointestinal stromal tumors should be considered. If the epithelioid cell component is predominant, the main consideration should be a carcinoid tumor, although the enlarged nuclei of the ganglion-like cells may suggest a carcinoma. Familiarity with the entity and a careful search for the different components will lead to a correct diagnosis in most cases. Immunohistochemical staining is helpful in difficult cases; positive staining for pancreatic polypeptide suggests the diagnosis of a gangliocytic paraganglioma as op-posed to a carcinoid tumor, since periampullary carcinoids that produce this substance are rare.

PARAGANGLIOMA

Most tumors reported as "paragangliomas" of the ampulla or periampullary duodenum (89,91, 92) have been gangliocytic paragangliomas, especially those with the descriptive name "non-chromaffin paraganglioma." It is not clear that any cases of classic paraganglioma have been found in this region. One possibly "pure" duodenal paraganglioma has been reported (90); the 56-year-old man presented with gastric discomfort and had a 0.5 cm mass in the first portion of the duodenum. The tumor had the typical "zell-ballen" arrangement of epithelioid cells, and spindle cells and ganglion cell were absent. Immunohistochemistry to further characterize this tumor was not available. Paragangliomas that affect the small intestine usually originate in the mesentery rather than in the bowel wall (88).

REFERENCES

General

1. Burke AP, Federspiel BH, Sobin LH, Shekita KM, Helwig EB. Carcinoids of the duodenum. A histologic and immunohistochemical study of 65 tumors. Am J Surg Pathol 1989;13:828–37.
2. Solcia E, Sessa F, Rindi G, et al. Classification and histogenesis of gastroenteropancreatic endocrine tumors. Eur J Clin Invest 1990;20:72–81.
3. Stamm B, Hedinger CE, Saremaslani P. Duodenal and ampullary carcinoid tumors A report of 12 cases with pathological characteristics, polypeptide content and relation to the MEN I syndrome and von Recklinghausen's disease (neurofibromatosis). Virchows Arch [A] 1986;408:475–89.

Carcinoid Tumors

4. Attanoos R, Williams GT. Epithelial and neuroendocrine tumors of the duodenum. Semin Diag Pathol 1991;8:149–62.
5. Bapat RD, Relekar RG, Kanbur AS, Someshwar V, Vora IM. Neurofibromatosis associated with periampullary carcinoid tumour of duodenum. Indian J Gastroenterol 1989;8:306–7.
6. Barber PV. Carcinoid tumour of the ampulla of Vater associated with cutaneous neurofibromatosis. Postgrad Med J 1976;52:514–7.
7. Burke AP, Federspiel BH, Sobin LH, Shekita KM, Helwig EB. Carcinoids of the duodenum. A histologic and immunohistochemical study of 65 tumors. Am J Surg Pathol 1989;13:828–37.
8. Dancygier H, Klein U, Leuschner U, Hubner K, Classen M. Somatostatin-containing cells in the extrahepatic biliary tract of humans. Gastroenterology 1984;86:892–6.
9. Dawson BV, Kazama R, Paplanus SH. Association of carcinoid with neurofibromatosis. South Med J 1984;77:511–3.
10. Dayal Y, Tallberg K, Nunnemacher G, DeLellis RA, Wolfe HJ. Duodenal carcinoids in patients with and without neurofibromatosis. Am J Surg Pathol 1986;10:348–57.
11. Dixon JM, Chapman RW, Berry AR. Carcinoid tumour of the ampulla of Vater presenting as acute pancreatitis. Gut 1987;28:1296–97.

12. Hatzihtheoklitos E, Buchler MW, Friess H, et al. Carcinoid of the ampulla of Vater. Clinical characteristics and morphologic features. Cancer 1994;73:1580–8.
13. Hough DR, Chan A, Davidson H. Von Recklinghausen's disease associated with gastrointestinal carcinoid tumors. Cancer 1983;51:2206–8.
14. Johnson L, Weaver M. Von Recklinghausen's disease and gastrointestinal carcinoids. JAMA 1981;245:2496.
15. Kapur BM, Sarin SK, Anand CS, Varma K. Carcinoid tumour of ampulla of Vater associated with viscero-cutaneous neurofibromatosis. Post Med J 1983;59:734–5.
16. Klein A, Clemens J, Cameron J. Periampullary neoplasms in von Recklinghausen's disease. Surgery 1989;106:815–9.
17. Lee HY, Garber PE. Von Recklinghausen's disease associated with pheochromocytoma and carcinoid tumor. Ohio State Med J 1970;66:583–6.
18. Liu K, Mergener K, Feldman JM, Gottfried MR. Carcinoids of the ampulla of Vater: a unique subset of gastrointestinal carcinoid tumors [Abstract]. Mod Pathol 1997;10:59A.
18a. Makhlouf HR, Burke AP, Sobin LH. Carcinoid tumors of the ampulla of Vater. A comparison with duodenal carcinoid tumors. Cancer 1999;85:1241–9.
19. Mulder CJ, Festen HP, Mertens JC, et al. Carcinoid tumor of the ampulla of Vater presenting with biliary obstruction: report of four cases. Gastrointest Endosc 1987;33:385–7.
20. Noda Y, Watanabe H, Iwafuchi M, et al. Carcinoids and endocrine cell micronests of the minor and major duodenal papillae. Their incidence and characteristics. Cancer 1992;70:1825–30.
21. Ranaldi R, Bearzi I, Cinti S, Suraci V. Ampullary somatostatinoma. An immunohistochemical and ultrastructural study. Pathol Res Pract 1988;183:8–16.
22. Ricci JL. Carcinoid of the ampulla of Vater. Local resection or pancreaticoduodenectomy. Cancer 1993;71:686–90.
23. Sanchez-Sosa S, Angeles Angeles A, Orozco H, Larriva-Sahd J. Neuroendocrine carcinoma of the ampulla of Vater. A case of absence of somatostatin in a vasoactive intestinal polypeptide, bombesin, and cholecystokinin-producing tumor. Am J Clin Pathol 1991;95:51–4.
24. Solcia E, Sessa F, Rindi G, et al. Classification and histogenesis of gastroenteropancreatic endocrine tumors. Eur J Clin Invest 1990;20:72–81.
25. Stamm B, Hedinger CE, Saremaslani P. Duodenal and ampullary carcinoid tumors. A report of 12 cases with pathological characteristics, polypeptide content and relation to the MEN I syndrome and von Recklinghausen's disease (neurofibromatosis). Virchows Arch [A] 1986;408:475–89.
26. van Basten JP, van Hoek B, de Bruine A, Arends JW, Stockbrugger RW. Ampullary carcinoid and neurofibromatosis: case report and review of the literature. Neth J Med 1994;44:202–6.

Glandular Carcinoid Tumor

27. Attanoos R, Williams GT. Epithelial and neuroendocrine tumors of the duodenum. Semin Diag Pathol 1991;8:149–62.
28. Burke AP, Federspiel BH, Sobin LH, Shekita KM, Helwig EB. Carcinoids of the duodenum. A histologic and immunohistochemical study of 65 tumors. Am J Surg Pathol 1989;13:828–37.
29. Burke AP, Sobin LH, Shekitka KM, Federspiel BH, Helwig EB. Somatostatin-producing duodenal carcinoids in patients with von Recklinghausen's neurofibromatosis. A predilection for black patients. Cancer 1990;65:1591–5.
30. Dayal Y, Nunnemacher G, Doos WG, DeLellis RA, O Brien MJ, Wolfe HJ. Psammomatous somatostatinomas of the duodenum. Am J Surg Pathol 1983;7:653–64.
31. Dayal Y, Tallberg KA, Nunnemacher G, DeLellis RA, Wolfe HJ. Duodenal carcinoids in patients with and without neurofibromatosis. A comparative study. Am J Surg Pathol 1986;10:348–57.
32. Griffiths DF, Jasani B, Newman GR, Williams ED, Williams GT. Glandular duodenal carcinoid—a somatostatin rich tumour with neuroendocrine associations. J Clin Pathol 1984;37:163–9.
33. Lee HY, Garber PE. Von Recklinghausen's disease associated with pheochromocytoma and carcinoid tumor. Ohio State Med J 1970;66:583–6.
34. Marcial MA, Pinkus GS, Skarin A, Hinrichs HR, Warhol MJ. Ampullary somatostatinoma: psammomatous variant of gastrointestinal carcinoid tumor—an immunohistochemical and ultrastructural study. Report of a case and review of the literature. Am J Clin Pathol 1983;80:755–61.
35. Ranaldi R, Bearzi I, Cinti S, Suraci V. Ampullary somatostatinoma. An immunohistochemical and ultrastructural study. Pathol Res Pract 1988;183:8–16.
36. Sawady J, Katzin WE, Mendelsohn G, Aron DC. Somatostatin-producing neuroendocrine tumor of the ampulla (ampullary somatostatinoma). Evidence of prosomatostatin production. Am J Clin Pathol 1992;97:411–5.
37. Simmons TC, Henderson DR, Gletten F, Pascua L, Greene C. The association of neurofibromatosis, psammomatous ampullary carcinoid tumor, and extrahepatic biliary obstruction [Letter]. J Clin Gastroenterol 1987;9:490–2.
38. Stamm B, Hedinger CE, Saremaslani P. Duodenal and ampullary carcinoid tumors. A report of 12 cases with pathological characteristics, polypeptide content and relation to the MEN I syndrome and von Recklinghausen s disease (neurofibromatosis). Virchows Arch [A] 1986;408:475–89.
39. Stommer PE, Stolte M, Seifert E. Somatostatinoma of Vater's papilla and of the minor papilla. Cancer 1987;60:232–5.
40. Swinburn BA, Yeong ML, Lane MR, Nicholson GI, Holdaway IM. Neurofibromatosis associated with somatostatinoma: a report of two patients. Clin Endocrinol 1988;28:353–9.
41. Taccagni GL, Carlucci M, Sironi M, Cantaboni A, Di Carlo V. Duodenal somatostatinoma with psammoma bodies: an immunohistochemical and ultrastructural study. Am J Gastroenterol 1986;81:33–7.
42. Wheeler MH, Curley IR, Williams ED. The association of neurofibromatosis, pheochromocytoma, and somatostatin–rich duodenal carcinoid tumor. Surgery 1986;100:1163–9.

Gastrin-Producing Carcinoid Tumor

43. Donow C, Pipeleers-Marichal M, Schröder S, Stamm B, Heitz PU, Klöppel G. Surgical pathology of gastrinoma. Site, size, multicentricity, association with multiple endocrine neoplastic type 1, and malignancy. Cancer 1991;68:1329–34.

44. Mukai K, Grotting JC, Greider MH, Rosai J. Retrospective study of 77 pancreatic endocrine tumors using the immunoperoxidase method. Am J Surg Pathol 1982;6:387–99.

45. Solcia E, Sessa F, Rindi G, et al. Classification and histogenesis of gastroenteropancreatic endocrine tumors. Eur J Clin Invest 1990;20:72–81.

46. Weichert RF, Roth LM, Krementz ET, Hewitt RL, Drapanas T. Carcinoid-islet cell tumors of the duodenum. Report of twenty-one cases. Am J Surg 1971;121:195–205.

Adenocarcinoid Tumor

47. Abt AB, Carter SL. Goblet cell carcinoid of the appendix. An ultrastructural and histochemical study. Arch Pathol Lab Med 1976;100:301–6.

48. Burke AP, Lee YK. Adenocarcinoid (goblet cell carcinoid) of the duodenum presenting as gastric outlet obstruction. Hum Pathol 1990;21:238–9.

49. Jones MA, Griffith LM, West AB. Adenocarcinoid of the periampullary region: a novel duodenal neoplasm presenting as biliary tract obstruction. Hum Pathol 1989;20:198–200.

50. Kourea H, Albores-Saavedra J, Klimstra DS. The spectrum of neuroendocrine tumors of the periampullary region. In preparation.

51. Shah IA, Schlageter MO, Boehm N. Composite carcinoid-adenocarcinoma of ampulla of Vater. Hum Pathol 1990;21:1188–90.

52. Warkel RL, Cooper PH, Helwig EB. Adenocarcinoid, a mucin-producing carcinoid tumor of the appendix: a study of 39 cases. Cancer 1978;42:2781–93.

Gangliocytic Paraganglioma

53. Anders KH, Glasgow BJ, Lewin KJ. Gangliocytic paraganglioma associated with duodenal adenocarcinoma. Case report with immunohistochemical evaluation. Arch Pathol Lab Med 1987;111:49–52.

54. Aung W, Gallagher HJ, Joyce WP, Hayes DB, Leader M. Gastrointestinal hemorrhage from a jejunal gangliocytic paraganglioma. J Clin Pathol 1995;48:84–5.

55. Barbareschi M, Frigo B, Aldovini D, Leonardi E, Cristina S, Falleni M. Duodenal gangliocytic paraganglioma. Report of a case and review of the literature. Virchows Arch [A] 1989;416:81–9.

56. Buchler M, Malfertheiner P, Baczako K, Krautzberger W, Beger HG. A metastatic endocrine-neurogenic tumor of the ampulla of Vater with multiple endocrine immunoreaction—malignant paraganglioma? Digestion 1985;31:54–9.

57. Burke AP, Helwig EB. Gangliocytic paraganglioma. Am J Clin Pathol 1989;92:1–9.

58. Cohen T, Zweig SJ, Tallis A, Tuazon R, Reich R. Paraganglioneuroma of the duodenum. Report of a case with radiographic findings, angiographic findings, and a review of the literature. Am J Gastroenterol 1981;75:197–203.

59. Collina G, Maiorana A, Trentini GP. Duodenal gangliocytic paraganglioma. Case report with immunohistochemical study on the expression of keratin polypeptides. Histopathology 1991;19:476–8.

60. Cooney T, Sweeney EC. Paraganglioneuroma of the duodenum: an evolutionary hybrid? J Clin Path 1978;31:233–44.

61. Dahl E, Waugh JM, Dahlin DC. Gastrointestinal ganglioneuromas. Am J Pathol 1957;33:953–65.

62. Damron TA, Rahman D, Cashman MD. Gangliocytic paraganglioma in association with a duodenal diverticulum. Am J Gastroenterol 1989;84:1109–14.

63. Dookhan DB, Miettinen M, Finkel G, Gibas Z. Recurrent duodenal gangliocytic paraganglioma with lymph node metastases. Histopathology 1993;22:399–401.

64. Guarda LA, Ordonez NG. Gangliocytic paraganglioma of the duodenum: report of cytologic, histologic, immunohistochemical, and ultrastructural features of a case. Diagn Cytopathol 1987;3:314–9.

65. Guarda LA, Ordonez NG, del Junco GW, Luna MA. Gangliocytic paraganglioma of the duodenum: an immunocytochemical study. Am J Gastroenterol 1983;78:794–8.

66. Hamid QA, Bishop AE, Rode J, et al. Duodenal gangliocytic paragangliomas: a study of 10 cases with immunocytochemical neuroendocrine markers. Hum Pathol 1986;17:1151–7.

67. Hashimoto S, Kawasaki S, Matsuzawa K, Harada H, Makuuchi M. Gangliocytic paraganglioma of the papilla of Vater with regional lymph node metastasis. Am J Gastroenterol 1992;87:1216–8.

68. Inai K, Kobuke T, Yonehara S, Tokuoka S. Duodenal gangliocytic paraganglioma with lymph node metastasis in a 17-year-old boy. Cancer 1989;63:2540–5.

69. Kawaguchi K, Takizawa T, Koike M, Tabata I, Goseki N. Multiple paraganglioneuromas. Virchows Arch [A] 1985;406:373–80.

70. Kepes JJ, Zacharias DL. Gangliocytic paragangliomas of the duodenum. A report of two cases with light and electron microscopic examination. Cancer 1971;27:61–70.

71. Kermarec J, Duplay H, Lesbros F. Paragangliome gangliocytique du duodenum. Une observation avec etude ultra-structurale. Arch Anat Cytol Path 1976;24:261–8.

72. Kheir SM, Halpern NB. Paraganglioma of the duodenum in association with congenital neurofibromatosis. Possible relationship. Cancer 1984;53:2491–6.

73. Konok GP, Sanchez-Cassis G. Gangliocytic paraganglioma of the duodenum. Can J Surg 1979;22:173–5.

74. Ljungberg O, Jarnerot G, Rolny P, Wickbom G. Human pancreatic polypeptide (HPP) immunoreactivity in an infiltrating endocrine tumour of the papilla of Vater with unusual morphology. Virchows Arch [A] 1981;392:119–26.

75. Lukash WM, Hyams VJ, Nielsen OF. Neurogenic neoplasms of the small bowel: benign nonchromaffin paraganglioma of the duodenum. Report of a case. Am J Dig Dis 1966;11:575–9.

76. Perrone T. Duodenal gangliocytic paraganglioma and carcinoid. Am J Surg Pathol 1986;10:147-50.

77. Perrone T, Sibley RK, Rosai J. Duodenal gangliocytic paraganglioma. An immunohistochemical and ultrastructural study and a hypothesis concerning its origin. Am J Surg Pathol 1985;9:31–41.

78. Qizilbash AH. Benign paraganglioma of duodenum. Case report with light and electron microscopic examination and brief review of literature. Arch Pathol 1973;96:276–80.

79. Reed R, Caroca PJ, Harkin JC. Gangliocytic paraganglioma. Am J Surg Pathol 1977;1:207–16.

80. Sando WC, Mills SE, Rodgers BM. Duodenal gangliocytic paraganglioma occurring in adolescence. J Pediatr Gastroenterol Nutr 1986;5:659–64.

81. Scheithauer BW, Nora FE, Lechago J. Duodenal gangliocytic paraganglioma. Clinicopathologic and immunocytochemical study of 11 cases. Am J Clin Pathol 1986;86:559–65.

82. Smithline AE, Hawes RH, Kenyon KK, Cummings OW, Kumar S. Gangliocytic paraganglioma, a rare cause of upper gastrointestinal bleeding. Endoscopic ultrasound findings presented. Dig Dis Sci 1993;38:173–7.

83. Sonneland PR, Scheithauer BW, Lechago J, Crawford BG, Onofrio BM. Paraganglioma of the cauda equina region. Clinicopathologic study of 31 cases with special reference to immunocytology and ultrastructure. Cancer 1986;58:1720–35.

84. Stephens M, Williams GT, Jasani B, Williams ED. Synchronous duodenal neuroendocrine tumours in von Recklinghausen's disease—a case report of co-existing gangliocytic paraganglioma and somatostatin-rich glandular carcinoid. Histopathology 1987;11:1331–40.

85. Taylor HB, Helwig EB. Benign nonchromaffin paraganglioma of the duodenum. Virchows Arch Path Anat 1962;335:356–66.

86. Van Campenhout E. Contribution a l'etude de l'histogenese du pancreas chez quelques mammiferes. Les complexes sympathico-insulaires. Arch Biol (Liege) 1927;37:121–71.

87. Van Campenhout E. Etude sur le developpement et la signification morphologique des ilots endocrines du pancreas chez l'embryon de mouton. Arch Biol (Liege) 1925;35:45–88.

Paraganglioma

88. Burke AP, Helwig EB. Gangliocytic paraganglioma. Am J Clin Pathol 1989;92:1–9.

89. Kheir SM, Halpern NB. Paraganglioma of the duodenum in association with congenital neurofibromatosis. Possible relationship. Cancer 1984;53:2491–6.

90. Matilla A, Rivera F, Fernandez-Sanz J, Galera H. Nonchromaffin paraganglioma of the duodenum. Virchows Arch [A] 1979;383:217–23.

91. Qizilbash AH. Benign paraganglioma of duodenum. Case report with light and electron microscopic examination and brief review of literature. Arch Pathol 1973;96:276–80.

92. Williams SJ, Lucas RJ, McCaughey RS. Paraganglioma of the duodenum: a case report. Surgery 1980;87:454–8.

22

BENIGN AND MALIGNANT MESENCHYMAL TUMORS AND OTHER MALIGNANT TUMORS OF THE AMPULLARY REGION

BENIGN MESENCHYMAL TUMORS

Only a small number of benign mesenchymal neoplasms have been reported in the ampulla, probably because there is minimal mesenchymal tissue present. More frequently, a periampullary duodenal mesenchymal tumor extends into the ampulla, causing biliary obstruction and presenting clinically as an ampullary mass. Most benign periampullary mesenchymal tumors are of smooth muscle or adipose tissue origin, although other tumor types have been reported.

BENIGN GASTROINTESTINAL STROMAL TUMORS

Leiomyoma

Benign gastrointestinal stromal tumors (GIST) are the most common mesenchymal tumors originating in the duodenum (2,7), and they may involve the ampulla. Because these tumors, even those that contain rare mitotic figures, may metastasize, the diagnostic term "benign" should be restricted to those hypocellular tumors that are less than 4 cm in diameter and lack significant mitotic activity (7). Histologically, the cells are arranged in interlacing fascicles or bundles (fig. 22-1). With immunohistochemistry, stromal tumors arising in the small intestine often are shown to contain actin, but those arising in the duodenum are usually devoid of muscle markers (7). Tumors that contain actin are classified as leiomyomas. We have observed only one leiomyoma among 172 ampullary tumors.

Lipoma

Lipomas are commonly found in the submucosal or subserosal layers of the small intestine, including the duodenum. Generally, patients are asymptomatic, although tumors located in the submucosa may cause ulceration of the overlying mucosa with consequent hemorrhage. Although some lipomas may surround the ampullary orifice, obstructive jaundice is unusual because of their soft consistency.

Hemangioma and Lymphangioma

Benign vascular tumors may involve the duodenum (2). Two examples of lymphangioma involving the ampulla have been reported (1,5). Both tumors caused obstructive jaundice. Cavernous lymphatic channels were present in the submucosa around the ampulla, accompanied by scattered lymphoid aggregates.

Neurogenic Tumors

Neurofibroma. Neurofibromas associated with von Recklinghausen's disease are found in every anatomic site, and the ampulla is no exception. However, despite the common involvement of the gastrointestinal tract, clinically detected ampullary neurofibromas are unusual (10). Most of the clinically evident cases have caused jaundice (11), obstructive pancreatitis (9), or pancreatic exocrine insufficiency (13).

Histologically, these ampullary neurofibromas resemble their counterparts found in other sites. Interestingly, two other ampullary tumors have been reported with a higher frequency in patients with von Recklinghausen's disease than neurofibromas: glandular carcinoid tumor and gangliocytic paraganglioma. Therefore, an ampullary tumor endoscopically identified in a patient with von Recklinghausen's disease cannot be considered a neurofibroma without a confirmatory biopsy (12). While the distinction from a benign gangliocytic paraganglioma may not be clinically important, glandular carcinoid tumor is a malignant neoplasm.

Ganglioneuroma. Ganglioneuromas occur throughout the gastrointestinal tract, especially in association with neurofibromatosis. In the periampullary region, however, the majority of tumors reported as "ganglioneuromas" have contained carcinoid-like (or paraganglioma-like) elements (3), which qualifies them as gangliocytic paragangliomas. In only two reported cases have ganglioneuromas in the second part of the duodenum lacked the epithelioid elements of a gangliocytic paraganglioma (6,8). These two tumors occurred

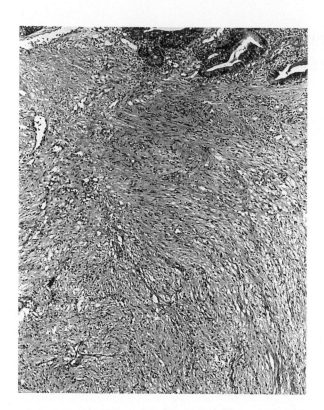 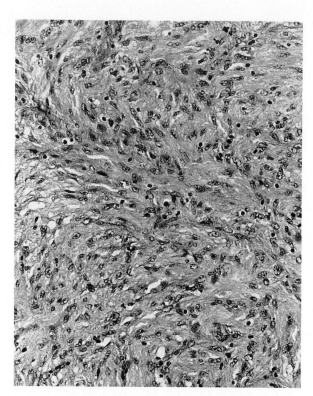

Figure 22-1
LEIOMYOMA OF THE PERIAMPULLARY DUODENUM
Left: At low power, the tumor is relatively hypocellular and circumscribed, abutting but not invading the overlying mucosa (top).
Right: The cells are arranged in vague fascicles. At higher power, the nuclei are relatively uniform and only mildly atypical; no mitotic figures are identified.

in patients with no evidence of neurofibromatosis and neither one involved the ampulla.

MALIGNANT MESENCHYMAL TUMORS

Primary sarcomas of the ampulla are exceptionally rare. In most instances, a sarcomatoid neoplasm involving the ampulla represents a spindle cell undifferentiated carcinoma or, if truly mesenchymal, has arisen in the periampullary duodenal wall (20). Most of the latter cases are gastrointestinal stromal tumors. In addition, a few case reports of other primary sarcomas of the periampullary region have appeared.

Leiomyosarcoma and Malignant Gastrointestinal Stromal Tumors

Three types of malignant GIST have been described in the small intestine: leiomyosarcoma, gastrointestinal autonomic nerve tumor, and GIST not otherwise specified (15). Although any of the three may occur in the duodenum, we have only encountered leiomyosarcomas involving the ampulla (18); they represented 1.2 percent of ampullary tumors in our material.

Compared to leiomyomas, leiomyosarcomas are larger, more cellular, and mitotically more active (16). Both spindle cell (fig. 22-2A,B) and epithelioid types occur. Location in the ampulla does not have any special clinical or pathologic significance, other than the potential for obstructive jaundice and the greater difficulty of surgical removal, compared to elsewhere in the small intestine.

Immunohistochemistry may be helpful in classifying these tumors: leiomyosarcomas stain for actin, gastrointestinal nerve tumors stain for S-100 protein and neuron-specific enolase (although inconsistently), and GISTs not otherwise specified express only vimentin (15,19). Electron microscopy is often necessary to confirm the diagnosis of gastrointestinal autonomic nerve

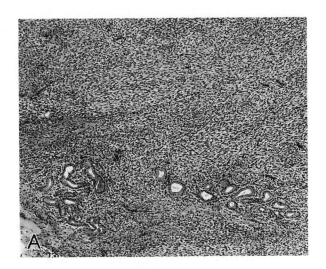

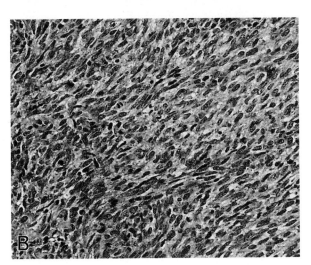

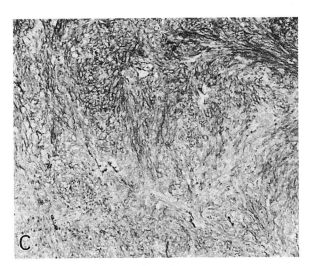

Figure 22-2
SPINDLE CELL LEIOMYOSARCOMA
INVOLVING THE AMPULLA
A: At low power, the tumor is very cellular and infiltrates diffusely around periampullary ductules (bottom).
B: Although the spindle cells do not show marked atypia, there are innumerable mitotic figures.
C: Positive immunohistochemical staining for actin is consistent with the smooth muscle nature of this GIST.

tumor and may also provide evidence of muscle differentiation in GISTs having nonspecific features by immunohistochemistry.

Rhabdomyosarcoma

Although less common than in the biliary tree, embryonal rhabdomyosarcomas have been reported in the ampulla (14,17). Both reported cases occurred in children (ages 3 and 6.5 years), in whom the tumors presented with biliary obstruction. Grossly, the tumors appeared to originate in the very distal bile duct, in one case projecting into the duodenal lumen. Histologically, the tumors resembled botryoid rhabdomyosarcoma of other sites, with nests of small

cells in a myxoid stroma undermining the ampullary epithelium (fig. 22-3). Diagnostic "strap cells" were also present. Although one case was diagnosed at autopsy (17), the other patient underwent pancreatoduodenectomy followed by chemotherapy and external radiation and was alive without disease at 5 years (14).

Kaposi's Sarcoma

Ampullary Kaposi's sarcoma has been reported in association with the acquired immunodeficiency syndrome (AIDS) (21,22). Jaundice was the presenting symptom. In one patient there was associated sclerosing cholangitis due to biliary cryptosporidiosis (22).

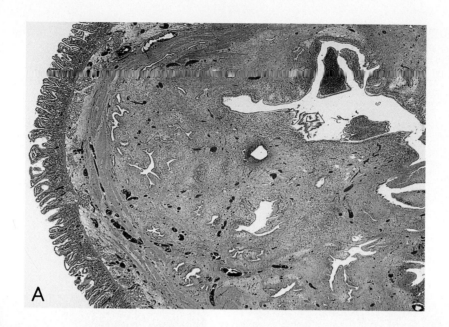

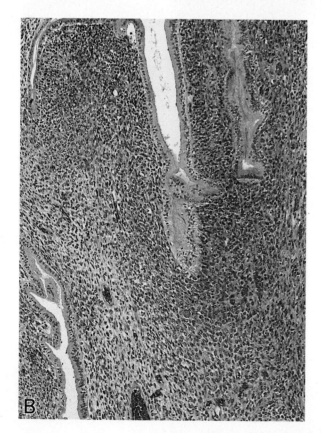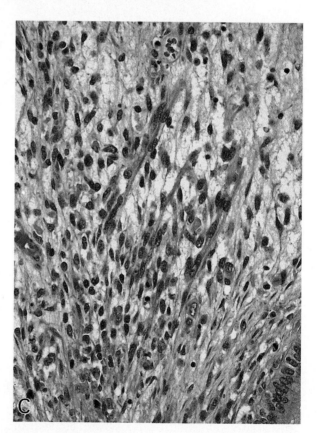

Figure 22-3
EMBRYONAL RHABDOMYOSARCOMA OF THE AMPULLA

A: The tumor obliterates the intra-ampullary portion of the distal common bile duct but does not involve the overlying duodenal mucosa.

B: There is a condensation of tumor cells around the remaining epithelial elements of the ampulla, the so called cambium layer.

C: Although many of the tumor cells are nondescript spindle cells or primitive-appearing mesenchymal cells, scattered elongate "strap cells" are identifiable. (Courtesy of Dr. Thomas Giordano, Ann Arbor, MI.).

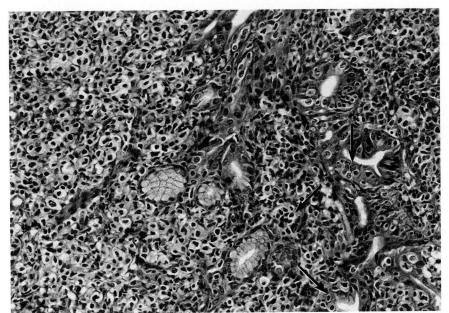

Figure 22-4
MALIGNANT LYMPHOMA
INVOLVING THE AMPULLA
In this MALT type diffuse lymphoma, the tumor cells have relatively abundant cytoplasm and a focal plasmacytoid configuration. Lymphoepithelial lesions involving periampullary ductules are noted (arrows).

OTHER MALIGNANT TUMORS

Lymphoma

Lymphomatous involvement of the ampulla usually occurs as a manifestation of disseminated disease. The few examples of primary lymphoma of the ampulla have been low-grade B-cell lymphomas (23–25). One displayed features of a mucosa-associated lymphoid tumor (MALT) type lymphoma with additional involvement of the duodenum (fig. 22-4) (24). The clinical course has been indolent.

REFERENCES

Benign Mesenchymal Tumors

1. Artaza T, Potenciano JM, Legaz M, Muñoz C, Talavera A, Sanchez E. Lymphangioma of Vater's ampulla: a rare cause of obstructive jaundice. Endoscopic therapy. Scand J Gastroenterol 1995;30:804–6.
2. Coit DG. Cancer of the small intestine. In: DeVita VT Jr, Hellman S, Rosenberg SA, eds. Cancer: principles and practice of oncology. Philadelphia: JB Lippincott, 1993:915–28.
3. Dahl E, Waugh JM, Dahlin DC. Gastrointestinal ganglioneuromas. 1957;33:953-65.
4. Franquemont DW, Frierson HF Jr. Muscle differentiation and clinicopathologic features of gastrointestinal stromal tumors. Am J Surg Pathol 1992;16:947–54.
5. Friedrich HJ, Schramon H, Peckholz I. Kavernöses lymphangiom der papilla vateri als ursache eines verschlubikterus. Zentradbl Chir 1985;110:1263–5.
6. Gemer M, Feuchtwanger MM. Ganglioneuroma of the duodenum. Gastroenterology 1966;51:689–93.
7. Goldblum JR, Appelman HD. Stromal tumors of the duodenum. A histologic and immunohistochemical study of 20 cases. Am J Surg Pathol 1995;19:71–80.
8. Goldman RL. Ganglioneuroma of the duodenum. Relationship of nonchromaffin paraganglioma of the duodenum. Am J Surg 1968;115:716–9.
9. Kahrilas PJ, Hogan WJ, Geenen JE, Stewart ET, Dodds WJ, Arndorfer RC. Chronic recurrent pancreatitis secondary to a submucosal ampullary tumor in a patient with neurofibromatosis. Dig Dis Sci 1987;32:102–7.
10. Klein A, Clemens J, Cameron J. Periampullary neoplasms in von Recklinghausen's disease. Surgery 1989;106:815–9.
11. Meyer GW, Griffiths WJ, Welsh J, Cohen L, Johnson L, Weaver MJ. Hepatobiliary involvement in von Recklinghausen's disease. Ann Intern Med 1982;97:722–3.
12. Simmons TC. Ampullary neurofibroma [Letter]. Dig Dis Sci 1988;33:1500–1.
13. Wormsley, KG, Logan WF, Sorrell VF, Cole GC. Neurofibromatosis with pancreatic duct obstruction and steatorrhoea. Postgrad Med J 1967;43:432–5.

Malignant Mesenchymal Tumors

14. Caty MG, Oldham KT, Prochownik EV. Embryonal rhabdomyosarcoma of the ampulla of Vater with long-term survival following pancreaticoduodenectomy. J Ped Surg 1990;25:1256–8.

15. Erlandson RA, Klimstra DS, Woodruff JM. Sub-classification of gastrointestinal stromal tumors based on evaluation by electron microscopy and immunohistochemistry. Ultrastr Pathol 1996;20:373–93.

16. Goldblum JR, Appelman HD. Stromal tumors of the duodenum. A histologic and immunohistochemical study of 20 cases. Am J Surg Pathol 1995;19:71–80.

17. Isaacson C. Embryonal rhabdomyosarcoma of the ampulla of Vater. Cancer 1978;41:365–8.

18. Jones BA, Langer B, Taylor BR, Girotti M. Periampullary tumors: which ones should be resected. Am J Surg 1985;149:46–52.

19. Lauwers GY, Erlandson RA, Casper ES, Brennan MF, Woodruff JM. Gastrointestinal autonomic nerve tumors. A clinicopathological, immunohistochemical and ultrastructural study of 12 cases. Am J Surg Pathol 1993;17:887–97.

20. Michelassi F, Erroi F, Dawson PJ, et al. Experience with 647 consecutive tumors of the duodenum, ampulla, head of the pancreas, and distal common bile duct. Ann Surg 1989;210:544–56.

21. Rene E, Chevalier T, Godeberge B, Bonfils S. Gastrointestinal manifestations of AIDS. Ann Gastroenterol Hepatol 1985;21:389–91.

22. Seitz JF, Giovannini M, Wartelle C, Monges G, Dhiver C, Gastaut JA. Kaposi's sarcoma of Vater's ampulla associated with sclerosing cholangitis caused by cryptosporidium in a patient with AIDS [Letter]. Gastroenterol Clin Biol 1990;14:889–91.

Other Malignant Tumors

23. Barek L, Orron D. Non-Hodgkin's lymphoma presenting as periampullary mass with obstructive jaundice. J Comput Tomogr 1986;10:89–92.

24. Pawade J, Lee CS, Ellis DW, Vellar ID, Rode J. Primary lymphoma of the ampulla of Vater. Cancer 1994;73:2083–6.

25. Zhu L, Slee GR, Domenico DR, Mao C, Howard JM. B-cell lymphoma of ampulla of Vater: observation for six years. Pancreas 1995;10:208–10.

23
TUMOR-LIKE LESIONS OF THE AMPULLARY REGION

Tumor-like lesions of the periampullary region are important because confusion with carcinoma may result in unnecessary radical surgery. The lesions discussed below all can simulate periampullary carcinoma, either by producing biliary obstruction or by presenting as a mass endoscopically.

PAPILLARY HYPERPLASIA

Papillary hyperplasia is a poorly described proliferative lesion that involves the ampullary mucosa. The epithelium of the ampulla is markedly papillary and is lined by a single layer of cytologically bland, cuboidal to columnar (biliary type) epithelial cells (fig. 23-1). Papillary hyperplasia accentuates the normally present papillae of the valve of Wirsung. There is no proliferation of smooth muscle in papillary hyperplasia. We have seen this condition associated with inflammatory processes adjacent to ampullary tumors, and as an incidental finding in pancreatoduodenectomy specimens removed for nonampullary lesions. We are not aware of a case of papillary hyperplasia causing biliary obstruction or clinical confusion with carcinoma. On endoscopic biopsy, however, it would be possible to misinterpret this lesion as an adenoma.

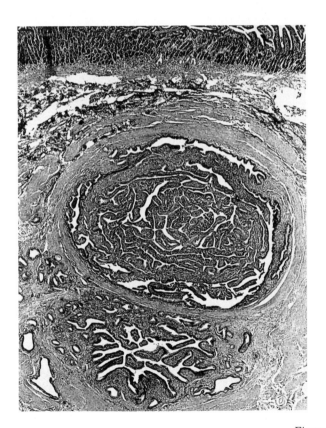 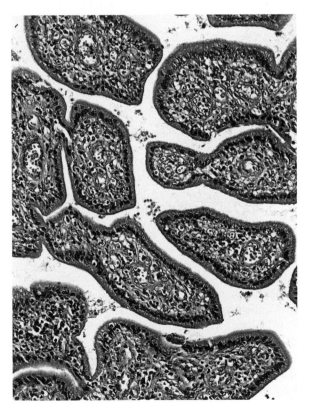

Figure 23-1
PAPILLARY HYPERPLASIA OF THE AMPULLARY EPITHELIUM

Left: In this florid example, the lumen of the ampulla is partially occluded by papillary formations, and the tumor resembles an adenoma at low power.

Right: At high power, the papillae are simple and lined by a single layer of cytologically bland, biliary type epithelial cells showing minimal nuclear pseudostratification. The fibrovascular cores of the papillae contain a mixed inflammatory infiltrate.

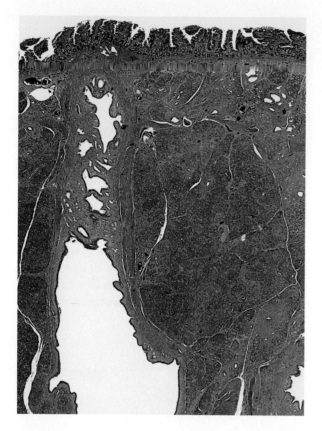 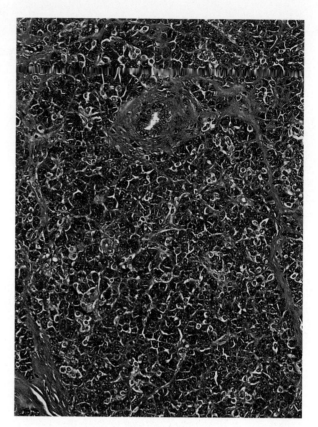

Figure 23-2
PANCREATIC HETEROTOPIA
Left: Lobules of well-developed pancreatic tissue surround the ampulla and compress the common bile duct. The overlying duodenal mucosa is intact.
Right: In this example, only ductal and acinar cells are evident.

HETEROTOPIC TISSUES

Pancreatic Heterotopia

Pancreatic heterotopia is a common incidental finding in the duodenal submucosa, where some cases represent remnants of the minor papillae. Most patients are asymptomatic. Although heterotopic pancreatic tissue is rarely encountered in the ampulla (2–4), this location may result in symptoms, bringing the patient to clinical attention. Nodules of heterotopic pancreatic tissue may contain all of the normal pancreatic elements (ducts, acini, and islets) but more commonly they lack an endocrine component (fig. 23-2). When acini are few the lesion may resemble an adenomyoma. Although presumably congenital in nature, most cases have presented in adulthood.

Gastric Heterotopia

One report exists of biliary obstruction due to heterotopic gastric mucosa at the ampulla (1). An 83-year-old male developed jaundice and upper gastrointestinal hemorrhage and was found to have fundic type gastric mucosa (including chief and parietal cells) within the ampulla.

ADENOMYOMATOUS HYPERPLASIA AND "ADENOMYOMA"

Adenomyomas are localized aggregates of pancreatobiliary type ducts and ductules arranged in a lobular configuration and accompanied by fascicles of smooth muscle. Histologically identical lesions occur in the gallbladder and bile ducts. Alternative terms include *myoepithelial hamartoma, adenomyomatous hamartoma, adenomyomatous hyperplasia,* and *adenomyosis*. Most adenomy-omas are nodular, tumor-like masses, although some exhibit an ill-defined diffuse configuration (often termed *adenomyomatous hyperplasia* or *adenomyosis*).

The median age of patients with adenomyoma of the ampulla is 66 years (5,6,8,9). Abdominal pain and obstructive jaundice are frequent, and chole-lithiasis is sometimes noted (6). Because a small number of cases of adenocarcinoma have been found in association with periampullary ad-enomyomas (5,6), the latter lesion has been re-garded as potentially preneoplastic (7). It is not yet clear whether adenomyomas themselves carry a significant increased risk for malignant transformation or whether the rare cases of car-cinoma associated with adenomyomas have been over-represented in the literature. The primary clinical significance of adenomyoma is its dis-tinction from carcinoma, which may be compli-cated because endoscopic biopsies may show only benign ductules and smooth muscle, normal constituents of the ampulla (10).

Adenomyomas are generally small (less than 1 to 2 cm) nodules located in the submucosa adjacent to the distal common bile duct (fig. 23-3A). In the diffuse type (adenomyomatous hyperplasia), there may be a poorly defined thickened area within the ampulla. Often the common bile duct is dilated proximal to the lesion. The nodular type shows a well-circumscribed mass of smooth muscle and fibrous tissue containing lobules of small ducts surrounded by clusters of smaller ductules (fig. 23-3B,C). The ducts and ductules are lined by cytologically bland cuboidal epithelium resem-bling the normal lining of the pancreatic and bil-iary ducts (fig. 23-3D). Between the epithelial lob-ules lie interlacing bundles of smooth muscle. In some cases, inflammatory cells may be conspicu-ous in the stroma. The diffuse type exhibits similar constituents, although the ductules may not be arranged in lobules and the lesion may blend imperceptibly with the surrounding normal struc-tures. As such, the diffuse type of adenomyoma (adenomyomatous hyperplasia) may be difficult to distinguish from normal ampullary ductules and smooth muscle showing proliferative changes, in response to inflammation, for example.

A number of theories exist about the origin of adenomyomas. They may represent examples of heterotopic pancreatic tissue in which the acinar

and endocrine elements are absent (fig. 23-4), especially when nodular in configuration. The similar anatomic distribution of the two lesions, the lobular configuration of the ducts and ductules, and the finding of fascicles of smooth muscle within typical examples of pancreatic heterotopia support this view. Other observers favor the interpretation of a proliferative lesion of the ductules of Beale, with reactive proliferation of smooth muscle. A hamartomatous nature has been favored by many authors. Finally, some authors regard ad-enomyomas as truly neoplastic (9).

BRUNNER'S GLAND HYPERPLASIA

Proliferation of Brunner's glands may occur in either a localized or diffuse fashion. Although originally designated as "Brunner's gland adeno-mas," these lesions are now regarded as hyper-plastic or hamartomatous. Often localized, Brunner's gland hyperplasia assumes a polypoid configuration simulating a neoplasm (13). In-volvement of the ampulla is uncommon, al-though several examples have been recorded (12,14). Symptoms are generally minimal and may include abdominal pain, pyloric obstruc-tion, or hemorrhage. Exceptionally, a peri-ampullary lesion may induce obstructive jaun-dice, simulating a carcinoma (14). Histologically, Brunner's gland hyperplasia generally does not exceed 1 cm. The lesion is submucosal and con-sists of lobules of cytoarchitecturally normal Brunner's glands associated with ducts and fas-cicles of smooth muscle (fig. 23-5).

HAMARTOMATOUS POLYPS

Both juvenile polyps and Peutz-Jeghers pol-yps may occur in the duodenum (11), and al-though specific examples involving the ampulla have not been reported, there is no reason they should not occur.

FIBROINFLAMMATORY LESIONS

"Pseudotumor"

The term "pseudotumor" has been used for tumor-like lesions composed of inflammatory cells and reactive mesenchymal tissues. In some loca-tions (such as the lung), inflammatory pseudo-tumor refers to a specific clinicopathologic entity

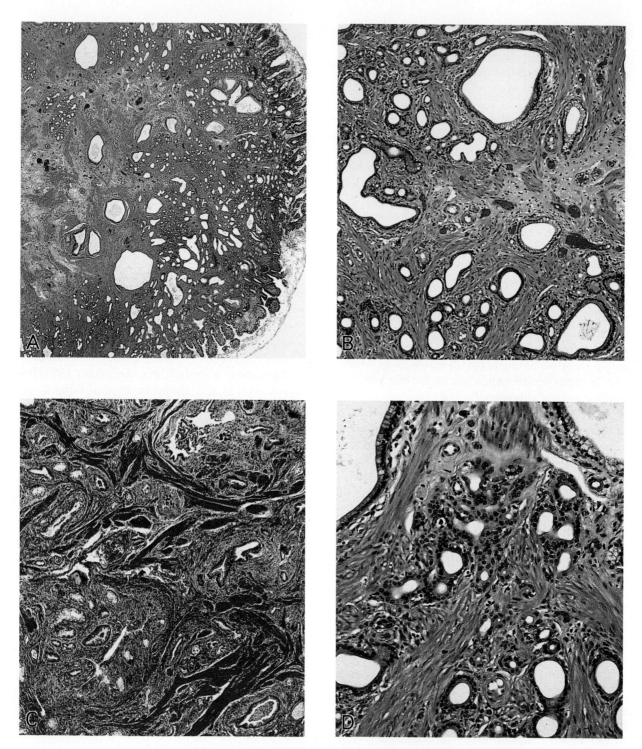

Figure 23-3

PERIAMPULLARY ADENOMYOMA (OR ADENOMYOMATOUS HYPERPLASIA)

A: At low power, there is a vaguely nodular collection of ductules, some of which are dilated, surrounded by a fibromuscular stroma.

B: The ductules are organized in loose lobular aggregates having central dilated, branched ductules surrounded by smaller tubular ductules.

C: Staining with Masson trichrome highlights the smooth muscle bundles surrounding the ductules.

D: Cytologically, the epithelial cells resemble those of normal biliary ductules, with a single layer of cuboidal to low columnar cells having round, uniform nuclei.

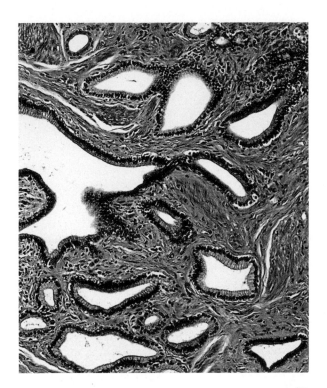

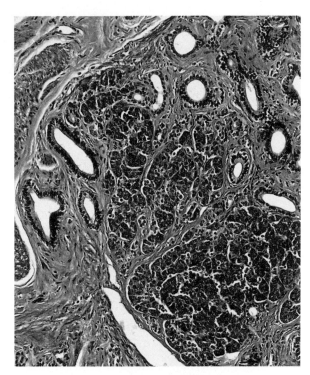

Figure 23-4
PERIAMPULLARY ADENOMYOMA

Left: This adenomyoma exhibits typical features in most of the lesion.

Right: In some areas, however, there are collections of pancreatic acinar cells, suggesting that the adenomyoma may represent a focus of pancreatic heterotopia having predominantly a ductal cell component.

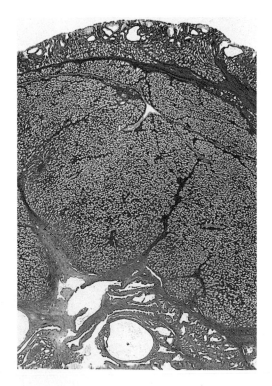

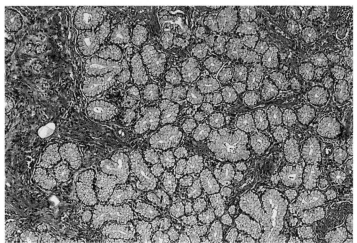

Figure 23-5
BRUNNER'S GLAND HYPERPLASIA

Left: Large lobules of Brunner's glands are present within the submucosa.

Above: The hyperplastic Brunner's glands resemble their normal counterparts, and fascicles of smooth muscle are present within the lesion (left).

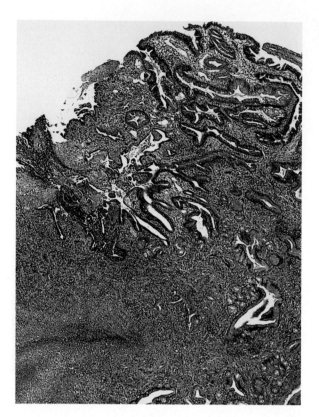
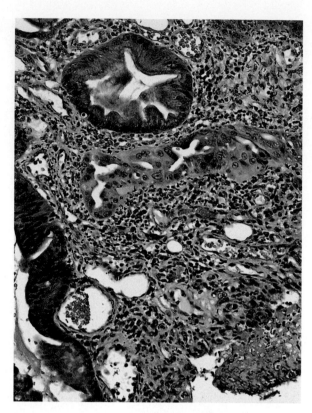

Figure 23-6
INFLAMMATORY PSEUDOTUMOR

Left: Fibroinflammatory lesions involving the ampulla may result in a tumor-like mass, descriptively designated a pseudotumor. This lesion consists of a rich inflammatory infiltrate containing reactive myofibroblasts.

Right: The adjacent epithelium of the ampulla exhibits reactive changes, resulting in atypia which may be mistaken for an adenoma or carcinoma on endoscopic biopsy.

with well-defined features, although in many instances, the term is used descriptively to encompass any pseudoneoplastic lesion of presumed inflammatory nature. The latter appears to be true of the ampulla, where most reported pseudotumors have lacked detailed pathologic descriptions. Ten pseudotumors of the ampulla which simulated ampullary neoplasms clinically and endoscopically have been described (16). The patients averaged 71 years of age. Six had gallstones (two within the common bile duct), suggesting a causal relationship with the inflammatory process. Histologically, the cases showed a mixed inflammatory infiltrate involving the ampullary epithelium (fig. 23-6). Reactive epithelial atypia was occasionally marked, raising a suspicion of carcinoma in two patients. Patients were treated by endoscopic sphincterotomy without recurrence of symptoms.

Myofibroblastic Proliferation

We have observed two examples of a tumor-like lesion consisting of a poorly defined nodule of proliferating, plump myofibroblastic cells in a background of mixed inflammatory cells (fig. 23-7). Due to the resemblance of the lesions to pseudosarcomatous myofibroblastic proliferations occurring elsewhere, we interpreted them as reactive rather than neoplastic.

Sclerosing Cholangitis

Sclerosing cholangitis can clinically simulate adenocarcinoma when it occurs in the extrahepatic bile ducts. Only exceptionally is the involvement distal enough within the common bile duct to raise the consideration of an ampullary carcinoma (15).

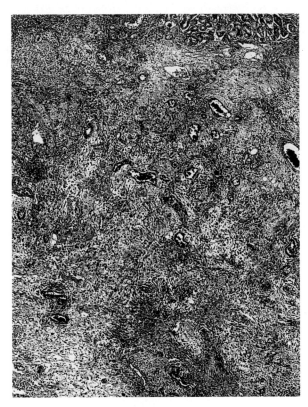
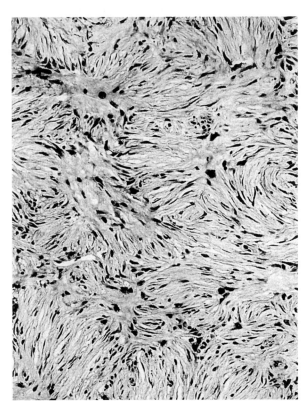

Figure 23-7
TUMOR-LIKE MYOFIBROBLASTIC PROLIFERATION INVOLVING THE AMPULLA
Left: The lesion contains abundant inflammatory cells and small vessels, and shows an extensive myofibroblastic proliferation.
Right: The myofibroblasts exhibit a storiform configuration, raising the alternative possibility of a low-grade myofibroblastic neoplasm.

Lithiasis

Gallstones may occasionally become lodged within the ampullary portion of the distal common bile duct and may clinically simulate a neoplasm. In addition, a firm mass is palpable at surgery, raising suspicions of carcinoma. Of course, the pathologic diagnosis is not problematic if a resection is performed, but endoscopic biopsies only reveal nonspecific inflammatory and reactive changes.

REFERENCES

Papillary Hyperplasia and Heterotopic Tissues

1. Blundell CR, Kanun CS, Earnest DL. Biliary obstruction by heterotopic gastric mucosa at the ampulla of Vater. Am J Gastroenterol 1982;77:111–4.
2. Laughlin EH, Keown ME, Jackson JE. Heterotopic pancreas obstructing the ampulla of Vater. Arch Surg 1983;118:979–80.
3. Tsunoda T, Eto T, Yamada M, et al. Heterotopic pancreas: a rare cause of bile duct dilatation. Report of a case and review of the literature. Jpn J Surg 1990;20:217–20.
4. Weber CM, Zito PF, Becker SM. Heterotopic pancreas: an unusual cause of obstruction of the common bile duct. Am J Gastroenterol 1968;49:153 9.

Adenomyomatous Hyperplasia and so-called Adenomyoma

5. Al Jitawi SA, Hiarat AM, Al-Majali SH. Diffuse myoepithelial hamartoma of the duodenum associated with adenocarcinoma. Clin Oncol 1984;10:289–93.
6. Bergdahl L, Andersson A. Benign tumors of the papilla of Vater. Am Surg 1980:563–6.
7. Cattell RB, Pyrtek LJ. Premalignant lesions of the ampulla of Vater. Surg Gynecol Obstet 1950;90:21–30.

8. Huang HL, Liu CL, Yang TL, Lin HJ. Adenomyoma of the papilla of Vater: a case report. Chung Hua I Hsueh Tsa Chih (Taipei) 1993;51:386–8.
9. Ulich TR, Kollin M, Simmons GE, Wilczynski SP, Waxman K. Adenomyoma of the papilla of Vater. Arch Pathol Lab Med 1987;111:388–90.
10. Venu RP, Rolny P, Geenen JE, Hogan WJ, Komorowski RA. Ampullary hamartoma: endoscopic diagnosis and treatment. Gastroenterology 1991;100:795–8.

Brunner's Gland Hyperplasia and Hamartomatous Polyps

11. Attanoos R, Williams GT. Epithelial and neuroendocrine tumors of the duodenum. Semin Diag Pathol 1991;8:149–62.
12. Fuller JW, Cruse CW, Williams JW. Hyperplasia of Brunner's glands of the duodenum. Am Surg 1977;43;246–50.

13. Silva S, Chandrasoma P. Giant duodenal hamartoma consisting mainly of Brunner's glands. Am J Surg 1977;133:240–3.
14. Skellenger ME, Kinner BM, Jordan PH. Brunner's gland hamartomas can mimic carcinoma of the head of the pancreas. Surg Gyn Obstet 1983;156:774–6.

Fibroinflammatory Lesions

15. Beachley MC, Lankau CA Jr. Sclerosing cholangitis simulating periampullary carcinoma: case report. Mil Med 1976;141:475–6.

16. Leese T, Neoptolemos JP, West KP, Talbot IC, Carr-Locke DL. Tumours and pseudotumours of the region of the ampulla of Vater: an endoscopic, clinical and pathological study. Gut 1986;27:1186–92.

24
SECONDARY TUMORS OF THE AMPULLARY REGION

Secondary involvement of the ampulla may occur by hematogenous metastases or, more commonly, by direct extension from an adjacent site.

DIRECT EXTENSION FROM ADJACENT SITES

Because the ampulla is closely juxtaposed to the duodenum, common bile duct, and head of pancreas, it is frequently involved by tumors arising in these sites. As previously discussed, distinguishing a primary duodenal carcinoma invading the ampulla from an ampullary primary extending onto the duodenum may be impossible. Fortunately, the therapy and prognosis of the two lesions are similar (2). A more significant problem involves the distinction of a carcinoma of the pancreas or bile duct from an ampullary primary. Both tumors frequently invade the duodenum and ampulla and may appear as an ulcerated luminal mass by endoscopy. Biopsies may reveal fragments of an adenocarcinoma without sufficient distinguishing features to enable the pathologist to identify the primary location. The problem is complicated by the fact that pancreatic carcinomas may extend along the basement membrane of the overlying mucosal surfaces, simulating an in situ growth pattern (fig. 24-1). In some cases, the resemblance of the carcinoma to adenomatous intestinal type

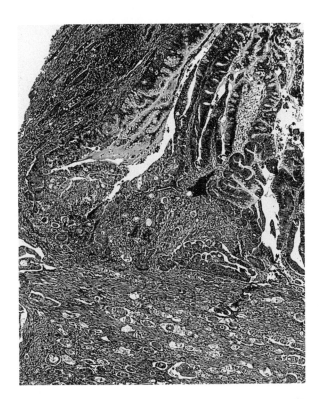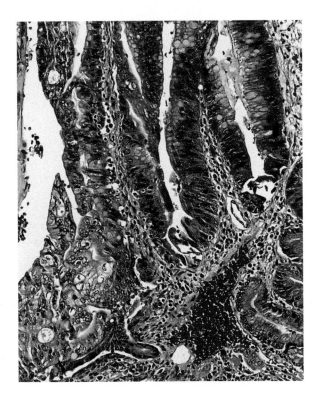

Figure 24-1
EXTENSION OF INVASIVE PANCREATIC CARCINOMA ALONG THE
BASEMENT MEMBRANE OF THE DUODENUM, SIMULATING A PAPILLARY ADENOMA

Left: The underlying pancreatic tumor is a typical ductal adenocarcinoma which has invaded through the duodenal wall onto the periampullary duodenal mucosa.

Right: At high power, foci of obvious carcinoma are seen spreading along the villous basement membrane (left), whereas adjacent villi exhibit a better differentiated population of cells with cytoarchitectural features very similar to those of periampullary adenoma.

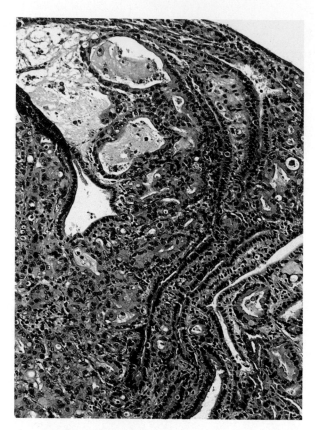

Figure 24-2
INVOLVEMENT OF THE AMPULLA
BY DIRECT EXTENSION OF A
PANCREATIC DUCTAL ADENOCARCINOMA
There is carcinoma interspersed between strips of benign ampullary ductal epithelium and no evidence of a preexisting adenoma.

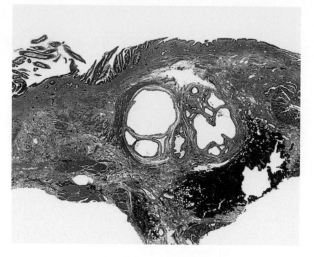

Figure 24-3
INVOLVEMENT OF THE AMPULLA BY AN
INTRADUCTAL PAPILLARY-MUCINOUS
NEOPLASM OF THE PANCREAS
At low power, the papillary fronds of the IPMN extend along the pancreatic duct (top). The histologic appearance is identical to that of a primary adenoma of the ampulla, and ampullary involvement may reflect diffuse adenomatous changes throughout the pancreatic ductal system including the ampulla and occasionally the bile duct as well.

mucosa is striking. Features that should raise the possibility of an underlying pancreatic or biliary carcinoma rather than an ampullary primary include the presence of invasive carcinoma within a portion of unremarkable (or simply inflamed) mucosa with no adenomatous mucosa present (fig. 24-2), growth along the villous basement membrane of nonintestinal type carcinoma cells, and the presence of a pancreatobiliary type carcinoma in an ampullary biopsy. Any of these findings can occur with an ampullary primary as well, but their presence should suggest that the ampullary nature of the tumor needs to be confirmed by other means.

Noninvasive tumors of the biliary or pancreatic ducts can also extend into the ampulla. In the pancreas, intraductal papillary-mucinous neoplasms may grow as multiple papillary nodules involving long segments of dilated ducts and extend to the ampulla (fig. 24-3) (7). Intraductal papillary-mucinous neoplasms resemble intestinal type papillary adenomas or papillary carcinomas of the ampulla; hence, if the extent of the lesion is not recognized it could be misinterpreted as an ampullary primary on endoscopic biopsy. Intraductal oncocytic papillary neoplasms of the pancreas may also extend along the ducts to involve the ampulla (1).

METASTASES

Hematogenous metastasis to the ampulla is rare. When present, ampullary metastases are generally a manifestation of widespread disease. Primary presentation with ampullary involvement is exceptional. One series of metastases to the upper gastrointestinal tract found one ampullary metastasis from osteogenic sarcoma among 14 patients with metastases to esophagus, stomach, or duodenum who had no evidence of involvement elsewhere (3).

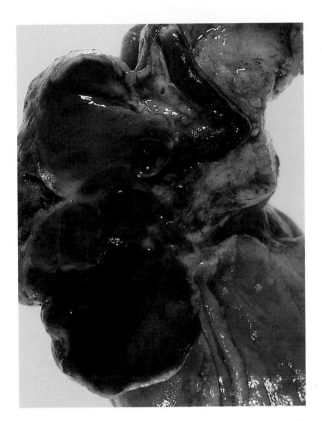

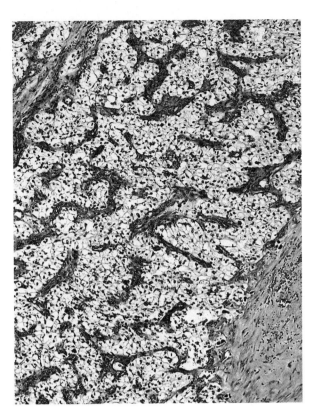

Figure 24-4
METASTATIC RENAL CELL CARCINOMA INVOLVING THE PERIAMPULLARY REGION
Left: Grossly, the tumor forms a large exophytic fleshy mass projecting into the duodenal lumen. A finger-like extension of tumor is present within the pancreatic duct and extends in retrograde fashion to involve the minor papilla, which is patent in this individual.
Right: Histologically, this is a typical renal cell carcinoma with a clear cell appearance.

One tumor which has been repeatedly reported to metastasize to the ampulla is renal cell carcinoma (fig. 24-4) (4–6,10). The ampullary involvement may occur many years after removal of the primary and patients may represent the only site of recurrence (4,6,10). The tumor is often polypoid (fig. 24-4, left) and patients may present with upper gastrointestinal hemorrhage. One patient presented with malabsorption (5). Surgical excision of the metastasis, if solitary, has been associated with survival for several years (4). Histologically, metastatic renal cell carcinoma has a highly characteristic appearance, but may be confused with the rare primary clear cell carcinoma of the ampulla, a tumor that generally makes mucin, in contrast with renal cell carcinoma.

Other tumors that metastasize to the ampulla include melanoma (8) and mammary carcinoma (fig. 24-5), especially lobular carcinoma, which may simulate a signet ring cell carcinoma (9).

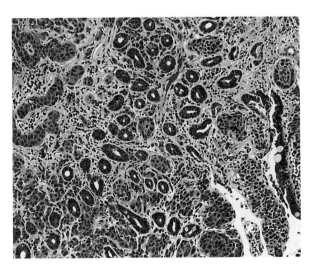

Figure 24-5
METASTATIC MAMMARY CARCINOMA
INVOLVING THE AMPULLA
Small nests of tumor cells are present between non-neoplastic duodenal glands.

REFERENCES

1. Adsay NV, Adair CF, Heffess CS, Klimstra DS. Intraductal oncocytic papillary neoplasms of the pancreas. Am J Surg Pathol 1996;20:980–94.

2. Howe JR, Klimstra DS, Moccia RD, Conlon KC, Brennan MF. Factors predictive of survival in ampullary carcinoma: results in 123 patients between 1983–1995. Ann Surg 1997;228:87–94.

3. Kadakia SC, Parker A, Canales L. Metastatic tumors to the upper gastrointestinal tract: endoscopic experience. Am J Gastroenterol 1992;87:1418–23.

4. Leslie KA, Tsao JI, Rossi RL, Braasch JW. Metastatic renal cell carcinoma to ampulla of Vater: an unusual lesion amenable to surgical resection. Surgery 1996;119:349–51.

5. McKenna JI, Kozarek RA. Metastatic hypernephroma to the ampulla of Vater: an unusual cause of malabsorption diagnosed at endoscopic sphincterotomy. 1989;84:81–3.

6. Robertson GS, Gertler SL. Late presentation of metastatic renal cell carcinoma as a bleeding ampullary mass. Gastrointest Endosc 1990;36:304–6.

7. Solcia E, Capella C, Kloppel G. Tumors of the pancreas. Atlas of Tumor Pathology, 3rd Series, Fascicle 20. Washington, D.C.: Armed Forces Institute of Pathology, 1997;53–64.

8. Stauch S, Rosch W. Verschlussikterus durch pankreaskopfmetastase eines malignen melanoms. Bildgebung (Switzerland) 1987;56:115–7.

9. Taal BG, den Hartog Jager FC, Steinmetz R, Peterse H. The spectrum of gastrointestinal metastases of breast carcinoma. I. Stomach. Gastrointest Endosc 1992;38:130–5.

10. Venu RP, Rolny P, Geenen JE, Hogan WJ, Komorowski RA, Ferstenberg R. Ampullary tumor caused by metastatic renal cell carcinoma. Dig Dis Sci 1991;36:376–8.

25

PROSECTION OF THE PANCREATODUODENECTOMY SPECIMEN

SURGICAL RESECTION

Surgical resection of ampullary neoplasms consists of either local excision, including endoscopic polypectomy or local transduodenal surgical excision (ampullectomy), or pancreatoduodenectomy (Whipple resection).

The standard pancreatoduodenectomy specimen includes the distal stomach and pylorus along with the first, second, and third portions of the duodenum, the head of pancreas, and the distal common bile duct. The gallbladder and cystic duct may also be attached. A variation of the procedure known as the pylorus-preserving pancreatoduodenectomy leaves the entire stomach and pyloric sphincter intact, providing a better functional result without reducing the ability to encompass the entire tumor, at least for ampullary carcinoma.

The gross evaluation of the pancreatoduodenectomy specimen depends upon proper orientation. Occasionally, large amounts of omental adipose tissue are attached to the portion of stomach, and there may be fibrosis in the area of the pancreas along with numerous surgical sutures and clips, all of which may obscure the anatomy. Place the specimen in the normal anatomic position; from this aspect, the cut margins of the pancreatic and biliary ducts will not be visible. Note that the anterior aspect of the pancreas is covered by a smooth layer of peritoneum. Open the portion of intestine longitudinally along the aspect opposite the ampulla. Continue the incision to the proximal aspect of the gastric portion of the specimen. Proximal and distal mucosal margins may be submitted at this time. Examine the mucosal aspect of the ampulla of Vater. If a tumor is visible, note the gross configuration and whether it is exposed to the duodenal lumen or covered by intact mucosa of the papilla.

Turn the specimen over to view it from the posterior aspect. The remaining surgical margins include the cut distal pancreatic margin (including the pancreatic ductal margins), the cut common bile duct margin, and the soft tissue margins of the head of the pancreas, which can be divided into posterior and inferior pancreatic margins. The distal pancreatic and common bile duct margins should be shaved from the specimen and submitted en face. The inferior and posterior pancreatic margins may be inked at this time. The anterior aspect of the pancreas, while not a true cut surgical margin, may also be inked to determine whether tumor has spread to the peritoneal surface.

Gingerly attempt to insert probes along the common bile duct and the pancreatic duct from their distal aspect through the papilla. In cases of complete obstruction at the ampulla, it may not be possible to pass a probe. This is uncommon, however, and with gentle manipulation a probe is generally passable, especially along the common bile duct. Bear in mind that the pancreatic duct generally makes a right angle turn within the head of the pancreas, necessitating some rotational movements to pass a probe even through a normal duct. Once a pair of probes has been inserted into the respective ducts, the entire specimen can be bisected along the probes using scissors and scalpel where appropriate to reveal a longitudinal section of both ducts in parallel. The resulting cross section allows examination of the full length of the two ducts along with their orientation to the tumor. The size of the tumor should be measured in three dimensions, along with a gross assessment of depth of penetration. Remember that the distance an ampullary tumor invades into the pancreas is important for staging.

An effective method for sectioning ampullary tumors is to begin with a section parallel to the plane of transection described above (i.e., parallel to the pancreatic and biliary ducts). Such a section includes the tumor, the duodenal mucosa, the profiles of pancreatic and biliary ducts, as well as the head of pancreas, also showing the maximal depth of tumor penetration through the duodenal wall or into the head of pancreas. The remainder of the tumor can be sectioned radially from the ampulla, similar to the method for sectioning a "cone" biopsy of the uterine cervix. It is generally possible to include inked deep pancreatic margins and the anterior pancreatic surface in these sections. The peripancreatic tissues must be carefully examined for lymph nodes. Lymph nodes are commonly identified along the common bile duct in the anterior and posterior pancreatoduodenal regions, along the posterior and inferior aspects of the head of the pancreas, and in the adipose tissue of the greater and lesser curvature of the stomach. Additionally, lymph nodes are often detected incidentally in random sections of the pancreatic tissue, as peripancreatic lymph nodes are often very closely associated with the parenchyma.

THE SURGICAL PATHOLOGY REPORT

The surgical pathology report of an ampullectomy or pancreatoduodenectomy specimen for ampullary carcinoma should include all of the information necessary for TNM staging and other items as follows:

1. Whether the specimen is received fresh or formalin fixed, and whether it has been previously opened.
2. What structures are present (distal stomach, pylorus, duodenum, gallbladder, portion of bile duct, head of pancreas, segment of portal vein, etcetera) and the dimensions of each.
3. Characteristics of the external surface, especially the anterior peritoneal aspect of the head of the pancreas; circumference and patency of pancreatic and biliary ducts; and presence of stones, strictures, or stents.
4. Appearance of the ampulla from the luminal aspect of the duodenum, including the location and gross classification of the tumor. Size, color, and consistency of the tumor.
5. Histologic type, grade, and stage of the tumor. Extension into sphincter of Oddi, duodenal submucosa, muscularis propria, head of pancreas, and periduodenal soft tissues should be stated. The extent of pancreatic invasion should be measured.
6. Presence and location of associated adenoma or dysplastic epithelium, along with the degree of dysplasia. If an intraductal papillary carcinoma component is present, the proportion of invasive carcinoma should be indicated.
7. Presence or absence of vascular or perineural invasion.
8. Presence or absence of tumor at the surgical margins and peritoneal surfaces.
9. Status of lymph nodes at all sampled locations.
10. Presence of pathologic changes in other structures: pancreas, duodenum, gallbladder, etcetera.
11. Results of ancillary studies (immunohistochemistry, electron microscopy) if performed.

Index*

Gallbladder

*Numbers in boldface indicate table and figure pages.

Extrahepatic Bile Ducts

Ampullary Region

◇◇◇